Medical Etnics *and* Humanities

Edited by

Frederick Adolf Paola, MD, JD
Medical Director
Physician Assistant Program, Southwest Florida
Professor
College of Allied Health and Nursing, Health Professions Division
Nova Southeastern University

Affiliate Associate Professor of Medicine
University of Florida College of Medicine

Robert Walker, MD
Associate Professor
College of Medicine, Internal Medicine
University of South Florida

Lois LaCivita Nixon, PhD, MAT, MLitt, MPH
Professor
College of Medicine and Internal Medicine
University of South Florida

JONES AND BARTLETT PUBLISHERS
Sudbury, Massachusetts
BOSTON   TORONTO   LONDON   SINGAPORE

World Headquarters

Jones and Bartlett Publishers
40 Tall Pine Drive
Sudbury, MA 01776
978-443-5000
info@jbpub.com
www.jbpub.com

Jones and Bartlett Publishers
Canada
6339 Ormindale Way
Mississauga, Ontario L5V 1J2
Canada

Jones and Bartlett Publishers
International
Barb House, Barb Mews
London W6 7PA
United Kingdom

Jones and Bartlett's books and products are available through most bookstores and online booksellers. To contact Jones and Bartlett Publishers directly, call 800-832-0034, fax 978-443-8000, or visit our website, www.jbpub.com.

Substantial discounts on bulk quantities of Jones and Bartlett's publications are available to corporations, professional associations, and other qualified organizations. For details and specific discount information, contact the special sales department at Jones and Bartlett via the above contact information or send an email to specialsales@jbpub.com.

This publication is designed to provide accurate and authoritative information in regard to the Subject Matter covered. It is sold with the understanding that the publisher is not engaged in rendering legal, accounting, or other professional service. If legal advice or other expert assistance is required, the service of a competent professional person should be sought.

Production Credits

Publisher: David Cella
Acquisitions Editor: Kristine Johnson
Associate Editor: Maro Gartside
Production Manager: Julie Champagne Bolduc
Production Assistant: Jessica Steele Newfell
Senior Marketing Manager: Barb Bartoszek
Manufacturing and Inventory Control Supervisor: Amy Bacus

Composition: SNP Best-set Typesetter Ltd., Hong Kong
Cover Design: Kristin E. Parker
Cover Image: © Timothy R. Nicols/ShutterStock, Inc.
Printing and Binding: Malloy, Inc.
Cover Printing: Malloy, Inc.

Library of Congress Cataloging-in-Publication Data
Paola, Frederick A.
    Medical ethics and humanities / Frederick Adolf Paola, Robert Walker, Lois LaCivita Nixon.
        p. ; cm.
    Includes bibliographical references and index.
    ISBN 978-0-7637-6063-2 (pbk. : alk. paper)
    1. Medical ethics. 2. Physicians' assistants. I. Walker, Robert, 1957– II. Nixon, Lois LaCivita.
III. Title.
    [DNLM: 1. Ethics, Medical. 2. Bioethical Issues. 3. Humanities. 4. Physician Assistants—education. W 50 P211m 2010]
    R724.P225 2010
    174.2–dc22
                                                                                                    2009005390

6048
Printed in the United States of America
13 12 11 10 09   10 9 8 7 6 5 4 3 2 1

CONTENTS

PREFACE

The morality of aspiration . . . is the morality of the Good Life, of excellence, of the fullest real-
ization of human powers . . . [A] man might fail to realize his fullest capabilities . . . [but]
in such a case he was condemned for failure, not for being recreant to duty; for shortcoming,
not for wrongdoing . . . Where the morality of aspiration starts at the top of human achieve-
ment, the morality of duty starts at the bottom . . . It is the morality of the Old Testament and
the Ten Commandments. It speaks in terms of "thou shalt not," and, less frequently, of "thou
shalt." It does not condemn men for failing to embrace opportunities for the fullest realiza-
tion of their powers . . . [but rather] for failing to respect the basic requirements of social
living . . . If we look for affinities among the human studies, the morality of duty finds its
closest cousin in the law, while the morality of aspiration stands in intimate kinship with aes-
thetics . . . [There] is an invisible pointer that marks the dividing line where the pressure of
duty leaves off and the challenge of excellence begins . . . This line of division serves as an
essential bulwark between the two moralities. If the morality of duty reaches upward beyond
its proper sphere the iron hand of imposed obligation may stifle experiment, inspiration, and
spontaneity. If the morality of aspiration invades the province of duty, men may begin to
weigh and qualify their obligations by standards of their own and we may end with the poet
tossing his wife into the river in the belief—perhaps quite justified—that he will be able to write
better poetry in her absence.[1]

This is, as you might guess from the title, a book about medical ethics and humanities.
Ethics refers to moral philosophy (or the *philosophy of morality*), and medical ethics, consequently, refers to moral philosophy as it relates to the practice of medicine. *Morality* is used
herein "normatively to refer to a code of conduct that, given specified conditions, would
be put forward by all rational persons."[2]

By *humanities* we mean those academic disciplines united by a commitment to the qualitative study of the human condition. The term *medical humanities* may be defined:

> . . . broadly to include an interdisciplinary field of humanities (literature, philo-
> sophy, ethics, history, and religion), social science (anthropology, cultural studies,
> psychology, and sociology), and the arts (literature, theater, film, and visual arts)

xiii

and their application to medical education and practice. The humanities and arts provide insight into the human condition, suffering, personhood, [and] our responsibility to each other, and offer a historical perspective on medical practice.[3]

The organization of this book, *Medical Ethics and Humanities*, is fairly straightforward. Section I is intended to introduce the reader to various ways of approaching ethics and to provide a framework for later material. It begins with a philosophical discussion of ethical theory (Chapter 1), followed by chapters on biomedical ethical principles (Chapter 2), the moral rules (Chapter 3), casuistry/case-based reasoning (Chapter 4), and professionalism and the internal morality of medicine (Chapter 5).

Section II explores topics in the provider–patient relationship, including confidentiality (Chapter 6), competency (Chapter 7), and informed consent (Chapters 8 and 9).

Section III deals with ethical issues across the lifespan, such as ethics and genetics (Chapter 10), human reproduction and birth (Chapter 11), pediatric ethics (Chapter 12), death (Chapter 13), and end-of-life decision making (Chapter 14).

Section IV, following up on the law–morality nexus explored earlier in the text (see, for example, Chapter 3), explores legal topics relevant in a text on medical ethics, including health law and medical malpractice (Chapter 15) and professional relationships and the allocation of responsibility among medical providers (Chapter 16).

Because of the strong nexus between medical ethics and the medical humanities, the text concludes with Section V, which deals with the humanities in medicine. It reflects the strong historical commitment of the University of South Florida's College of Medicine to the medical humanities. Chapter 17 provides an introduction to the medical humanities, followed by chapters dealing with some of what the medical humanities have to tell us about human reproduction and birth (Chapter 18), the human lifespan (Chapter 19), and human aging and death (Chapter 20).

This book grew out of courses taught between 1996 and the present at the University of South Florida College of Medicine (*profession of medicine* and *ethics and humanities*) and between 2005 and the present at the Nova Southeastern University Physician Assistant Program (*legal and ethical issues in health care*). We hope that course directors and students alike will regard the book favorably, and we look forward to feedback from readers regarding ways in which it might be improved in future editions.

References

1. Fuller LL. *The Morality of Law*. New Haven, CT: Yale University Press; 1969.
2. Gert B. The definition of morality. In: The Stanford Encyclopedia of Philosophy. Available at: http://www.science.uva.nl/~seop/entries/morality-definition. Accessed March 5, 2008.
3. Medical Humanities, NYU School of Medicine. Available at http://medhum.med.nyu.edu. Accessed February 12, 2009.

ACKNOWLEDGMENTS

The editors would like to take this opportunity to thank all of the contributing authors for their hard work. Likewise, we are grateful for the helpful comments of our reviewers, who helped shape the final product:

Ralph Baergen, PhD, MPH
Department of Philosophy
Idaho State University

Missy M. Bennett, EdD
Associate Professor
Department of Teaching and Learning
Georgia Southern University

Bill Bondeson, PhD
Curators Professor of Philosophy and
    Medicine
University of Missouri

Michael J. Booker, PhD
Professor of Philosophy
Jefferson College

Jennifer Davis-Berman, PhD
Professor of Social Work
Department of Sociology, Anthropology,
    and Social Work
University of Dayton

Roy A. Guizado, MS, PA-C
Chair, Department of Physician Assistant
    Education
Associate Professor of Physician Assistant
    Education
Western University of Health Sciences

Barbara Head, PhD, RN, CHPN, ACSW
Assistant Professor
Interdisciplinary Program for Palliative
    Care and Chronic Illness
University of Louisville

Peter G. Holub, DPM, MS, EdS
Ethics Writer, *Internet Journal of Allied
    Health Sciences and Practice*
Assistant Professor, Bioethics and Medical
    Professionalism
College of Allied Health and Nursing
Nova Southeastern University

Paul R. Johnson, PhD
Professor
Department of Liberal Arts
D'Youville College

Dana Nadalo, MHS, PA-C
Academic Faculty
Physician Assistant Program
School of Allied Health Sciences
Baylor College of Medicine

Luis A. Ramos, MS, PA-C
Assistant Professor and Program Director
Master of Physician Assistant Studies
Chatham University

Ralph Rice, PA-C
Associate Professor and Associate Director
Department of Physician Assistant
   Studies
Wake Forest University School of
   Medicine

Dana Sayre-Stanhope, EdD, PA-C
Associate Professor and Division Director
Physician Assistant Program
Department of Family and Preventive
   Medicine
Emory University School of Medicine

Madhu Singh, PhD
Department of Psychology
Tougaloo College

Robert J. Solomon, MS, PA-C, DFAAPA
Professor and Academic Coordinator
Towson University/CCBC
Essex Physician Assistant Program
School of Health Professions
The Community College of Baltimore
   County

Peter M. Stanford, MPH, PA-C
Clinical Assistant Professor
Physician Assistant Department
University of Maryland Eastern Shore

Of course, we could not have completed this project without the guidance and assistance of Maro Gartside, associate editor, and Kristine Johnson, our editor, of Jones and Bartlett Publishers. Finally, we wish to express our deepest gratitude and affection to our families, without whose nurturing love and patient endurance this book could not have been born.

CONTRIBUTORS

Maria L. Cannarozzi, MD, FAAP
Assistant Professor
College of Medicine, Internal Medicine, and
    Pediatrics
University of South Florida

Charles M. Culver, MD, PhD
Professor
Medical Education
Barry University

Bernard Gert, PhD
Stone Professor of Intellectual and Moral
    Philosophy
Dartmouth College
Adjunct Professor
Psychiatry
Dartmouth Medical School

Daniel P. Maher, PhD
Associate Professor
Philosophy
Assumption College

James P. Orlowski, MD
Chief of Pediatrics, Chairman of Ethics
University Community Hospital

Hana Osman, PhD
Assistant Professor
College of Public Health
University of South Florida

Kyrus Patch, MSPAS, PA-C
Assistant Professor
Physician Assistant Program
Nova Southeastern University

Yvette E. Pearson, PhD
Assistant Professor
Philosophy
Old Dominion University

Susan Schmerler, MS, JD
St. Joseph's Regional Medical Center

Section I

Introduction to the Study of Ethics

Chapter 1

Theory in Bioethics

"Little men," he once said, "spend their days in pursuit of [wealth, fame and worldly possessions]. I know from experience that at the moment of their deaths they see their lives shattered before them like glass. I've seen them die. They fall away as if they have been pushed, and the expressions on their faces are those of the most unbelieving surprise. Not so, the man who knows the virtues and lives by them."

—Mark Helprin, *Winter's Tale*

Chapter Learning Objectives
At the conclusion of this chapter the reader will be able to:

1. Define the term *bioethics*

2. Compare and contrast private and public moral justification

3. Understand the necessity of critically examining one's moral opinion as it relates to competing opinions

4. Distinguish between the critique of moral opinion developed by classical philosophy and the dismissal of opinion by modern philosophy

5. Understand the two contrary pressures brought to bear by Descartes on moral reasoning

6. Understand that science does not exist and occupy a place of importance in our lives independent of moral judgment about the good

7. Know the tenets of Aristotle's philosophy and be able to apply those tenets to the study of bioethics

8. Know the tenets of Thomas Aquinas's philosophy and be able to apply those tenets to the study of bioethics

9. Know the tenets of Immanuel Kant's philosophy and be able to apply those tenets to the study of bioethics

10. Know the tenets of John Stuart Mill's philosophy and be able to apply those tenets to the study of bioethics

11. Understand why it is important to consider various ethical theories in bioethics

If *bioethics* is the discipline devoted to the articulation of good decisions in the practice of health care, it seems to be an inherently practical discipline. In the context of caring for the sick, which calls for intelligent action with some urgency, nothing could be more irrelevant and more disruptive than to become preoccupied with theoretical questions relating to our action. If we needed absolutely clear answers to questions such as "What is a human being?" or "What is disease?" before we could treat a sick person, we could be paralyzed by doubts. It makes little sense to insist that the sick person prove his or her humanity by a theoretically compelling argument before receiving the attention of health care professionals. And yet, despite this obvious priority of practical concerns to theoretical concerns, we find persistent interest in the theoretical foundations of bioethics. Controversy over the best resolution to practical difficulties—such as what to do about embryonic stem cell research or physician-assisted suicide—pushes people to look for secure and compelling rational arguments in support of the decisions or policies they endorse. Reasoned argument, as distinct from any other basis on which people might prefer or embrace a particular line of action, supports the moral integrity and legitimacy of action.

There is an ambiguity contained in the claim that the integrity of moral[1] choices depends on their rationality. The ambiguity may be recognized in the fact that bioethics literature abounds with arguments in favor of and against actions such as abortion and yet no person seeking an abortion or declining to seek one is required to give a compelling argument in support of that decision. Generally speaking, personal decisions in the arena of bioethics are decided on the basis of reasoned arguments, religious beliefs, personal preferences, or any other grounds that are persuasive to the people making the decision. No outside assessment of the merits of these decisions takes place as a matter of course. By contrast, when we try to determine what sorts of options public policy ought to permit individuals to elect in their own circumstances, people are most energetic in bringing forth rational argumentation to support what they understand to be good or right. And, more important, we see energetic criticism and attempted refutations of the positions and arguments advanced by others. Personal decisions in health care, like other moral choices, are generally regarded as private, and we make these choices while enjoying significant freedom from scrutiny and from any burden of justification. Decisions about issues such as embryonic stem cell research, by contrast, are decisions about the appropriate or morally good public policy, and for these decisions we require a different form of justification, one that is more thoroughly rational in its approach. This helps to explain why bioethics tends to become involved in, if not reduced to, debates about public policy.

The discrepancy between these two kinds of moral justification, one private and one public, can be seen to be prepared and defended by, for example, Immanuel Kant. At the risk of oversimplifying a tremendously complex argument, we note that Kant distinguishes between what can be believed and what can be known. According to Kant, answers to ultimate questions in which human beings have an interest, such as the existence of God and the immortality of the human soul, can be believed, but not known. To prevent anyone's dogmatic imposition of belief on one side or the other of these controversial matters, Kant urged the free public expression of all such beliefs, provided that they be subject to reasoned criticism. Each person would be free to believe what he or she wishes for any reasons the individual finds subjectively satisfying, but no one would be permitted to impose any belief on others unless it could be shown to be objectively (i.e., rationally) justified. Our common life, then, would be ruled by reason and not by prejudice, dogmatism, or sectarian strife. Kant's approach, on the basis of an epistemological critique of our knowing powers, circumscribes or eliminates troublesome controversies by declaring them insoluble for human reason and, at the same time, preserves individual liberty to believe as one sees fit (provided one does not to claim to *know* the truth).[2]

Although few people study Kant's arguments in this area, the protection of individual freedoms or rights or autonomy against unjust abridgement by others or by government is deeply rooted in our political and legal structures, our moral education, and our social life. In fact, contemporary bioethical approaches tend to begin somewhere after the point Kant left off. That is, most bioethical literature takes for granted some version of the epistemological limits argued for by Kant and other modern philosophers.[3] The two main elements of modernity—the new natural science as the standard for human knowing and the new moral and political structures of democratic liberalism—tend to be presupposed within the mainstream of bioethics. It is easy to see that this epistemological depreciation of certain kinds of human thought trades on the authority of modern science. For this reason, in order to understand the role of theory in bioethics, it is helpful to take a broad view, one that also considers premodern approaches to the relation between theory and moral practice. It is only from this perspective that one can discern the challenges to any adequate theory in bioethics. The aim of this introduction is not to repeat the sorts of conventional introductions that can be found in other anthologies. Here, the aim is to acquaint the reader with the substantive questions and difficulties that must be addressed if we are to think seriously about the role of ethical theory in guiding the use of scientific medicine.

The Place of Theory in Bioethical Reasoning

Moral Opinion and Moral Philosophy

None of us comes to the examination of moral theory innocently and, as it were, untouched by moral reasoning. This presents a great obstacle to initiating a systematic or scholarly investigation of ethics. Although moral questions might be explicitly raised for the first time in such an investigation, that investigation cannot be the first exposure to moral thinking and expressions of moral approval and disapproval. When we raise moral questions or begin to study bioethics and moral philosophy generally, we cannot do so except as people who have already been deeply affected by the complex tradition of moral discourse. We inhabit a world decisively shaped by the moral and political judgments of those who are around us and those who came before us. Although there are individuating aspects of each person's moral experience, which combine to render everyone's moral formation somehow unique, there are also common features that we absorb by sharing a language, a political and legal system, and a more or less common way of life.

When we come to the discipline of bioethics, we have already been educated morally, to some extent, and have learned to use words like *rights* and *good* and *evil* and *autonomy* and *justice*. We already know or think we know the difference between a moral issue and non-moral issue, and we have declared and constituted ourselves morally by our actions. When we engage in moral discourse, we embrace, to varying degrees, moral distinctions that arise in and draw their sense from developed philosophical and theological traditions. This language is easier to use than it is to understand, and our habitual use of words such as *justice* or *rights*, without having to define what they mean, may hide the fact that we do not always know the full meaning, provenance, and adequacy of the moral opinions we use and endorse. The opinions we casually absorb without considered judgment also shape our actions and thus establish our moral character. In action and in speech, one person may appeal to rights and another to nature or natural law, but both may be only vaguely aware of what that language and associated distinctions were originally devised to express. Thus, ordinary moral discussions proceed by appeal to uncritically accepted distinctions and opinions we find ready-made for us in the discourse we learn from others.

In these circumstances, the study of moral philosophy serves first of all as a critical reflection on uncritically accepted moral discourse. This reflection helps to illuminate the content of our own moral thinking, speaking, and acting. It can lead us to clarify what we think and also to refine and improve our opinions. We might reconsider and eventually abandon as untrue or incoherent some moral opinion we have previously held and acted upon. This process is not simple and does not occur necessarily or automatically. In fact, most of us have a certain resistance to a searching examination of our own opinions. They are, after all, *our* opinions, and we do not merely hold them but also endorse them and have come to be attached to them. We live our lives by reference to these expressions of our grasp of the difference between good and bad, the important and the trivial, and praiseworthy and blameworthy action.

All human beings live by reference to an understood discrimination between what is good and what is bad, but one never finds complete agreement about these matters. The diversity of human judgment about good and bad is as ubiquitous and necessary as the fact of those judgments themselves. If we do not take for granted the impossibility of knowing the truth, it seems necessary to examine the truth of the competing opinions. This examination raises serious difficulties, but the price for avoiding it may prove to be very high. At the very least, it amounts to living thoughtlessly, at the mercy of whatever combination of opinions happens to have coincided in our moral formation. There is no characteristic pain or other signal that identifies our opinions as unexamined. It is quite possible to live as others live and never examine the opinions by which one lives. Plato's dialogues are perhaps the best illustration of the complexity and the questionableness embedded in moral opinions that are, on the surface, both clear and obvious. Plato's dialogues show both the ease with which people use moral terms they only half understand and the resistance such people exhibit to the process of clarifying and perhaps improving their opinions. There seems to be a persistent human tendency to avoid the effort needed to examine one's moral opinions, and yet Plato's dialogues imply that living such an unexamined life amounts to failing to live as a human being.

To have one's life affected by and informed by opinions whose truth or goodness one has not had a chance to examine is a characteristic difficulty encountered by all human beings. René Descartes expressed the admixture of unreason and error that inevitably afflicts us all unawares:

> And hence I also thought that, because we have all been children before being men, and because it was necessary for us to be governed for a long time by our appetites and our preceptors, which were often contrary to one another, and neither of which perhaps counseled us always for the best, it is almost impossible for our judgments to be so pure and solid as they would have been if we had had the entire use of our reason from our birth and had always been conducted only by it.[4]

Descartes grasped the difficulty in which we all find ourselves, but he rejected the solution that had traditionally been thought to be necessary. The traditional solution is the Socratic solution, namely, the critical and thoroughgoing examination of the opinions we have inherited. Socratic philosophy, as presented in Plato's dialogues, takes prephilosophical opinion as its starting point and subjects it to rational scrutiny with the goal of replacing that opinion with knowledge. We all naturally begin with the practical concern to live our lives well, but we are surrounded by a multiplicity of opinions regarding how to live well. Classical moral philosophy, which here means ancient Greek moral philosophy, aims to provide a thoughtful consideration of and resolution of the question or problem of how one ought to live.

The alternative solution, defended by Descartes, has altered the situation such that today we do not face precisely the same contrast between ordinary moral opinion and moral philosophy that Socrates illuminated. Our encounter with these issues is profoundly reconfigured by the presence of modern natural science. The intellectual architects of modern science, people such as Descartes and Francis Bacon, intended to alter this relationship by introducing a new kind of science that would both be more certain and more useful than the science or philosophy that had preceded. In fact, when Descartes alluded to the power of inherited opinion in the passage quoted earlier, he did so in order to express dissatisfaction with this tradition precisely because it seems to culminate in nothing but uncertainty and endless disputes. Descartes hoped to replace the then-dominant scholastic and speculative philosophy with a practical one, which would know the forces and actions of material nature in order to render us "like masters and possessors of nature." Descartes specifically pointed to the fruits this would bear in our concern for the conservation of health, which he identified as the primary good and the foundation of all other goods in this life. The clarity with which Descartes grasped these relationships and the power of the argument he proposed make it almost impossible to overstate the importance of his *Discourse on Method* for understanding the character of contemporary bioethics.

Modernity and Ethical Theory

The central element of Descartes' project, to reorient the relation between science and practical life, has been successfully accomplished for the most part, even if major elements of his philosophical and scientific thinking have been ignored or discarded. For this reason alone, Descartes' argument would command our attention. But we must also attend to the crucial fact that the argument Descartes advances in favor of his new scientific method and of his project as a whole is a rhetorical and popular argument directed not to philosophers and scholars, but to the public. Descartes envisions science that enjoys popular support because the goal (or a significant part of the goal) of that science is humanitarian, in the sense that it aims at the "relief and benefit of man's estate," to use Francis Bacon's phrase.[5] Modern science is conceived by its founders and presented to the public as beneficial especially to the nonscientists, and this practical benefit is advanced to win credit for the modern scientific and philosophic project. This attitude toward science, which is very widely—albeit not universally—accepted, is accompanied by a confidence or a trust in science as the most secure kind of human knowing. This respect for science as the most authoritative form of human knowledge reshapes how we now face the philosophical investigation of the moral opinions we inherit.

It is worth considering the structure of Descartes' argument in its broad outlines. As already noted, he expressed dissatisfaction with the traditional education he had received because it was both uncertain and not useful for life. Descartes proposed to educate himself by beginning with a resolute demand for certain knowledge on the strength of a rigorous method. The method involved the doubt of any opinion, however probable, unless it could be proved to be certainly true in accord with his method. He planned to begin from absolutely certain metaphysical foundations and then to proceed to physics and the other sciences. The key point for our present purposes is the significance of the rejection of all doubtful opinions as uncertain. Descartes did not, in Socratic fashion, accept probable opinions for examination; instead, he cast them aside as if they were false, lest they corrupt his judgment by bringing him to admit as true anything that was less than completely certain. Descartes illustrates how the demand for absolute certainty in all our judgments makes it impossible to attend to the pressing business of life. His solution was to construct a merely provisional moral code consisting of a few practical rules to govern his action while he sought rigorous certainty in his thoughts. He embraced these maxims as useful, but uncertain, that is, as quite possibly untrue and quite certainly not known to be true, but eminently beneficial nonetheless. He presented the moral code as *provisional*, implying that his philosophical pursuit of the truth would lead him to examine the truth of these moral maxims in due order and ultimately to establish moral philosophy on the same indubitably certain theoretical foundations as the rest of his science.[6] In the *Discourse* itself, as Descartes outlines the content and structure of his physics, he points out that on the basis of the laws he has discerned in nature he has discovered truths more useful and more important than all he had learned previously. The clear implication is that his physics is even more useful and more important than his provisional morality.

It goes without saying that Descartes' physics proved to be flawed and that the metaphysical theses he advanced have not been universally accepted, but the structural relationship he articulated between natural science, practical benefit, and moral reasoning has largely carried the day.[7] In fact, soon after Descartes, John Locke argued that metaphysical knowledge of the sort Descartes declared to be foundational was impossible.[8] Immanuel Kant would declare that our ultimate metaphysical ignorance was no impediment to our universal and necessary knowledge of natural science. Kant helped to formulate the distinction between matters about which we may have belief from matters about which we may have knowledge.[9] Simplifying matters considerably, we may describe the present configuration of these structural relations as follows. Science, and what can claim the name of science, enjoys the mantle of objectivity and universality, whereas moral beliefs, by contrast, represent personal values or private commitments. Science can claim to be the knowable truth, recognized by all, whereas moral beliefs remain uncertain, controversial, and without authority to command deference. It is of the utmost importance to emphasize that we are speaking here of the popular estimation of science and are ignoring the numerous, substantial controversies within science about its meaning, its realism, its limits, and so on. Science occupies what may be described as a fixed point of reference around which competing moral beliefs must orient themselves. Argumentation within the realm of bioethics is more or less required to take whatever scientific medicine establishes as the objective truth, unbiased by moral bias or prejudice. This is essentially the relation established on the strength of Descartes' argument for certainty in the sciences.

Descartes also established a second relation between the knowledge of nature and practical utility. In place of merely speculative knowledge, he argued that the knowledge of truths that proved useful offered the greatest benefit to mankind. Descartes appealed to and strengthened the belief that knowledge should be useful as he argued that the path to genuine utility in action lay in the certainty or security of one's foundations. This relation obtains today in our distinction between theoretical and applied sciences, wherein we expect that true theory provides the foundation for effective practice. In Cartesian fashion, just about every academic discipline seeks secure foundations in order to free itself from uncertain presuppositions and pave the way toward fruitful results. Descartes' argument in the *Discourse on Method* has created the landscape within which our contemporary discussions of bioethics take place.

Today, if we try to examine, in quasi-Socratic fashion, the moral opinions with which we have been raised, our efforts are complicated by the authority of science precisely because it presents itself as objectively independent of the vagaries and uncertainties of human opinion. In its apparent cognitive superiority to ordinary moral opinion, science becomes the most significant feature of our moral education. The fact of modern science, its omnipresence especially but not exclusively in the form of the technology that permeates our lives, provides a common point of reference for people whose ethnic, cultural, political, and religious ways of life are otherwise tremendously diverse. The structure established or inspired by Descartes manifests itself in the tendency for all bioethical discussions to begin with a review of the scientific facts, which are presupposed to be the common point of reference whose truth is more securely grasped than is the truth of any moral thesis.

Consequences for Bioethics

The consequences of the influence of Descartes on bioethics are not hard to discern. There are two contrary pressures brought on moral reasoning. The first pressure stems from the distinction between science and what science establishes on the one hand against moral beliefs on the other. Moral beliefs or maxims were relegated to the realm of uncertain opinion by Descartes. He embraced a code of morality as useful, although uncertain—that is, not known or not knowable. This attitude survives in our present-day reinterpretation of moral beliefs as commitments or values that derive their authority from having been accepted or endorsed by us. We no longer expect there to be a knowable moral truth. We expect rather to negotiate moral compromise within a pluralistic set of diverse moral views. We do not expect the good to be knowable in the way that scientifically accessible facts are knowable. The second pressure tends in the opposite direction and inclines us to refashion ethics in imitation of modern science. Thus, there has been tremendous interest in securing the foundations of bioethics as a way of overcoming the endless controversy and disagreement that characterizes morality. On this view, bioethics, like business ethics or legal ethics, is a form of applied ethics, which is conceived as dependent upon more fundamental and universal theoretical ethics.

At this point it may be helpful to note how these two pressures are reflected in two senses of the word *theory* in contemporary usage. In each case, *theory* takes its meaning by being contrasted with something else. In the first use, theory is equivalent to what is uncertain or what is supposed to be true, although the actual state of affairs may well be different. We say that a given act leads to such and such a result "in theory." The contrasting phrase is "in reality" or "in practice." In physics, subatomic particles are regarded as "theoretical entities" until they are proven to be real. Theories are proposed or constructed as possibly true descriptions, though they may ultimately prove to be misconceived or untrue. Theory, in this meaning, is an idealized account that may or may not accurately reflect what actually obtains. In a second contrast, we distinguish the theoretical sciences from the applied sciences. In this use, theory enjoys greater epistemological stability and provides the foundation for reliable practice. In this view, ethical theory tends to be conceived as having no direct or inherent link to particular practical determinations or judgments.[10] This approach conceives ethical theory as prior to and the ultimate source of legitimacy for particular ethical judgments. This yields a superficial similarity to the classical approach to moral philosophy insofar as ordinary moral judgments are understood to be in need of a more rigorous rational support. The difference is that the contemporary approach reproduces Descartes' doubt of ordinary opinion. Ordinary moral judgments are treated as uncertain to the extent that they lack theoretical, rational foundations. Whatever cannot be so established is regarded as *unknowable*, although, as Kant argued, people are free to *believe* what they wish about such matters. The classical approach takes ordinary moral opinion as primary and seeks to improve, refine, or correct it, but not to replace it with a perfectly rational, foundational theory.

The critical attitude toward ordinary moral opinion pervades contemporary bioethics because of the centrality of science to modern medicine. To quote a recent textbook on bioethics: "The extent to which contemporary medicine has become effective in the treatment of disease and illness is due almost entirely to the fact that it has become scientific medicine."[11] Scientific knowledge about chemical and biological operations provides the foundation for effective medical practice. Insofar as medicine is scientific, it tends to carry with it the suspicion or doubt of all opinions that are not scientifically known.[12] A sign of this appears clearly in the standards of experimental design in clinical trials to protect against bias and to prove conclusively the superior effectiveness of one treatment modality over another. Unsystematic clinical experience is not insignificant, but the randomized controlled clinical trial remains, as it is often called, the gold standard. In this context, it is reasonable to expect that the cognitive status of moral opinions, which are not even open to scientific proof, would be depreciated still more.

The difficulty created by this situation is the familiar problem of the modern world, which became undeniably clear in the twentieth century. The problem is the existence of a very powerful science of nature, including a very powerful medical science, in the absence of a correspondingly powerful knowledge of how to use that power well. Our science that enables us to manipulate nature seems to be available only at the price of our remaining ignorant, or at least uncertain, of what the right or good use of that power happens to be. The contemporary schools of ethical thought have never enjoyed the same success in overcoming controversy and disagreement that the sciences have. Whether this failure of these ethical schools is due to their having arisen hand in hand with modern science is impossible to examine in the present circumstances. We note that the power of modern science in general and scientific medicine in particular urges us to look for knowable ethical standards.

One of the sources we ought to consider is classical moral philosophy. Classical philosophy is often thought to have been refuted by modern philosophy, but when we consider how Descartes and others successfully introduced and promoted what has come to be modern science, a more complicated picture emerges. The argument in favor of modern science is not a scientific argument, but what can best be characterized as a moral argument. Descartes' moral argument promoted a new kind of science that would be more certain and more useful than its classical predecessor. Therefore we have to distinguish (1) the "prescientific" moral argument by which Descartes introduced and popularized the new science from (2) the merely useful, provisional morality that follows from the standards of the new science.[13] Once we make this distinction, two important things become clear.

First, when Descartes advances his argument for the goodness of the new conception of science, he is essentially engaged in a moral argument with classical philosophy about the proper goals of human knowledge. The full title of Descartes' work is *Discourse on the Method for Rightly Conducting One's Reason and for Seeking Truth in the Sciences.* This moral conflict with classical philosophy precedes the introduction of the new science. The fact that Descartes' argument was successful means that the pursuit of science today depends on a prior acceptance of the argument (or its conclusion) that the new science is good. Thus, science does not exist and occupy a place of importance in our lives independent of a moral judgment about the good. It is a sort of illusion to suppose that science stands independent of particular moral judgments about what is good and what is bad. Science is not morally neutral and above the fray of competing moral judgments. Our grasp of the moral significance of the science that shapes our medicine, then, requires that we face this argument.

Second, whereas Descartes' argument for the goodness of science is mostly overlooked and taken for granted, the subordinate status of moral belief (in his provisional moral maxims) has been taken to mean that all moral beliefs are comparatively uncertain. Because this structural relationship has been widely accepted as true, the fact that the natural science of classical philosophy has been shown to be untrue has been taken to mean that classical moral philosophy has also been undermined. However much it may be true that Descartes intended to establish moral science on the foundations of his physics and metaphysics, it is not true that all of classical moral philosophy depends directly on foundations established in physics and metaphysics.[14] It would be more accurate to say that, in the classical approach, knowledge of what we are is worked out together with knowledge of the good that perfects us. We come to know what it is to be human as we come to know what it is to live well. The rejection of ancient physics, in whole or in part, on the strength of modern science does not directly entail the failure of ancient moral thought. The argument between Descartes and the tradition about the proper character and goal of science takes place and must be addressed on the prescientific plane.

The best approach to understanding the role of moral theory in bioethics must consider the contrast between classical and modern conceptions of moral reasoning. The first part of this chapter has attempted to sketch the relation between "theory" and moral reasoning and scientific medicine. The second part of this chapter considers four approaches to ethical theory: two classical and two modern. Each of the theories is examined primarily by reference to a principal work of a single author. This necessarily involves some simplification of issues that are both complicated and controversial. It is not possible to give a comprehensive account of each author or school. The goal is to introduce these schools in order to clarify the depth of the difficulties that confront us as we try to reason intelligently about bioethics today.

Four Theories

Aristotle: *Nicomachean Ethics*

It is unusual to consider Aristotelian moral philosophy in the context of bioethics. At most, adherents of virtue ethics invoke the name and doctrine of Aristotle when they try to address bioethical questions by reference to virtues that medical practitioners especially ought to embody.[15] There is more to be drawn from Aristotle's account if we approach his thought from the perspective of a person who is trying to make decisions about the place of health in relation to happiness and well-being in life as a whole. For the purposes of this chapter, we will consider Aristotle's *Nicomachean Ethics*,[16] which is a philosophical articulation of the structure and character of human happiness, understood as the best way of life.

Aristotle understands happiness as the proper fulfillment of human beings. All human beings agree on the name *happiness* as what they seek finally in all their activities, but they disagree on the content of that happiness. Some identify it with being honored, some with pleasure, and so on. The disagreement necessitates an inquiry into what genuinely completes human life, for it is obvious that we might anticipate finding happiness in some activity or some possession, only to be disappointed. The difference between what people desire and what actually fulfills them opens up the space for investigating of what happiness consists. For Aristotle, happiness is the specifically human completion. He conceives of happiness as the excellent or virtuous performance of properly human activities. This means that happiness does not consist in mere bodily health or in the enjoyment of sensual pleasures, which are operations we share with plants and animals. The properly human virtues involve the excellent operation of reason. Rationality and speech are proper to human beings, and human happiness cannot exist apart from the virtuous cultivation of our rationality.

There are two classes of virtues, the moral virtues and the intellectual virtues. The *moral virtues* consist in habitual dispositions to feel and act rightly with respect to characteristically human concerns. Thus, courage is the virtue needed to act well in the presence of feelings of fear and confidence. Temperance or moderation is the virtue that enables people to act well under the influence of bodily pleasures and pains. The several virtues involve a specific harmony between the irrational, appetitive part of the soul, which is the seat of the emotions, and the rational, thinking part of the soul. The virtue or perfection of the rational part of the soul related to the moral virtues is called *prudence* or *practical wisdom* (*phronesis* in Greek). This partly intellectual, partly moral virtue discriminates the appropriate action in particular circumstances, which comes to light as a relative mean between extremes. The proper action is a relative mean because it is not uniformly the same for all persons, but is flexible, in the way that the amount of food and exercise right for each person varies considerably; however, it is always a mean between too much and too little. The moral virtues include an irrational component, or, perhaps more clearly, they are constituted in part by having one's desires and feelings shaped such that, for example, the temperate person desires to act in the way that his or her practical wisdom also directs. Thus, a morally virtuous person is characterized by habitually correct desire, which means that reason and desire both incline the person together to the same virtuous deed.

The *intellectual virtues* perfect human beings insofar as they know and understand (VI, esp. 3–7). Theoretical wisdom, the peak of the intellectual virtues in Aristotle's account, involves contemplation of necessary and universal truths. Aristotle presents this as the highest human activity and the activity that most fully completes human beings as human beings. This chapter is not the place to go into a detailed explication of Aristotle's argument in this area. It is, nevertheless, appropriate to point out that Aristotle envisions the primary form of human happiness as somehow exceeding the happiness that is available through the active life of moral virtue. His *Nicomachean Ethics* culminates in a twofold doctrine of human happiness, which consists either in morally virtuous activity or in intellectually virtuous activity. Aristotle does not fully articulate the relation between these two forms of happiness, but he does give primacy to the intellectual form as higher and more self-sufficient than the moral form (X.7 and X.8).

After this broad and sweeping summary, it is helpful to add a few points that are especially relevant to contemporary bioethics. First, when Aristotle identifies happiness as the "end" of human life, this must be carefully distinguished from things with which it might be confused. The term *end*, which translates the Greek word *telos*, primarily means the fulfillment or completion of a thing and not merely the outcome or termination or result of some activity. The end is the perfection of something and not merely what happens to it last. So, when we say in English that some person or project "met with a bad end," we do not mean by *end* what Aristotle means by *telos*. More important, *end* should not be confused with *purpose*, which is a misinterpretation as detrimental to understanding Aristotle as it is common.[17] Briefly, the end of a thing is the proper fulfillment of that thing according to its nature. The fulfillment of the dog is not the fulfillment of the horse. A purpose is anything that can be the target of human choosing. We might use a dog or a horse for various purposes (and even for the same purpose), and these purposes may or may not be congruent with the end of each animal. An end is independent of our willing, whereas purposes are constituted by our willing. So, for example, the end of a deer is vital activity as a deer, roaming through forests and generating offspring. It is not the fulfillment of the deer when a human being makes it his purpose to turn the deer into venison. The end of a shoe is attained when it is worn by someone who is walking or running, but the shoe might also serve a multitude of purposes, such as propping open a door or killing a spider. Again, the art of medicine has as its end health, but it may also be used for the purpose of earning money or fame. In the most important case, Aristotle claims that the human being has an end that is independent of the various purposes one might pursue in life. This enables him to distinguish between what someone does with his or her life and what would genuinely fulfill that person as a human being. One could make bodily pleasure one's life purpose, but it would not, according to Aristotle's argument, change the fact that one's end is something different. The successful attainment of many great and diverse bodily pleasures would not render one happy, because one would still have failed to achieve one's end as human.

This distinction between end and purpose is especially helpful in bioethics because it provides a principle in light of which we can discriminate appropriate limits to the use of medical expertise. Medical knowledge is open to multiple uses; it can be turned to the purposes of the healer, the torturer, the interrogator, the executioner, and many others. If it is true that medicine and the physician have as their natural end the production, preservation, and restoration of health, it becomes possible to reject certain purposes as incompatible with the nature of medicine. Thus, whatever one thinks of the morality of suicide or assisted suicide, the distinction between ends and purposes makes it possible to mount an argument that the physician's involvement is incompatible with the nature of the medical profession. This sort of argument helps to preserve medicine from becoming a mere instrument at the service of any and all purposes for which its expertise might be useful. Some purposes can be pursued congruently with the ends of things, or at least without destroying them, but others are in conflict with those ends, and the pursuit of such purposes corrupts the thing in question. It is especially important for bioethicists and for medical practitioners to consider these relationships today as the horizons open up for expanding medical knowledge in the direction of various "enhancements" that aim to make people not merely healthy, but "better than well."[18]

A second point to emphasize is how this understanding of human happiness illuminates our thinking about human health. Aristotle identifies health as the perfection or virtue appropriate to the nutritive part of the soul, the part operative in nutrition, metabolism, and reproduction. He then promptly excludes this part of the soul and health from any constitutive role in his account of properly human excellence or happiness.[19] This exclusion often sounds strange to contemporary ears, for we seem to think that health has greater moral significance. Even if we agree with Aristotle that a human being does not deserve moral praise on account of having good digestion, it is fairly common to attach *some* moral significance to taking care of one's health, which proves to be something Aristotle too eventually acknowledges.[20] Aristotle explicitly de-emphasizes the significance of bodily well-being in his account of human happiness as human excellence in the highest sense. For him, although life itself (and thus also health) is recognized as good (IX.9), the goodness of life and health are not fully understandable in isolation from the goods for which they are occasionally sacrificed. In this respect, Aristotle's moral thought is a helpful counterbalance to contemporary bioethics, which often tries to resolve bioethical questions by reference to the goodness of health and in abstraction from any specific appraisal of what health is good for. It is reasonable to expect bioethics to be distorted if it tries to proceed solely on the basis of the near-universal agreement that health is good while ignoring the great differences in the goods that are higher than health.

Third, Aristotle presents his moral philosophy as practical rather than theoretical. This means we undertake moral philosophy not simply in order to know, but in order to become good (see I.3 and II.2). Moral philosophy is pursued in order to improve our lives, not in order to contemplate truths about human nature. There is a theoretical consideration of the human soul (by which Aristotle means the animating principle of the human body), but it belongs to the biological part of the science of nature (physics). Ethics also considers the human soul, but only insofar as it is appropriate for a practical inquiry into human action (see I.13). The important point for our purposes is that Aristotle's distinction between theoretical and practical sciences is not identical with the contemporary distinction between theoretical and applied sciences. For Aristotle, the practical sciences do not depend on the theoretical sciences. The starting point for his ethics is being raised in good habits, which conveys the essential awareness of morally decent action (see I.3 and I.4). One does not begin with an abstract grasp of the good and deduce moral precepts or action guides from that first principle. One begins, rather, with what is first for us, which is the moral distinction between good and bad as it is grasped in ordinary opinion. This grasp is not perfect, but it is the starting point for the philosophical reflection on the adequacy of ordinary moral opinion. Obviously, this means that Aristotelian moral philosophy does not rest on the secure foundations that were so emphasized by Descartes. Aristotle seems to think that these starting points, imprecise and imperfect as they may be, are the necessary beginning points for ethics. This conflict between Aristotle and Descartes is central to Descartes' argument for a new kind of science with more certain foundations.

A fourth point of emphasis is Aristotle's concentration on moral character over particular acts. Aristotle's ethics concentrates on the character of a human being and the kind of life a person leads rather than on the particular acts he or she might perform. Whereas some contemporary approaches to ethics might focus on the rightness or wrongness of particular kinds of acts, such as abortion, capital punishment, or lying, Aristotle mostly ignores this sort of thing and speaks instead of the character of a human being as constituted by the repetitive performance of virtuous or vicious actions. If one's character is temperate or generous, one reliably acts in that way. The significance of any single action is diminished in comparison to the character one establishes over time and can be expected to exhibit in the future. This tends to make Aristotle's ethics less than completely helpful in the context of bioethics, where the acts that are in dispute tend not to be acts that form part of one's ordinary moral life. Actions undertaken in the context of medical care tend to be episodic and not the sorts of thing that constitute moral character in Aristotle's sense.

Finally, we return to the significance of practical wisdom for Aristotle's account. In Aristotle's view, the standard for moral goodness is the virtuous human being. The character and the judgment of the excellent moral agent form and express the indispensable standard for good and bad. There is no moral rule book and no process of reasoning that substitutes for the exemplary character and prudence of the virtuous human being. "For the morally decent man judges each matter correctly and in each matter the truth appears to him. For the noble and pleasant things are peculiar in accord with each character, and perhaps the morally decent man differs from others most by seeing the truth in each, being as it were the rule and measure of them" (III.4).[21] Aristotle negotiates the pervasive conflict of moral opinions by identifying the prudent human being as the standard for recognizing what is genuinely good. This person's character, the settled way in which the passions are habitually structured, permits him or her to see the moral truth of things. Recognition of what is good in human action does not belong to all human beings equally. The privileged perspective belongs to the practically wise. To the obvious objection that the practically wise cannot be recognized as wise by those who do not already agree with them, Aristotle can only reply by restating that this reinforces the need for being brought up in good moral habits so that one will be able to see the truth in moral affairs. This nonegalitarian solution remains unsatisfactory to many today, but it seems to be the only position open to someone who holds that there is some nonobvious truth to know in moral matters. Aristotle articulates practical wisdom as a kind of excellence in moral perceptiveness, an ability to discriminate moral phenomena with greater than average perspicuity (VI, chapters 8–13). An analogy with other areas helps. Every person can see a painting or watch a sporting event and can discriminate, to varying degrees, the good and the bad, but a capable art critic can discern more of what is present in a given painting, and an intelligent sports analyst can articulate the order and the structure of what the athletes are doing. Every person sees the same phenomena, but not all perceive them with the same insight.

Thomas Aquinas: *Summa Theologiae*

Thomas Aquinas is usually presented as a proponent of natural law ethics. This is true to an extent, but it is misleading in the sense that natural law occupies a very small and subordinate part of Aquinas's account of moral reasoning. Aquinas is primarily a Catholic theologian who incorporates much of Aristotle's moral teaching into a more comprehensive and more systematic framework. Thus, in his *Summa Theologiae*[22] he begins the discussion of human action with a consideration of the ultimate end of man (or happiness), which is argued to consist primarily in the vision of God in heaven and secondarily in the imperfect or incomplete happiness available in this life (I-II, q. 3, a. 8). By "imperfect happiness" Aquinas means the sort of happiness Aristotle articulated, consisting either in intellectually or morally virtuous activity (I-II, q. 3, a. 6). Aquinas, like Aristotle, then considers the acts and the virtues that conduce to the end of human happiness. Like Aristotle, he conceives of happiness as an end that is independent of the particular purposes or desires that human beings happen to have. There is, in his view, a natural desire for happiness or a natural inclination toward human perfection, but this primarily means that human beings are oriented or ordered toward a particular end as their fulfillment, not that the content of human happiness can be discovered by simply heeding whatever appetites and desires one happens to have spontaneously. A natural inclination is an orientation toward some sort of perfection of one's nature. Thus, to say that human beings have a natural inclination for speech means that our nature is perfected by cultivating speech, not that all human beings feel an urge to speak or take pleasure in speaking.

Aquinas mentions the natural inclinations in his presentation of natural law (I-II, q. 94), but it should be noted that the content of the law is not derived from an examination of human desires. Aquinas's consideration of the various kinds of law (such as civil law and divinely revealed law, like the Ten Commandments) belongs to his treatment of the *extrinsic* principles of human action. The natural law is a "participation of the eternal law in the rational creature" (I-II, q. 91, a. 2).[23] The eternal law is the providential rule by which God governs all creation. Nonrational creatures are simply subject to this law, but a rational creature is subordinated to providence in a more excellent way, by being provident for itself and for others. Natural law, then, is the rational or human grasp of God's providential governance of all creation. We become aware of this not by deducing it from the structure of human nature or by analyzing human inclinations, but by reference to moral experience (see I-II, q. 94, a. 5, reply to third objection).[24] The central point here for our purposes is that Aquinas's teaching on natural law is an attempt to defend the intelligibility of the natural moral order without direct appeal to divine revelation. Aquinas does not, as a matter of fact, appeal to natural law as a way of distinguishing good acts from bad acts. Natural law does provide a way of speaking about the availability of moral truth to natural human reason without reliance on faith or revelation. Natural law is relevant less for identifying the goodness or badness of particular acts and more for emphasis on the nonsectarian view of the moral goodness that is promoted. This becomes important in contemporary health care in the conduct of Catholic health facilities. The moral principles that govern the delivery of Catholic health care are regarded not as belonging properly to the Catholic faith, but as natural, meaning that they are intelligible independently of specific political and cultural traditions as well as specific religious doctrines or beliefs.

The bulk of Aquinas's account of moral theology recasts and develops a largely Aristotelian account of the virtues. When Aquinas does want to account for the goodness or badness of particular human actions, he appeals not to natural law, but to the so-called three fonts: the moral object, the intention, and the circumstances of the action.[25] The moral object is both the most important element to clarify in this triad and the most difficult to grasp clearly. Simply stated, the *moral object* is what is chosen when we perform human acts. We can speak of the observable, physical component (the exterior act) as the material performance. The moral object is constituted by what we choose in a given material performance. For example, one person hands money to someone else. The moral object is determined by what is chosen in this performance: repaying a debt, giving a gift, making a loan, paying extortion, or whatever it may be. The moral object is not identical with what occurs materially. No one chooses a raw material performance; we always choose some act, determinate in its kind, which could also be chosen by other agents, for different reasons, and in different circumstances.

The aim with which a given act is chosen is called the *intention* or the *intended end*.[26] A single human action involves choosing a determinate kind of action or object with a particular intention or series of intentions. For example, a medical student chooses to study in order to pass classes in order to earn a degree in order to be able to practice medicine in order to heal the sick and so on. When we act, we choose an object as ordered to an intention: we give a gift with the aim of expressing affection; we vaccinate in order to develop immunity; we amputate for the sake of preserving life; we give analgesics with the intention of relieving pain. The willed action is a unity, distinguishable into a chosen object and an intention.

We might also distinguish an indefinite number of *circumstances* of any action, some of which are more relevant than others. Normally, circumstances contribute very little to the character of an action, but they can also be noteworthy. Whether the analgesics act quickly or not is a circumstance, usually of minor significance. Whether the left leg or the right leg is amputated is circumstantial; what is of essential importance is that the *diseased* leg be amputated. What is an insignificant circumstance in one context can be important in another. For example, in the context of many moral actions it is normally insignificant that one happens to be a physician, but that circumstance becomes central to the moral character of one's acts in the presence of sick people.

In Aquinas's view, all of our choices and intentions ultimately must be integrated into the pursuit of the final human end, happiness. The ultimate end is the standard that regulates everything that is done for the sake of that end. Thus, all of the elements of each moral action must be good, or at least morally neutral, for that action to be morally good. Acts and intentions that cannot be integrated with or that detract from the ultimate end are recognizable as bad acts and intentions. Acts and intentions that cohere with and tend to promote the ultimate end are recognizable as good acts and intentions. Typically, the circumstances are the least important component of moral actions. Normally, circumstances do not render an action good or bad; they merely increase or decrease the moral goodness or badness that is principally drawn from the object and the intention. Occasionally, again, what is ordinarily circumstantial can become so important as to change the character of an action. Reading the newspaper in order to be an informed citizen normally constitutes a good action, but if one does this while at work or when one ought to be doing something more serious, it constitutes a form of negligence. The three fonts of morality are reference points that can be discerned in any given act, but the act must be prudentially assessed as an integral whole in relation to one's comprehensive end as a human being.

This approach permits an emphasis on individual actions in their goodness and badness that is more amenable to customary questions in bioethics. It is this dimension of Aquinas's presentation that Catholic health facilities tend to rely on, as distinct from natural law, when they want to address the morality of acts such as abortion, euthanasia, sterilization, the various forms of fertility assistance, organ transplantation, and so on. Each of these can be analyzed as a moral object, in abstraction from the good intentions that people seek to accomplish through these actions. If these acts, as moral objects, promote the ultimate end, they are good, and if they detract from it or conflict with it or otherwise cannot be integrated into a reasoned pursuit of that end, they are bad according to their kind. They might, as a matter of fact, still be chosen by someone, on account of the good intentions that can be pursued through them, but the goodness of the intentions being sought is not sufficient to prevent the act as an integral whole from being morally bad. The formulaic principle is that the end intended does not justify the choice of evil means.

This kind of reasoning lies behind the familiar prohibitions that are associated with the delivery of health care in the Catholic context. It is important to note, however, that Catholic health facilities understand the various "prohibited procedures" not primarily as conflicting with theological beliefs, but as being incompatible with the naturally knowable end of all human beings, Catholic and non-Catholic alike. The case of abortion is particularly instructive as to how this sort of reasoning works. It is true that Catholic moral reasoning recognizes all deliberate abortion, from the first moment of conception, as an immoral act. It does not, however, do so on account of a theologically dogmatic account of the moment at which the human person or the rational soul comes to be. The official formulation prohibits the *practice* of all abortion even as it reaffirms our *philosophical* uncertainty as to the precise moment at which the human person comes to be. Ignorance about the theoretical question of when the human person comes to be is coupled with practical certainty about the incompatibility with human happiness of killing what may well be an innocent person.[27]

The object-intention-circumstances approach also forms the basis for what is often called the *principle of the double effect*.[28] This principle is actually nothing more than a somewhat complicated set of distinctions aiming to clarify the lines of responsibility for actions that we deliberately perform. Normally, we are responsible for what we deliberately choose to do and for what we intend to achieve through what we choose. Nevertheless, the actual results of our activity are not identical with what we properly or directly will. In many cases the actual results differ from what we intended, such as when a vaccination actually triggers an illness instead of fostering immunity. Sometimes we do accomplish what we intend, but there are additional consequences, causally related to what we have chosen or intended, that lie outside what we directly will. For example, the scarring that is consequent upon surgery is neither directly chosen as a means nor intended as the aim of the surgeon's activity. It is an unavoidable consequence of what is directly willed. Again, the impaired ability to walk that follows as a result of amputating a leg is a foreseeable consequence of the amputation, which is what is directly chosen as a means of preserving life. The impairment is said to be indirectly voluntary, which identifies it as something that follows as a result of what is voluntarily done, although it is not itself pursued voluntarily. The principle of double effect is sometimes called the *principle of the indirect voluntary*. Although this principle has many critics, it attempts to articulate the ordinary recognition that we are responsible not only for what we will but also for what we foresee or should foresee as a consequence of what we will, although we are only indirectly responsible for this. A physician who performs a tubal ligation is directly responsible for the sterilization of the woman, whereas one who performs a hysterectomy to remove a cancerous uterus is indirectly responsible for subsequent infertility.

The significance of the difference between being directly responsible and being indirectly responsible is not trivial. In Aquinas's view, we are obliged not to choose or intend what is evil and we are obliged not to permit too much evil to arise through our actions. Nevertheless, if we were obliged to prevent every evil that might arise from our actions, we would hardly be able to act. The resulting attitude is not unlike the traditional medical principle of *primum non nocere*. One must consider not only the treatment one applies and the intended goal of that treatment but also the side effects and other merely possible outcomes that the patient risks enduring because of the treatment applied. The oversimplified formula of how to calculate all of these possible outcomes states that one must be sure to do, on balance, more good than harm. Aquinas would not countenance this formulation, which is essentially utilitarian. The more precise formulation of the principle of double effect claims instead that one must be sure that the good that one aims to achieve is so serious as to warrant risking the bad consequences that might ensue. Thus, it is inaccurate to say that the principle of double effect requires that the good effects must outweigh the bad effects. With that formula, one could never know whether an action was good or bad until after it had been performed. Also, one would be left saying that, in the case of vaccinations for example, it was good to vaccinate all of those who were benefited by the vaccine in the long run, but it was bad to vaccinate all of those who were harmed by it. Thus, the very same action that was chosen would be in one case good and in another bad, but only in view of the consequences that actually ensued in each case. The principle of double effect enables one to recognize actions as good and choiceworthy for the sake of serious goods aimed at through them, despite the awareness or expectation that serious evils could also follow. Thus, it is reasonable and prudent to choose, say, measles vaccination for the sake of the benefits that are likely to follow from it and in order to prevent the evils that are likely to follow from refusing it, even though a particular person might be seriously harmed by vaccination. It remains a morally good choice—albeit one with serious, unfortunate consequences—because the good that was sought was serious enough to risk that outcome. There does remain indirect responsibility for this outcome. For this reason, we are obligated not to expose ourselves to serious risks except for the sake of equally or more serious goods; similarly, vaccine manufacturers are morally obligated to make their products as free as possible from dangerous side effects.

Finally, we note that the principle of double effect is often formulated as encapsulated in several theses:

1. The act (or object) chosen must be morally good or indifferent.
2. The intention aimed at must be good.
3. The good effect must not be accomplished by means of the bad effect.
4. The good effect (or intention) must be at least as serious as the evil effect that may result.

Just a few comments are in order. With respect to the first point, we should note that indifferent acts are those that are not essentially ordered to the promotion of human happiness or to its detraction. These are acts such as walking, sleeping, reading, or hammering. As characterized, they are indeterminate in their goodness or badness because they do not essentially conduce to happiness or conflict with it. These sorts of acts depend for their goodness and badness on the intentions with which they are chosen and on the circumstances in which they are chosen. The third thesis specifies that any evil that is foreseen must not be chosen as the means by which one accomplishes the good one intends to do, but at most may be *permitted* as a consequence of what is done deliberately. If the good cannot be achieved except by means of the evil, it is not merely an effect, but a means that is directly willed. For example, in the case of euthanasia, the death of the patient is not merely a side effect of the relief of suffering; death is the means by which suffering is relieved.[29] The fourth point is often mischaracterized as requiring, as has been stated, that the good consequences must outweigh the evil. In fact, the principle of double effect is supposed to prevent the need to resort to such calculations to determine the goodness or badness of our choices.

Although this presentation of Thomistic ethical theory has emphasized the role of natural reason or philosophy, it must be recognized that the Christian theological dimension is ineradicable from Aquinas's thought. This transtemporal concern for the complete human good, as available only by divine grace, exerts significant influence on Thomistic thought and on bioethical reasoning in the Catholic context. Specifically, Catholic moral reasoning, however much it emphasizes the sanctity of human life, is characterized also by recognition of the limitation of the goodness of the preservation of bodily life. For this reason, Catholic faith ultimately interprets both suffering and death in light of God's providence. Not only expert medical care but also the availability of the sacraments and pastoral care constitute an integral part of Catholic health care. It is, after all, this view of the ultimate meaning and end of human life that inspired the foundation of Catholic hospitals. These institutions provide health services in light of the Catholic grasp of moral principles not only for Catholics but for all people as a way of displaying rather than imposing this understanding of the goodness of human life and health.[30]

Immanuel Kant: *Foundations of the Metaphysics of Morals*

In contrast to the two preceding moral theories, Kant emphatically separates the demands of morality from the search for happiness.[31] He did this in order to defend or restore dignity to human beings as capable of rising above selfish concern for the satisfaction of their desires and pursuing instead their duty. He spoke of the widely or universally experienced conflict between, on the one hand, our wishes and inclinations, the full satisfaction of which he called happiness, and, on the other hand, the stern commands of our duty, the fulfillment of which promises nothing to our needs and desires. Given this understanding of happiness—the satisfaction of one's desires, whatever they happen to be—Kant saw that interpreting morality as the rational discernment of the path to subjective satisfaction made morality nothing more than rational selfishness. We might find this view of moral reasoning defended in John Locke's *An Essay Concerning Human Understanding*, which interprets happiness as the longest-lasting experience of pleasure in whatever sources one happens to find pleasure. Moral reasoning, on this view, is calculation in the pursuit of happiness.[32] Kant argues that making morality serve our inclinations corrupts morality from the start. Moral dignity arises either from the fulfillment of one's duty as one's duty, without regard for—and perhaps even in conflict with—one's wishes, or at least from the capacity to act from one's duty rather than from inclination.[33] Kant elevates morality to the highest human pursuit. All of the interests of reason, he argued, must be subordinated to reason's ultimate interest, which is moral.[34] All of Kant's critical philosophy, then, is ultimately ordered toward the promotion of morality.

The instrumentality of philosophy for moral goodness does not mean that philosophy or, for that matter, any serious cultivation of the mind is necessary in order to do one's duty. Kant regards the recognition of one's duty as relatively simple, something that is plain to ordinary human understanding. The role of philosophy is to protect ordinary moral attitudes regarding one's duty from threats that would undermine our efforts to do what we all know we ought to do. The first sort of threat is the reinterpretation of morality as mere calculation of the path to satisfaction of one's desires. The second sort of threat arises from modern natural science. As Kant understands it, modern science presents nature as a "heteronomy of efficient causes, for every effect is possible only according to the law that something else determines the efficient cause to its causality" (63–64). "Heteronomy of efficient causes" means that nature amounts to a mechanistic system in which the action of any given thing now and in the future is rigorously determined by prior causes. Because human beings too are part of an act within the order of nature, this threatens morality if the human will itself is determined by external efficient causes. If nature is rigorously deterministic, there would be no genuine room for human freedom, which is presupposed by all moral agency (73–74).

Kant was willing to grant that nature is the realm of universal and necessary efficient causality in order to secure scientific knowledge in this realm against skeptical doubts arising from people like David Hume. The price he had to pay was the admission that we cannot know that we are in fact free moral agents. In his view, we must nevertheless regard ourselves as free or presuppose ourselves as free, not insofar as we belong to the material realm of appearances, but insofar as we conceive ourselves to belong to a supersensible realm in which freedom is possible. Kant's position is not that we must simply hope that

we are free, but that insofar as we take ourselves seriously as moral agents we all do necessarily regard ourselves as free and the source of our own actions whenever we act: "Now
I say that every being which cannot act otherwise than under the Idea of freedom is thereby
really free in a practical respect. That is to say, all laws which are inseparably bound with
freedom hold for it just as if its will were proved free in itself by theoretical philosophy"
(65). Freedom from determination to activity by foreign causes is the necessary presupposition we all make when we take ourselves to be moral agents. By regarding ourselves
as free, we must also regard ourselves as bound to obey moral duty: "Therefore a free will
and a will under moral laws are identical" (64).

To be a moral agent is to be the kind of agent that ought to act out of respect for the
moral law and not out of self-interest. We are moral agents properly speaking because of
our rational dimension, not because of other features that characterize us as human (the
body, emotions, sexuality, sociality, and so on). In fact, in Kant's view, morality applies to
all rational beings as such and is independent of the specific constitution of human
nature. It is not an exaggeration to say that whereas the tradition conceives of human
beings as belonging to the genus animal and being specifically differentiated by the presence of reason, Kant conceives of us as belonging to the genus of rational being and being
specifically differentiated as terrestrial. Kant conceives of moral agency as rational autonomy, by which he means reason is the law or the source of the law by which one lives. This
law, however, is universal because every rational being as such legislates identically with
every other rational being, because as rational they do not differ. That is, autonomous
action involves acting in independence of every foreign or heteronomous principle of the
will. The chief candidates for heteronomous principles of the will are the inclinations,
external efficient causes, and subordination to some divine law that promises rewards or
threatens punishment. Kant's emphasis on the abstraction from human nature seems
excessive, but it should be noted that he devoted considerable attention to human nature
in other works.[35]

The formal character of Kant's view of autonomous action is captured by his presentation of what he calls the *categorical imperative*. Kant distinguishes imperatives as either
hypothetical or categorical. Hypothetical imperatives command only on the condition (or
the hypothesis) that we seek some goal. Thus, the command to "break eggs" is hypothetical in the sense that it binds only those who in fact want to make omelets. Generally,
Kant calls hypothetical imperatives "rules of skill." These are imperatives that dictate how
to accomplish various tasks, but by which we are bound only *if* we want to attain what
the task accomplishes. Some hypothetical imperatives are known by the special name
"counsels of prudence" because these imperatives tell us what to do in order to become
happy.[36] Kant assumes that all human beings are driven by "a necessity of nature" to seek
happiness and, thus, we can be sure that all in fact do seek happiness (32). This purpose
belongs to all as a matter of the factual constitution of human nature. Our inclinations
lead us to seek happiness, and the counsels of prudence are the accumulated experiential
wisdom of how to satisfy the inclinations more or less reliably.

Over against these imperatives Kant presents the categorical imperative as the sole unconditionally binding moral imperative. This imperative commands without regard to the specific material content of an action and without regard to its intended result. The goodness of moral action does not depend on accomplishing specific purposes in the material realm, but only on willing in the right way. For Kant, this simply means conformity to the universality of law as necessary. The categorical imperative has no specific content; it expresses unconditional acceptance of law as such. "There is, therefore, only one categorical imperative. It is: Act only according to that maxim by which you can at the same time will that it should become a universal law" (38). Kant presents this as an analogy with the universal laws of nature. We are to use the formulation of the categorical imperative to test the morality of any principle (or "maxim") we might adopt by supposing that what we embrace in our choice were to become a universal and necessary law of nature. What if everybody not only did but had to do what I am doing? That is, what if everybody committed suicide when life became difficult? What if everybody made false promises when it was convenient to do so? Kant considers these and other examples to illustrate that the formal character of universality is the mark of a morally upright maxim, whereas making an exception to accommodate one's own interest is the mark of violation of one's duty. Adopting maxims that fail the categorical imperative is ultimately to be at odds with oneself as a rational agent because one takes as one's maxim something that cannot be coherently willed as a universal law for all rational agents.

In an effort to spell out its meaning more fully, Kant gives two other formulations of the same categorical imperative. One of these formulations has won great currency in contemporary bioethics, although it is usually interpreted in isolation from and often in conflict with the rest of Kant's account. The second formulation of the imperative is: "Act so that you treat humanity, whether in your own person or in that of another, always as an end and never as a means only" (46). Kant's view is that human beings, as rational, are persons and stand higher in dignity than mere things. He does not claim, as he is sometimes loosely interpreted to claim, that a human person may never be treated as a means. He says, consistently, that a person should always be treated as an end and not *merely* or *only* as a means. Clearly, this qualification is important, for example, in medical research. Human subjects of research are necessarily the means by which medical scientists come to learn how to produce benefits that may, but often do not, benefit the subjects themselves. The Kantian standard could permit such research, but it requires that the subjects be treated during the experiment as persons and not as mere things, not as the chemical components of an experimental drug are treated. Things, in contrast to persons, may be treated solely by reference to their instrumentality for accomplishing human purposes.

In addition to the emphasis on human dignity in the form of the requirement of treating human beings as ends in themselves, Kant's ethical theory has influenced bioethics especially by his emphasis on autonomy. What Kant meant by autonomy is the capacity to conduct oneself in accord with universal rational principles and not the liberty or license to conduct oneself as one sees fit. Autonomy is nevertheless often invoked in contemporary ethical debates as if whatever a human being were to choose for himself or herself were justified by the fact of its being chosen, irrespective of what the choice might be.[37] Kant's clause in the second formulation of the categorical imperative—that one must treat humanity as an end "whether in your own person or in that of another"—illuminates the basis for duties to oneself.[38]

Kant takes it to be a great problem that it is possible for human beings to be subject to a categorical imperative. How is it possible that human beings, driven as we are by needs and inclinations, can also be bound by the unconditional command of morality? We cannot show from experience that we are in fact capable of acting in accord with it, because we can never be sure that any given agent has indeed acted solely out of duty to the pure moral law and not out of some form of (perhaps hidden) self-interest. The necessary presupposition of ourselves as autonomous (even though we cannot show how we are free) is meant to solve this problem, but it still leaves another problem unsolved: Why should anyone be moral? That is, assuming that it is possible for us to act in conformity with pure duty, why should we (66)? Kant regards this as a related problem, and he states only that human beings do in fact take an interest in moral laws.

> The subjective impossibility of explaining the freedom of the will is the same as the impossibility of discovering and explaining an interest which man can take in moral laws. Nevertheless, he does actually take an interest in them, and the foundation of this interest in us we will call the moral feeling. This moral feeling has been erroneously construed by some as the standard for our moral judgment, whereas it must be regarded rather as the subjective effect which the law has upon the will to which reason alone gives objective grounds. (77-78)

Kant regards this interest in morality as "pure" because it arises only when the universal validity of the maxim is reason's determining ground. This makes it different in kind from any interest we might happen to take in what can be accomplished through the actions we perform. Kant takes the interest in morality as a fact of reason and claims "an explanation of how and why the universality of the maxim as law (and hence morality) interests us is completely impossible for us men" (78-79). This problem may be the necessary result of the separation of morality from happiness.[39]

John Stuart Mill: *Utilitarianism*

Kant's ethics is often called *deontological* because it emphasizes unconditional duties, irrespective of the consequences of our actions and of what we intend to accomplish in the world through our actions. For Kant, neither the success nor the failure of our efforts in the world is morally relevant; acting from the motive of duty is morally decisive. Mill's utilitarian ethics[40] is, in part, a specific reaction to Kant and his apparent unconcern for the consequences of our willing. Mill emphasizes the end or the consequences of human activity, and therefore his ethics is called *consequentialist*.[41] Mill argues that the end of all human action and first principle of morality is the greatest happiness principle, also known as the principle of utility. Mill goes so far as to say that the principle of utility is indispensable even to Kant, who claims to derive morality without reference to consequences. Mill objects that Kant's application of the categorical imperative only works if we evaluate maxims by reference to the consequences that would ensue if those maxims were adopted universally (4).

Mill explains that *utility* or *the greatest happiness principle* "holds that actions are right in proportion as they tend to promote happiness; wrong as they tend to promote the reverse of happiness. By happiness is intended pleasure and the absence of pain; by unhappiness, pain and the privation of pleasure" (7). Only pleasure and freedom from pain are desirable as ends in themselves; other things are desirable as the means to pleasure or because pleasure inheres in them. Mill distinguishes higher and lower pleasures; in this way, the question of quality as well as quantity of pleasure becomes relevant. The comparison and the ranking are to be made by those who are "competently acquainted" with both pleasures. "Of two pleasures, if there be one to which all or almost all who have experience of both give a decided preference, irrespective of any feeling of moral obligation to prefer it, that is the more desirable pleasure" (8). Mill's use of this standard of judgment is somewhat difficult to interpret because he both seems to appeal to the judgment of those who experience pleasures and pains, but also rejects some people as not competent to judge. "It is better to be a human being dissatisfied than a pig satisfied; better to be Socrates dissatisfied than a fool satisfied. And if the fool, or the pig, are of a different opinion, it is because they only know their own side of the question" (10). Mill appeals, then, to a standard of judgment that is analogous to Aristotle's prudent human being, but he also conceives this competent judgment as being much more widespread and easily acquired than Aristotle suggested. He appeals explicitly to the democratic standard of majority opinion to decide any disagreement among competent judges (11).[42]

There is in this conception a certain similarity to the Aristotelian and the Thomistic account of the relation between morality and happiness, but important differences emerge when we note that Mill's view is that the end in question is not the agent's own happiness but the greatest amount of happiness for all (11). In the course of dealing with an objection of whether a human being can, in any realistic sense, aim at such an expansive goal, Mill claims that human happiness is within our grasp if we marshal our efforts systematically.

> Yet no one whose opinion deserves a moment's consideration can doubt that most of the great positive evils of the world are in themselves removable, and will, if human affairs continue to improve, be in the end reduced within narrow limits. Poverty, in any sense implying suffering, may be completely extinguished by the wisdom of society combined with the good sense and providence of individuals. Even that most intractable of enemies, disease, may be indefinitely reduced in dimensions by good physical and moral education and proper control of noxious

influences, while the progress of science holds out a promise for the future of still more direct conquests over this detestable foe. . . . All the grand sources, in short, of human suffering are in a great degree, many of them almost entirely, conquerable by human care and effort. (15)

On closer inspection, then, Mill's first principle of morality—the pursuit of the maximum happiness for all mankind—proves to be a new formulation of the moral argument in favor of the scientific mastery of nature first explicitly articulated by Bacon and Descartes. The basic moral obligation of mankind is, in Mill's view, to take part in the humanitarian effort toward the relief and benefit of man's estate.

Mill emphasizes that in the pursuit of the greatest happiness, one's own happiness does not occupy any privileged position. Rather, one must be "as strictly impartial as a disinterested and benevolent spectator" (17). Mill presents this as congruent with or identical to the Christian teaching embodied in the command to love one's neighbor as oneself, although it should be noted that Mill wants to defend utilitarianism by reason and not by theological authority (4–5). He does not expect each human being to be pursuing the happiness of all of humankind constantly. Most actions will be more parochial. All the same, the standard of utility requires us to be certain that, while we benefit those who are near and dear, we do not violate the rights of anyone else (19).

Mill draws an instructive contrast between his view and Kant's by distinguishing between the "rule of action" and the "motive" of action (18–19). By "rule of action" Mill seems to mean what we will or what it is right for us to will, whereas by "motive" he means the feeling that brings us to will as we do. Thus, one might refrain from stealing because it is one's duty not to steal, or one might refrain from stealing out of fear of being caught. In each case, a person follows the right rule of action and acts for or in keeping with the greatest happiness of all, but the moral worth of that person (as distinct from the moral goodness of the deed) is judged differently in each case. Mill emphasizes the importance of doing the good action and does not think that the act is corrupted if its motive is impure. This leads Mill to distinguish between "intention" and "motive." Motive, he says, is the feeling that makes the agent will what he or she wills. The intention, he says, is "what the agent *wills to do* [emphasis in the original]," and the moral goodness or badness of an action depends entirely upon the intention.[43] A difficulty remains, however, in the difference between what we will to do and the multiplicity of consequences that may actually result from our willing. Where Kant ignored the moral significance of the actual consequences and Thomistic ethics attempts to distinguish between direct and indirect responsibility, Mill's utilitarianism sometimes emphasizes "what the agent wills to do" and sometimes emphasizes the actual results, which may have been unintentional, of what we will.[44]

At this point it is helpful to note another ambiguity in Mill's account that has subsequently been distinguished more clearly. Sometimes Mill speaks as if utilitarianism sanctions in each case the specific action that promotes the greatest happiness of the greatest number and sometimes he speaks as if it sanctions the rule that generally promotes the greatest happiness of the greatest number. These two positions are described as *act utilitarianism* and *rule utilitarianism*, respectively. A common objection against utilitarianism is that action does not permit us the time to calculate the consequences of our actions for all humankind. Mill responds to this in part by noting that the inherited experience of humankind is available to us in the form of various moral rules that guide us to prudential practices. For example, Mill appeals to the customary prohibition against lying and notes that, however useful particular lies might be, one must also recognize that such lies, chosen on account of a narrowly conceived expediency, actually work to undermine the trust human beings place in one another's word. In this way, those who lie actually deprive humankind of the goods made available through that trust and trustworthiness. Immediately, he qualifies this apparent endorsement of a utilitarian prohibition against lying: "Yet that even this rule, sacred as it is, admits of possible exceptions is acknowledged by all moralists; the chief of which is when the withholding of some fact (as of information from a malefactor, or of bad news from a person dangerously ill) would save an individual (especially an individual other than oneself) from great and unmerited evil, and when the withholding can only be effected by denial" (23). It should be noted that Kant, in particular, did not endorse the moral goodness of the useful lie and that this contrast with Mill illuminates the differences between them. These differences occupy bioethicists considering the question of a physician's obligation to disclose unpleasant or otherwise undesirable truths to patients.

The greatest happiness principle, at first sight, seems to answer much better than did Kant the question of why a human being should be moral, because moral standards are thereby reconnected with happiness, understood as pleasure, which is not something one needs to urge people to seek. Mill, nevertheless, recognizes the potential for conflict between an individual's pursuit of happiness and the general happiness: "Why am I bound to promote the general happiness? If my own happiness lies in something else, why may I not give that the preference?" (27). Mill replies that, if we abstract from external sanctions of reward or punishment that might arise from God or from men, we must recognize that the only genuinely *moral* sanction is the internal feeling that goes by the name of conscience or conscientiousness. "The internal sanction of duty, whatever our standard of duty may be, is one and the same—a feeling in our own mind; a pain, more or less intense, attendant on violation of duty, which in properly cultivated moral natures rises, in the more serious cases, into shrinking from it as an impossibility" (28). Mill sees that even if one agrees with Kant or with Aquinas that the ultimate standard of morality exists independently of human psychology, it is meaningless to speak of this standard as an operative moral sanction unless the human agent permits it to influence his or her action. In this sense, the only conceivable moral sanction is "entirely subjective, having its seat in human consciousness only" (29–30). What moves us can only be our appreciation of the moral standard as a standard for our action.

Mill thinks that we come to acquire these moral feelings of deference to the principle of utility primarily through education, although they have a natural basis in the social feelings of humankind. An improper education could corrupt our moral formation in very damaging ways. As a result, the moral formation of individuals is perhaps the most pressing social problem; again, Mill expresses optimism concerning the great progress that can be made through human institutions, provided that we begin early and cultivate the moral feelings of each toward the general happiness.

> If we now suppose this feeling of unity to be taught as a religion, and the whole force of education, of institutions, and of opinion directed, as it once was in the case of religion, to make every person grow up from infancy surrounded on all sides both by the profession and the practice of it, I think that no one who can realize this conception will feel any misgiving about the sufficiency of the ultimate sanction for the happiness morality. (33)

Mill concludes his discussion of the ultimate sanction of morality by pointing out that the cultivation of regard for the happiness of others must compete with the naturally much stronger selfish feelings, which, presumably, cannot be eradicated. Thus, he emphasizes the naturalness or apparent naturalness of a man's understanding himself as a social being, "which tends to make him feel it one of his natural wants that there should be harmony between his feelings and aims and those of his fellow creatures. . . . [T]o those who have it, [this feeling] possesses all the characters of a natural feeling. It does not present itself to their minds as a superstition of education or a law despotically imposed by the power of society" (34). In these remarks Mill seems to anticipate the potential for objections that were eventually made by Freud and others.[45] The general happiness might sometimes require renunciation of one's own happiness, but utilitarianism denies that renunciation itself is good. "A sacrifice which does not increase or tend to increase the sum total of happiness, it considers as wasted" (17).

The question of the sacrifice of the individual or of the minority for the greater general happiness raises what is perhaps the most consistent and troublesome objection to utilitarianism. The priority of the general happiness to that of the individual and the claim that it is the individual's obligation to seek the general happiness while regarding his or her own personal happiness as no more significant than that of any other single person together suggest alarming possibilities for the exploitation of individuals for the benefit of the general welfare. In the context of bioethics, one immediately thinks of the treatment of subjects of medical research or of the conscription of organs from living "donors." Kantianism, with its insistence that each instance of humanity be respected as an end in itself, seems to provide much sturdier restrictions on such activities.

Mill's treatment of justice, which occupies fully one-third of *Utilitarianism*, aims to respond in advance to these sorts of challenges. He begins by demonstrating that our grasp of "justice" is far from clear because of the multiplicity of applications of standards of justice. This discussion is reminiscent of some accounts of the difficulty of identifying what would be a just distribution of scarce medical resources. Is it just to treat everyone equally or, rather, in accord with what each variously deserves or needs? Mill appeals to a familiar distinction between perfect and imperfect duties. Perfect duties oblige always, whereas imperfect duties, such as charitable giving, "we are indeed bound to practice but not toward any definite person, nor at any prescribed time" (49). Others have rights to exact from us the fulfillment of our perfect duties. Imperfect obligations do not correspond to or give rise to a right in another to demand specific actions from us. The distinction between perfect and imperfect duties coincides exactly, Mill says, with that between justice and the *other* obligations of morality (50).

> I account the justice which is grounded on utility to be the chief part, and incomparably the most sacred and binding part, of all morality. Justice is a name for certain classes of moral rules which concern the essentials of human well-being more nearly, and are therefore of more absolute obligation, than any other rules for the guidance of life; and the notion which we have found to be of the essence of the idea of justice—that of a right residing in an individual—implies and testifies to this more binding obligation. (59)

The rules of justice are "more binding," but still not "absolutely binding," for the principle of the greatest happiness is still more fundamental than the rights to equal or impartial treatment.

> All persons are deemed to have a *right* to equality of treatment, except when some recognized social expediency requires the reverse. . . . It appears from what has been said that justice is a name for certain moral requirements, which, regarded collectively, stand higher on the scale of social utility, and are therefore of more paramount obligation, than any others, though particular cases may occur in which some other social duty is so important as to overrule any one of the general maxims of justice. (63)

Clearly, the adjudication of the competing pressures in each case requires an independent judgment of whether the greatest happiness is best served by following established rules or by making exceptions. The judgment must come from clear-sighted prudence or, at least, the opinion of the majority.

Conclusion

The preceding sketches of the moral thought of Aristotle, Aquinas, Kant, and Mill are necessarily incomplete. Even a brief survey manages to convey the substantive differences that separate them from one another. Recognizing those differences helps to indicate the depth and complexity that attends the search for an adequate bioethical theory. It also helps guard against a form of moral syncretism, in which we select what may be mutually incompatible principles, ideas, or standards as we find them convenient and try to fashion piecemeal solutions to practical difficulties as they arise. One form of this syncretism settles on a desirable solution and then sophistically constructs an argument to support that conclusion. For example, it is not impossible to find people who will embrace a utilitarian standard in order to support embryonic stem cell research, but a Kantian standard in order to oppose forcible removal of organs from prisoners. In the absence of a compelling reason why one does not embrace the same standard in the two cases, we suspect this approach of intellectual and moral vacuity.

Bioethics is especially susceptible to relying upon deracinated moral "tools" from different sources because, with the exception of Thomists in the Catholic health care arena, few people approach bioethics from the perspective of a comprehensive moral theory they have already embraced in its entirety. Most bioethical issues arise as practical problems for which we seek intelligent and good solutions. The moral discourse of our ordinary thinking readily furnishes us with a mixture of classical, Christian, and modern secular principles and concepts. It makes sense that we would use these as they seem appropriate for articulating solutions. Unless we exercise considerable caution, this might lead us to embrace an argument that is internally incoherent or otherwise ill-considered. Relying on thoughtlessly constructed arguments both undermines any particular solution we devise and tends to cast doubt on the whole enterprise of moral reasoning. A thorough skepticism about our ability to know moral truth is a serious moral position that needs to be considered, but the practical consequences of completely embracing the claim that no moral solution is knowably superior to any other ought to be sufficient to incline us at least to inquire seriously into the matter.

Utilitarianism always has a certain theoretical advantage insofar as it is very clearly true that one should think like a utilitarian in some cases—that is, when there is no moral difference between the means to be chosen. For example, if the goal is to treat cancer, one selects between competing medical interventions (chemotherapy, radiation, surgery, or some combination) by comparing the expected consequences of choosing each. We presuppose here that the means are morally equivalent. But is it always true that the available means are morally equivalent? If the goal is becoming the parent of a healthy baby, we might try sexual intercourse, artificial insemination, in vitro fertilization, cloning, adoption, or kidnapping. The necessity of giving a principled reason why the means are indifferent in the one case but not in the other requires us to consider moral questions in an intellectually serious and comprehensive way. This introduction has attempted to encourage that inquiry.

Chapter Summary

This chapter summarized the broad outlines of four ethical theories that stand at the center of the Western tradition. Each theory was examined by reference to the representative work of a single author: Aristotle's *Nicomachean Ethics*, St. Thomas Aquinas's *Summa Theologiae*, Immanuel Kant's *Foundations of the Metaphysics of Morals*, and John Stuart Mill's *Utilitarianism*. The two classical theories agree in identifying good moral action with the activity that is conducive to or constitutive of good living, which is identified with happiness. For these authors, inquiring into what action is morally good is a rational investigation into how to live as happily as possible, which means as virtuously as possible. Moral reasoning is simply the search for the kind of activity that is or leads to happiness. The two modern authors, by contrast, conceive of morality as a realm that is, in different ways, independent of the individual concern for happiness. Kant presents morality under the aspect of stern commands of duty that oblige us quite apart from and even in contempt of our selfish desires for happiness. The concern for happiness—which he conceives as the full satisfaction of whatever desires a person happens to have—is amoral, although this concern tends to interfere with our fulfillment of the moral law, in reference to which alone we can speak of human dignity. Mill conceives the principle of morality as the promotion of the greatest happiness, which consists in pleasure, of the greatest number of people. Moral obligation arises only in view of the general happiness, which may stand in tension with one's individual happiness. These four theories were introduced by examining the innovation exerting the greatest influence on both our medicine and our moral reasoning: modern science. This chapter described how any attempt to appreciate the role of theory in bioethics must address the prominence and authority of science.

Review Questions

1. What is the meaning of the term *bioethics*?

2. What is the difference between private and public moral justification?

3. How does one distinguish between classical and modern moral philosophy?

4. How does Descartes' *Discourse on Method* develop the landscape upon which contemporary bioethics is built?

5. According to Descartes, what are the two contrary pressures brought on moral reasoning?

6. How does Aristotle characterize a virtuous person?

7. According to Aristotle, what is the proper fulfillment of a human being?

8. What distinction does Aristotle make between an *end* and a *purpose*? How does this relate to issues in modern medicine such as physician-assisted suicide?

9. The philosophies of Aristotle and Thomas Aquinas are similar in many ways. How are they different from one another?

10. What are the characteristics of natural law according to Thomas Aquinas?

11. What are the three fonts Thomas Aquinas applies to the goodness or badness of a human action? Why are they important?

12. What is the principle of double effect? How can this principle be applied to modern bioethics?

13. Why did Immanuel Kant separate the demands of morality from the search for happiness?

14. What does Kant mean by the term *duty*?

15. What is utilitarianism?

16. What is the difference between a hypothetical imperative and a categorical imperative?

17. "Act only according to the maxim by which you can at the same time will that it should become a universal law" is an explanation of which imperative? What does it mean?

18. What is John Stuart Mill's first principle of morality?

19. John Stuart Mill argued that "It is better to be a human being dissatisfied than a pig satisfied." What does he mean by this statement?

20. Why is it important to understand the various ethical theories in bioethics?

Endnotes

1. Although it is sometimes useful to distinguish the terms *moral* and *ethical*, in this chapter they are used interchangeably.

2. See "The Discipline of Pure Reason" in Kant's *Critique of Pure Reason.*

3. The most prominent school of bioethical reasoning, the principlism of Tom Beauchamp and James Childress, substitutes the search for *coherent* moral beliefs in place of the search for *true* moral beliefs and postulates the insolubility in principle of fundamental moral disagreement. "Finally, available work using the method of coherence lacks the power to eliminate various conflicts among principles and rules. This insufficiency is not surprising, because all moral theories experience this problem, and coherence theory has no magical powers to settle these conflicts" (*Principles of Biomedical Ethics*, 5th ed. [Oxford: Oxford University Press, 2001], 401). H. Tristram Engelhardt, Jr., represents an interesting exception that proves the rule. He takes the epistemological insufficiency of secular reason as established, but he laments the fact and strives to defend both a contentless, consent-based, secular bioethics and the legitimacy of a plurality of content-full, private moralities that bind particular communities. See *The Foundations of Bioethics*, 2nd ed. (New York: Oxford University Press, 1996) and *The Foundations of Christian Bioethics* (Netherlands: Swets & Zeitlinger, 2000).

4. René Descartes, *Discourse on Method*, trans. with an interpretive essay by Richard Kennington, ed. Pamela Kraus and Frank Hunt (Newburyport, Mass.: Focus Publishing, 2007), 22. Subsequent references will be made to the pages of this text. French text in *Oeuvres de Descartes*, vol. 6, ed. Charles Adam and Paul Tannery (Paris: J. Vrin, 1964), 1–78.

5. See Richard Kennington, "Descartes and Mastery of Nature," *Organism, Medicine, and Metaphysics*, ed. Stuart F. Spicker (Dordrecht, Holland: D. Reidel Publishing, 1978), 201–23.

6. In Descartes' famous image of the tree of philosophy (preface to the French edition of *The Principles of Philosophy*), metaphysics forms the roots and physics the trunk, and the main branches are mechanics, medicine, and morals. "By 'morals' I understand the highest and most perfect moral system, which presupposes a complete knowledge of the other sciences and is the ulti-

mate level of wisdom." The fruit (the principal benefit of philosophy) hangs from the branches. *The Philosophical Writings of Descartes*, vol. 1, trans. John Cottingham, Robert Stoothoff, and Dugald Murdoch (Cambridge: Cambridge University Press, 1985), 186.

7. The distinction between philosophy and science, which we take for granted, became widely accepted only after Descartes. Even Newton thought of his *Principia* as belonging to "natural philosophy." Kant sharply distinguishes science from philosophy. See, for example, the discussion of demonstrations in *Critique of Pure Reason*, A734/B762–A738/B766.

8. Consider, for example, the doctrine of substance (book II, ch. 13) in Locke's 1689 *An Essay Concerning Human Understanding*.

9. See Transcendental Doctrine of Method, first section, "The Discipline of Pure Reason in its Dogmatic Use," and second section, "The Discipline of Pure Reason in its Polemical Use," in *Critique of Pure Reason*.

10. See, for instance, the presentation given in Tom L. Beauchamp and LeRoy Walters, eds., *Contemporary Issues in Bioethics*, 5th ed. (Belmont, Calif.: Thomson Wadsworth, 1999), 7–8.

11. Ronald Munson, *Intervention and Reflection: Basic Issues in Medical Ethics*, 8th ed. (Belmont, Calif.: Thomson Wadsworth, 2008), 7.

12. The title of an essay in a medical journal encapsulates this attitude. The full title is "An Anecdote Is an Anecdote Is an Anecdote . . . but a Clinical Trial Is Data." M. Donohoe and R. M. Rogers, *American Journal of Respiratory Critical Care Medicine* 149 (1994): 293–94.

13. In the prefatory paragraph to the *Discourse*, Descartes identifies the maxims of the provisional morality as drawn from the rules of his method. See also the fifth paragraph of the third part: "Besides, the three preceding maxims were founded only on my intention of continuing to instruct myself" (*Discourse on Method*, 30).

14. The issues here are enormously complex, and the situation may well be different for different authors. It seems safe to say that although Aristotle's ethics, for example, is not indifferent to metaphysics, the theoretical sciences do not precede and establish the starting point for practical sciences such as ethics and politics. Thomas Aquinas is a different and more difficult case, especially because he follows a theological order of presentation, beginning with God as the first principle of all things and descending to the created order.

15. See, for example, the chapter "Moral Character" in Tom L. Beauchamp and James F. Childress, *Principles of Biomedical Ethics*, 5th ed. (Oxford: Oxford University Press, 2001), 26–56.

16. *Nicomachean Ethics*, trans. W. D. Ross, rev. J. O. Urmson, in vol. 2 of *The Complete Works of Aristotle*, revised Oxford translation, ed. Jonathan Barnes (Princeton, N.J.: Princeton University Press, 1984). For the Greek text see L. Bywater, ed., *Aristotelis: Ethica Nicomachea* (Oxford: Oxford University Press, 1894). Subsequent references to *Nicomachean Ethics* will be made by citing the book and chapter with roman and Arabic numerals, respectively. In some cases, precise references to the Bekker line numbers will be made.

17. This distinction is clarified by Francis Slade, "Ends and Purposes," *Final Causality in Nature and Human Affairs*, ed. Richard F. Hassing (Washington, D.C.: The Catholic University of America Press, 1994), 83–85, and Robert Sokolowski, "What Is Natural Law? Human Purposes and Natural Ends," *Thomist* 68 (2004): 511. See also Aristotle's *Metaphysics* book IX, chapters 2 and 5.

18. President's Council on Bioethics, *Beyond Therapy: Biotechnology and the Pursuit of Happiness* (New York: ReganBooks, 2003).

19. See *Nicomachean Ethics* I.7 1097b34–1098a1 and I.13 1102b11–12. But also consider his recognition of the goodness of the life of the body and its indispensability for any form of excellence, for example, I.8, 1098b12–14, IX.9, 1170b1–2, VIII.7, 1159a5–12, and X.8, 1178b33–35.

20. For example, *Nicomachean Ethics* III.5, 1114a21–31.
21. The translation here is my own (III.4.1113a29–33).
22. Saint Thomas Aquinas, *Summa Theologiae* (Alba and Rome: Pauline Editions, 1962). For a translation containing most of the material treated here, see Saint Thomas Aquinas, *Treatise on Happiness*, trans. John A. Oesterle (Notre Dame, Ind.: University of Notre Dame Press, 1983). For the texts on natural law, see Saint Thomas Aquinas, *Political Writings*, ed. and trans. R. W. Dyson (New York: Cambridge University Press, 2002).
23. "*Et talis participatio legis aeternae in rationali creatura lex naturalis dicitur*" (I-II, q. 91, a. 2).
24. See Robert Sokolowski, "Knowing Natural Law," in *Pictures, Quotations, and Distinctions: Fourteen Essays in Phenomenology* (Notre Dame and London: University of Notre Dame Press, 1992), 277–91.
25. For confirmation of the importance of these three sources of morality, see *Catechism of the Catholic Church* (#1750). For Aquinas's presentation, see *Summa Theologiae* I-II, qq. 12, 13, 18, 19, and 20. See also Servais Pinckaers, *The Sources of Christian Ethics*, trans. Mary Thomas Noble (Washington, D.C.: The Catholic University of America Press, 1995) and David Gallagher, "Aquinas on Moral Action: Interior and Exterior Acts," *American Catholic Philosophical Quarterly*, Annual Supplement, LXIV (1990): 118–29.
26. Here *end* is not used in the precise sense in which we distinguished it from *purpose* earlier. Here, the end is the target of the human will and is therefore a purpose. We note again, however, that an end can in fact be targeted by deliberate human action, with the result that the same thing is, from different perspectives, an end and a purpose. Thus, health is the end of medical activity, and it can also be the case that the medical doctor aims at no purpose beyond restoring the health of a given patient.
27. See Congregation for the Doctrine of the Faith, *Declaration on Procured Abortion* (18 November 1974), especially footnote 19. This teaching is repeated in the Congregation's *Instruction on Respect for Human Life in its Origin and on the Dignity of Procreation* (22 February 1987) and in John Paul II, *The Gospel of Life* (25 March 1995), #58–63.
28. Aquinas gives a classic formulation of the basis of this in his discussion of homicide (II-II, q. 64, a. 7). Again, it should be noted that the extensive analysis and application of this principle in the secondary literature is magnificently out of proportion to the small scope given to this sort of reasoning by Aquinas.
29. See Congregation for the Doctrine of the Faith, *Declaration on Euthanasia* (5 May 1980).
30. See National Conference of Catholic Bishops, *Ethical and Religious Directives for Catholic Health Care Services*, 4th ed. (Washington, D.C.: United States Conference of Catholic Bishops, 2001). In addition to its historical importance, the examination of Catholic moral reasoning can be justified, if for no other reason, by the large number of Catholic health institutions in this country. All medical personnel in Catholic health facilities agree to deliver care in conformity to the moral principles articulated in the *Ethical and Religious Directives*.
31. Immanuel Kant, *Foundations of the Metaphysics of Morals*, 2nd ed., trans. Lewis White Beck (Upper Saddle River, N.J.: Prentice-Hall, 1997). Subsequent references to the pages of this work will be made parenthetically in the body of the text. German text: *Grundlegung zur Metaphysik der Sitten*, in *Kants Gesammelte Schriften*, vol. 4 (Berlin and New York: Walter de Gruyter, 1968).
32. See especially book II, chapters xx and xxi. Locke's doctrine of the pursuit of happiness, which is so important for American political life and thought, is specifically mentioned not in his political works, but in the *Essay*: "As therefore the highest perfection of intellectual nature, lies in a careful and constant pursuit of true and solid happiness; so the care of our selves, that we mistake not imaginary for real happiness, is the necessary foundation of our liberty" (book II

ch. xxi, §51). Happiness is real and true, but it is individual, and so it is a mistake to seek with Aristotle wherein the highest good might be found, for this is something different for different human beings (see book II, ch. xxi, §55). John Locke, *An Essay Concerning Human Understanding*, ed. Peter H. Nidditch (Oxford: Clarendon Press, 1975).

33. Kant characterizes human dignity in both ways. See *Foundations of the Metaphysics of Morals*, 2nd ed., trans. Lewis White Beck (Upper Saddle River, N.J.: Prentice-Hall, 1997), 57.

34. "Philosophy is the science of the relation of all knowledge to the essential ends of human reason. . . . Essential ends are therefore either the ultimate end or subordinate ends which are necessarily connected with the former as means. The former is no other than the whole vocation of man, and the philosophy which deals with it is entitled moral philosophy" (*Critique of Pure Reason*, trans. Norman Kemp Smith [New York: St. Martin's Press, 1965], 657–58 [A839/B867–A840/B868]).

35. In the preface to *Foundations*, Kant promises a practical anthropology to complement the rational consideration of moral philosophy he presents in this work. The nearest he came to completing this is the collection of his lectures on the subject in his fascinating *Anthropology from a Pragmatic Point of View*, trans. Robert B. Louden (Cambridge: Cambridge University Press, 2006). Here, Kant discusses the moral task of mankind as the progressive, historical effort to rise above the demands of our particular nature. The anthropology presents a mastery of nature argument as accomplished through the historical, progressive development of moral character.

36. We must note, however, that Kant argues that the indefiniteness of our concept of happiness requires that these imperatives amount to no more than counsels, not commands. Omniscience would be necessary to articulate the path to happiness, and "the task of determining infallibly and universally what action will promote the happiness of a rational being is completely unsolvable" (35).

37. Ronald Munson sketches what he says might constitute a Kantian argument in favor of suicide: "Our status as autonomous rational beings also endows us with an inherent dignity. If that status is destroyed or severely compromised, as it is when people become comatose and unknowing because of illness or injury, . . . [i]t may be more in keeping with our freedom and dignity for us to instruct others either to put us to death or to take no steps to keep us alive. . . . Voluntary euthanasia may be compatible with (if not required by) Kantian ethics" (*Intervention and Reflection*, 8th ed. [Belmont, Calif.: Thomson Wadsworth, 2008], 688). Contrast Kant's claim: "If in order to escape from burdensome circumstances he destroys himself, he uses a person merely as a means to maintain a tolerable condition up to the end of life. Man, however, is not a thing, and thus not something to be used merely as a means; he must always be regarded in all his actions as an end in himself. Therefore I cannot dispose of man in my own person so as to mutilate, corrupt, or kill him" (46).

38. For an especially helpful discussion of the distinction between what Kant meant by autonomy and what it has come to mean in contemporary bioethics, see Hadley Arkes, " 'Autonomy' and the 'Quality of Life': The Dismantling of Moral Terms," *Issues in Law and Medicine* 2 (1987): 421–33.

39. Two qualifications are important here. The first is that, as has been indicated, Kant means by happiness "the sum of satisfaction of all inclinations" (15), which he regards as a hopelessly vague notion. This is not what was meant by happiness according to Aristotle and Aquinas, each of whom identified it with the highest virtuous activity. The second point is that Kant does try to integrate morality and happiness insofar as he regards moral goodness as the condition of worthiness to be happy (9). There is, for Kant, no necessary connection between moral

goodness and well-being or happiness (59); the ideal that happiness be distributed in proportion to moral worth obtains, if anywhere, only in another world, a moral world (see *Critique of Pure Reason*, A807/B835–A812/B840).

40. John Stuart Mill, *Utilitarianism*, 2nd ed., ed. George Sheer (Indianapolis/Cambridge: Hackett Publishing, 2001). Subsequent references to pages of this edition will be made parenthetically in the body of the text.

41. Sometimes Mill's ethics is classed as "teleological" along with Aristotle's ethics, but because of the significant differences between an "end" (*telos*) and a "consequence" as the principle of moral reasoning, it is useful to distinguish the two schools of thought. The relevant differences should become clear in what follows.

42. A more complete account of Mill's understanding of happiness would need to consider his other works, especially *On Liberty*. There Mill discusses the relation between truth and utility and defends diversity in belief and in action.

43. It is difficult to bring this use of "intention" into line with the Thomistic use because Mill's use seems to be ambiguous between what Aquinas called "choice" and what he called "intention." The difficulty is complicated by Mill's use of "motive," which may refer to what we hope to gain through action (18). It seems safe to say that by "motive" Mill has in mind that psychological influence that leads us to will what we will, whereas the intention is either the act we perform or the act together with what is immediately accomplished in it.

44. Consider, for example, the treatment of the unintentional consequences of lying, mentioned in the next paragraph.

45. See, for example, *Civilization and Its Discontents*. In *On Liberty*, Mill shows himself to be especially attentive to the dangers of socially imposed compulsion.

Chapter 2

Principles of Biomedical Ethics

Ethics and equity and the principles of justice do not change with the calendar.

—D. H. Lawrence

Justice consists not in being neutral between right and wrong, but in finding out the right and upholding it, wherever found, against the wrong.

—Theodore Roosevelt

Chapter Learning Objectives

At the conclusion of this chapter the reader will be able to:

1. Understand the relationships among moral value judgments, moral rules or ideals, the principles of biomedical ethics, and ethical theory

2. List and explain the principles of biomedical ethics

3. List and recognize the requirements for autonomous choice

4. Define *competency* and *decisional capacity*

5. Recognize and distinguish the various types of controlling influences that undermine voluntariness

6. Recognize and distinguish nonmaleficence and beneficence

7. Explain the rule of the double effect and recognize instances in which it does and does not apply

8. Recognize and distinguish specific and general beneficence

9. Recognize situations in which beneficence is obligatory as opposed to ideal

10. Define *paternalism* and distinguish between weak (soft) and strong (hard) paternalism

11. Recognize instances in which strong (hard) paternalism might be justified

12. State the formal principle of justice

13. List several material principles of justice

14. Explain how utilitarian, egalitarian, and libertarian views of justice differ

In the following excerpt, Joan Gibson compares ethics to science in a way that is helpful to us here and, in the process, provides a framework for the topics discussed in Section I of this text.

[A] comparison between the giving of good reasons in science, which is called "explanation," and the giving of good reasons in ethics, which is called "moral justification," reveals striking procedural similarities bordering on identity. . . .

Answering the question "Why?" [in science] . . . is known as explanation: the accounting for observed phenomena at levels of increased abstraction, generalization, and simplification. Moving [in the opposite direction], once the "Why?"s are answered, generates the power of prediction about future similar observations and phenomena.

And so it is with giving good reasons for individual moral judgments. . . . Answering the "Why?" moving up the [ethics pyramid] is known as moral justification. Moving down the [ethics pyramid], once the "Why?"s are answered, yields decisions about similar, future moral value judgments that must be made. Answering "Why?" . . . requires that reasons be elucidated and organized. Truth in science as well as in ethics derives not so much from discovering isolated, once-and-for-all answers, but rather from continually articulating, evaluating and revising the reasons one gives for the continually modified propositions one asserts and the consistently reevaluated judgments one makes. Extrapolating into the future (. . . making [moral] decisions) is only as sound as the integrity of prior . . . moral justifications.[1]

Chapter 1 discussed the apex, as it were, of the metaphorical ethics pyramid—ethical theory. As we move down that pyramid, we will discuss ethics in an increasingly concrete or specific way—first at the level of moral principles (the focus of this chapter), then at the level of moral rules (the focus of Chapter 3), and finally at the level of moral decisions in individual cases (the focus of Chapter 4).

Different people think about or analyze problems in bioethics in different ways. Some may prefer to think through these problems in terms of the principles of biomedical ethics; others prefer the moral rules-based account of morality of Bernard Gert and associates (see Chapter 3); still others prefer the approach of casuistry (see Chapter 4). One of our purposes in this text, and in this section in particular, is to expose the reader to these various approaches.

Theory, Principles, Rules, and Moral Decisions

The focus of this chapter is on the principles of biomedical ethics, or *principlism*. Before embarking on a discussion of the principles themselves, let's consider the following question: What are moral principles? How do they relate to moral theory, moral rules, and moral decisions?

A *principle* may be defined as "a basic truth or a *general* law or doctrine that is used as a basis of reasoning or *a guide to action* or behavior."[2] Principles, like rules, are action guides, although, as the earlier excerpt should make clear, the guidance they provide is more abstract or general than that provided by rules. Gert and colleagues have written that "principles really are action guides that summarize and encapsulate a whole [moral] *theory* and thus, in a shorthand manner, assist a moral agent in making a moral decision."[3] Thus, deciding which moral principle (or principles) to invoke as an action guide will depend on the moral theory or theories to which one subscribes.[4]

The distinction between principles and rules can perhaps further be illustrated through the use of an example drawn from the literature on the philosophy of law. Consider the problem posed by a court's decision to deviate from precedent[5]—that is, to overrule its own prior decisions. Consider, for example, the important role that the *Roe v. Wade*[6] decision has played in American jurisprudence and politics since 1973. Should the Supreme Court reverse itself and overturn *Roe v. Wade*? If it did so, what would that say about the lawfulness of the original 1973 decision? Of the subsequent decision? The reluctance of the Court to reverse itself, and the reasons for that reluctance, were evident in the opening lines of the Court's opinion in *Planned Parenthood of Southeastern Pennsylvania v. Casey*,[7] a case in which it was thought that the Court might (though it did not) overrule *Roe v. Wade*: "Liberty finds no refuge in a jurisprudence of doubt. . . . After considering . . . the rule of *stare decisis* [*stare decisis* means "to abide by, or adhere to, decided cases"],[5(p978)] we are led to conclude this: The essential holding of *Roe v. Wade* should be retained and once again reaffirmed."[8]

There may be another way to look at the situation. Does a court that alters the law necessarily have to go outside the law to do so?

> Is it possible to argue that courts may *alter* the law while still being *bound* by the law? . . . Ronald Dworkin has developed a theory which seems to explain how that might be possible. . . . Dworkin argues that law does not consist solely of rules deliberately established in precedents and statutes. In his view, law also includes general principles which are implicit within the established black-letter provisions. Judges have the task of constructing a coherent moral theory that provides an appropriate abstract justification for the established rules and institutions. They may interpret and modify established rules in a way that brings them more closely into line with the overarching abstract justification. Thus, even when judges *modify* established legal rules they are doing so in the application of deeper legal principles.[9]

The Belmont Report

"The principles [of biomedical ethics] emerged from the work of the National Commission for the Protection of Human Subjects of Biomedical and Behavioral Research,"[3(p73)] which was created by an act of Congress in 1974. The commission was charged with "identify[ing] the basic ethical principles that should underlie the conduct of biomedical and behavioral research involving human subjects and . . . develop[ing] guidelines which should be followed to assure that such research is conducted in accordance with those principles."[10]

The commission identified three such basic principles as being "particularly relevant to the ethics of research involving human subjects: the principles of respect [for] persons, beneficence and justice."[11] The commission described these principles as follows:

1. *Respect for persons.* Respect for persons incorporates at least two ethical convictions: first, that individuals should be treated as autonomous agents, and second, that persons with diminished autonomy are entitled to protection. The principle of respect for persons thus divides into two separate moral requirements: the requirement to acknowledge autonomy and the requirement to protect those with diminished autonomy.

    An autonomous person is an individual capable of deliberation about personal goals and of acting under the direction of such deliberation. To respect autonomy is to give weight to autonomous persons' considered opinions and choices while refraining from obstructing their actions unless they are clearly detrimental to others. To show lack of respect for an autonomous agent is to repudiate that person's considered judgments, to deny an individual the freedom to act on those considered judgments, or to withhold information necessary to make a considered judgment, when there are no compelling reasons to do so.

    However, not every human being is capable of self-determination. The capacity for self-determination matures during an individual's life, and some individuals lose this capacity wholly or in part because of illness, mental disability, or circumstances that severely restrict liberty. Respect for the immature and the incapacitated may require protecting them as they mature or while they are incapacitated.

    Some persons are in need of extensive protection, even to the point of excluding them from activities which may harm them; other persons require little protection beyond making sure they undertake activities freely and with awareness of possible adverse consequence. The extent of protection afforded should depend upon the risk of harm and the likelihood of benefit. The judgment that any individual lacks autonomy should be periodically reevaluated and will vary in different situations.

    In most cases of research involving human subjects, respect for persons demands that subjects enter into the research voluntarily and with adequate information. In some situations, however, application of the principle is not obvious. The involvement of prisoners as subjects of research provides an instructive example. On the one hand, it would seem that the principle of respect for persons requires that prisoners not be deprived of the opportunity to volunteer for research. On the other hand, under prison conditions they may be subtly coerced or unduly influenced to engage in research activities for which they would not otherwise volunteer. Respect for persons would then dictate that prisoners be protected. Whether to allow prisoners to "volunteer" or to "protect" them presents a dilemma. Respecting persons, in most hard cases, is often a matter of balancing competing claims urged by the principle of respect itself.

2. *Beneficence.* Persons are treated in an ethical manner not only by respecting their decisions and protecting them from harm, but also by making efforts to secure their well-being. Such treatment falls under the principle of beneficence. The term "beneficence" is often understood to cover acts of kindness or charity that go beyond strict obligation. In this document, beneficence is understood in a stronger sense, as an obligation. Two general rules have been formulated as complementary expressions of beneficent actions in this sense: (1) do not harm and (2) maximize possible benefits and minimize possible harms.

    The Hippocratic maxim "do no harm" has long been a fundamental principle of medical ethics. Claude Bernard extended it to the realm of research, saying that one should not injure one person regardless of the benefits that might come to others. However, even avoiding harm requires learning what is harmful; and, in the process of obtaining this information, persons may be exposed to risk of harm. Further, the Hippocratic Oath requires physicians to benefit their patients "according to their best judgment." Learning what will in fact benefit may require exposing persons to risk. The problem posed by these imperatives is to decide when it is justifiable to seek certain benefits despite the risks involved, and when the benefits should be foregone because of the risks . . . .

    The principle of beneficence often occupies a well-defined justifying role in many areas of research involving human subjects. An example is found in research involving children. Effective ways of treating childhood diseases and fostering healthy development are benefits that serve to justify research involving children—even when individual research subjects are not direct beneficiaries. Research also makes it possible to avoid the harm that may result from the application of previously accepted routine practices that on closer investigation turn out to be dangerous. But the role of the principle of beneficence is not always so unambiguous. A difficult ethical problem remains, for example, about research that presents more than minimal risk without immediate prospect of direct benefit to the children involved. Some have argued that such research is inadmissible, while others have pointed out that this limit would rule out much research promising great benefit to children in the future. Here again, as with all hard cases, the different claims covered by the principle of beneficence may come into conflict and force difficult choices.

3. *Justice.* Who ought to receive the benefits of research and bear its burdens? This is a question of justice, in the sense of "fairness in distribution" or "what is deserved." An injustice occurs when some benefit to which a person is entitled is denied without good reason or when some burden is imposed unduly. Another way of conceiving the principle of justice is that equals ought to be treated equally. However, this statement requires explication. Who is equal and who is unequal? What considerations justify departure from equal distribution? Almost all commentators allow that distinctions based on experience, age, deprivation, competence, merit and position do sometimes constitute criteria justifying differential treatment for certain purposes. It is necessary, then, to explain in what respects people should be treated equally. There are several widely accepted formulations of just ways to distribute burdens and benefits. Each formulation mentions some relevant property on the basis of which burdens and benefits should be distributed. These formulations are (1) to each person an equal share, (2) to each person according to individual need, (3) to each person according to individual effort, (4) to each person according to societal contribution, and (5) to each person according to merit.

Questions of justice have long been associated with social practices such as punishment, taxation and political representation. Until recently these questions have not generally been associated with scientific research. However, they are foreshadowed even in the earliest reflections on the ethics of research involving human subjects. For example, during the 19th and early 20th centuries the burdens of serving as research subjects fell largely upon poor ward patients, while the benefits of improved medical care flowed primarily to private patients. Subsequently, the exploitation of unwilling prisoners as research subjects in Nazi concentration camps was condemned as a particularly flagrant injustice. In this country, in the 1940's, the Tuskegee syphilis study used disadvantaged, rural black men to study the untreated course of a disease that is by no means confined to that population. These subjects were deprived of demonstrably effective treatment in order not to interrupt the project, long after such treatment became generally available.

Against this historical background, it can be seen how conceptions of justice are relevant to research involving human subjects. For example, the selection of research subjects needs to be scrutinized in order to determine whether some classes (e.g., welfare patients, particular racial and ethnic minorities, or persons confined to institutions) are being systematically selected simply because of their easy availability, their compromised position, or their manipulability, rather than for reasons directly related to the problem being studied. Finally, whenever research supported by public funds leads to the development of therapeutic devices and procedures, justice demands both that these not provide advantages only to those who can afford them and that such research should not unduly involve persons from groups unlikely to be among the beneficiaries of subsequent applications of the research.[10]

As we shall see shortly, the principlism described by Beauchamp and Childress divides Belmont's principle of beneficence into two separate principles—the principle of beneficence and the principle of nonmaleficence.

The Principles of Biomedical Ethics

"Biomedical ethics has assumed a kind of 'principlist' orientation over the past 30 years";[1(p4)] stated otherwise, the dominant approach to biomedical ethics has been the approach espoused by Beauchamp and Childress in their classic textbook, *Principles of Biomedical Ethics*.[11] Beauchamp and Childress "believe that principles provide the most general and comprehensive norms . . . that guide actions. The difference [between rules and principles] is that rules are more specific in content and more restricted in scope than principles." Their approach is known as *principlism*, or the *four-principles approach* to biomedical ethics—or, more colorfully, as the Georgetown Mantra. The four principles are as follows: respect for autonomy; nonmaleficence; beneficence; and justice.

The Beauchamp and Childress text is probably the authoritative work on principlism, and it seems that most bioethical decisions are analyzed using the framework described therein. The popular text *Clinical Ethics: A Practical Approach to Ethical Decisions in Clinical Medicine*[12] employs the four principles in its practical approach.

Respect for Autonomy

Personal autonomy refers to self-governance, to "self-rule that is free from both controlling interference by others and from limitations, such as inadequate understanding, that prevent meaningful choice."[11(p58)] According to Beauchamp and Childress,

> The principle [of respect for autonomy] can be stated as a negative obligation and as a positive obligation. As a *negative* obligation: Autonomous actions should not be subjected to controlling constraints by others. . . . As a *positive* obligation, this principle requires respectful treatment in disclosing information and fostering autonomous decision-making."[11(p64)]

According to Beauchamp and Childress, the principle of respect for autonomy supports a number of more specific rules, including the following:

1. Tell the truth.

2. Respect the privacy of others.

3. Protect confidential information.

4. Obtain consent for interventions with patients.

5. When asked, help others make important decisions.[11(p65)]

In terms of the moral rules discussed in the next chapter of this book, the principle of respect for autonomy might be interpreted as another formulation of the moral rule "Do not deprive of freedom."[3(p78)]

In the medical context, because of the need for medical decisions to be made, the question with which we are most likely to be concerned is, Is this patient's choice (decision) an autonomous one? The earlier excerpt provides some clues to answering that question. First, in order to be an autonomous choice, a patient's choice must be *voluntary*. This is another way of saying that it must be free of "controlling constraints by others." Second, a patient's choice must be *informed*.

Of course, there is an aspect to patient autonomy that has nothing to do with any negative or positive obligations that might be owed patients by health care professionals (including physicians, physician assistants, and other allied health professionals), and so is not addressed in the previous excerpt. Some persons are simply not capable of making an autonomous choice. An example of such a person might be, for example, a neonate. The principal reason a neonate is incapable of autonomous choice (communication issues aside) is that he or she lacks *decision-making capacity*, or *competence*.[13] Where a choice is not autonomous because of decisional incapacity (i.e., incompetence), it follows that it may not be worthy of respect and that principles other than respect for autonomy may need to be invoked as a guide to action.

In summary, then, for a patient's choice to be an autonomous choice, the patient must make his or her choice *voluntarily* (free of controlling constraints), his or her choice must be adequately *informed*, and the patient must have *decision-making capacity* (i.e., he or she must be *competent*). Let's turn to a brief discussion of each of these requirements.

Voluntariness

According to Beauchamp and Childress, "a person acts voluntarily to the degree that he or she wills the action without being under the control of another's influence."[11(p93)] Beauchamp and Childress distinguish between influences that are controlling and those that are not. Controlling influences render acts nonautonomous because they are not voluntary. Noncontrolling influences do not vitiate the voluntariness of a person's choice.

Beauchamp and Childress discuss three types of influence. *Coercion* "occurs if and only if one person intentionally uses a credible and severe threat of harm or force to control another. . . . Coercion voids an act of autonomy; that is, coercion renders even intentional and well-informed behavior nonautonomous."[11(p94)]

Persuasion, on the other hand, refers to the process whereby "a person . . . come[s] to believe in something through the merit of reasons another person advances."[11(p94)] Stated otherwise, persuasion is "influence by appeal to reason."[11(p94)] Defined this way, persuasion is clearly not a controlling influence, because ultimately the final decision remains the patient's. Indeed, the entire informed consent process might be conceptualized as a process through which one person (the patient) comes to believe in something (that the intervention should be consented to or refused) through the merit of reasons advanced by the health care professional (HCP).

Finally, *manipulation* refers to "forms of influence that are neither persuasive nor coercive. The essence of manipulation is swaying people to do what the manipulator wants by means other than coercion or persuasion."[11(p95)] Beauchamp and Childress point out that, in the health care context, the principal form of manipulation is informational—that is, communicating information in a way that nonpersuasively increases the likelihood that its recipient will reach a certain conclusion. (For example, saying to a patient during the course of an informed consent discussion, "This treatment is usually successful" about a treatment that is successful 51% of the time is, strictly speaking, true, but is more likely to elicit consent from the patient than by communicating the same information by saying "This treatment fails almost half the time.") For this reason, we believe that it makes more sense to think about manipulation as implicating the informational arm of autonomy rather than the voluntariness arm.

Information and Informed Consent

This topic is dealt with in some detail in Chapters 8 and 9. Herein, we shall confine ourselves to the topic as it relates to principlism.

Regarding the *positive* obligation inherent in the principle of respect for autonomy, what information must an HCP convey to his or her patient? Probably most of us are familiar with the mantra admonishing us to discuss with patients the material or important "risks [of], benefits [of], and alternatives [to]" the clinical intervention under consideration, with the emphasis on the concept of materiality. By implication, the disclosure should, of course, include the HCP's recommendation.[11(p81)]

The question that naturally follows is, When is a fact a *material* fact? Retrospectively, the issue is likely to arise in the context of medical malpractice litigation, with the question for the jury being, Did the HCP fail to disclose to the patient material information? (This is discussed in Chapters 8, 9, and 15.) Prospectively, however, the question is, How do I as an HCP decide whether a particular fact is material and whether it should be disclosed to the patient? The moral obligations imposed by the principle of respect for autonomy are likely to be more exacting than the obligations of the law. Thus, the most common legal standard of disclosure is the

> "professional malpractice" standard, under which physicians are required to disclose to patients that information which would have been disclosed by the reasonable, minimally competent physician. . . . A substantial number of states use

the "material risk" or "reasonable patient" standard, which requires disclosure of risks that a reasonable patient would consider to be material in making a medical treatment decision. A small number of jurisdictions take an even more protective approach, requiring disclosure of information that a particular patient (as contrasted with a "rational" patient) would have wanted to make his or her decision.[14]

The latter standard is referred to as the *subjective standard*, and though it is the exception rather than the rule in the legal context, it is the "preferable *moral* standard of disclosure, because it alone acknowledges persons' specific informational needs."[11(p83)]

Where adequate disclosure has been made and the patient has had an opportunity to weigh the content of the disclosure in his or her decision making, the patient's subsequent choice may be said to be informed; alternatively, it may be said that the patient has given informed consent (or informed refusal, as the case may be). However, it is important to be aware that the term *informed consent* is sometimes used to signify something broader in scope; it is sometimes used as a synonym or alias for *autonomous choice*. Thus,

> Some commentators have attempted to define informed consent by . . . dividing [it] into an *information* component and a *consent* component. The information component refers to disclosure of information and comprehension of what is disclosed. The consent component refers to both a voluntary decision and an authorization to proceed. Legal, . . . philosophical, [and] medical . . . literatures . . . favor the following elements as the components of informed consent: (1) competence, (2) disclosure, (3) understanding, (4) voluntariness, and (5) consent. . . . One gives an informed consent to an intervention if (and only if) one is competent to act, receives a thorough disclosure, comprehends the disclosure, acts voluntarily, and consents to the intervention.[11(p79)] (Internal footnotes omitted)

Competency

As mentioned earlier, herein we employ the terms *competency* and *decisional capacity* interchangeably. As was true of informed consent, competency is discussed in detail elsewhere in this text (Chapter 7); herein, we limit ourselves to a discussion of the topic as it relates to the principle of respect for autonomy.

Competency (or *decisional capacity*) refers to one's ability to make a particular decision. To say that someone is competent to make a particular decision is shorthand for saying that we believe he or she should be allowed to make that decision under the circumstances that prevail. Note that competency is decision specific; I may believe that my three-year-old should be allowed to choose whether he wants chocolate or vanilla ice cream, but not whether he will or will not undergo life-saving surgery.

Byron Chell has written that generally "a person is labeled competent if (1) he or she has an understanding of the situation and the consequences of the decision, and (2) the decision is based upon rational reasons."[15] Case 2-A is taken from Chell's work.

Case 2-A

"An eighty-six-year-old female is informed that her leg is gangrenous and that an amputation is necessary to save her life. She refuses surgery, saying 'I am 86 and I have lived a good and full life. I do not want a further operation, nor do I want to live legless. I understand the consequence of refusing the amputation is death and I accept that consequence.' "[15(p120)] Is this patient competent to decide to refuse the surgery?

Analysis

The issue in this case is the patient's competency or decisional capacity. Does the patient understand her situation (i.e., that she has life-threatening gangrene)? Yes. Does she understand the consequences of her decision (i.e., that she will die without surgery)? Yes. Is her decision based on rational reasons? Most of us would probably conclude that the reasons for the refusal are rational under the situation—that having to undergo unwanted further surgery and having to live legless at the age of eighty-six might reasonably be adjudged to be a greater harm than death to an eighty-six-year-old. Her refusal should be honored.

If the patient refused surgery, insisting that she did not have gangrene, we could argue that she was incompetent because she lacked an understanding of the situation. If instead, while conceding that she had gangrene, she nevertheless refused surgery, insisting that the gangrene would be cured by a course of antibiotics, we could argue that she was incompetent because she lacked an understanding of the consequences of her decision. "If she were to say, 'I understand the [situation and the] consequences but I refuse the operation because the moon is full,' it is not likely she would be considered competent. . . . Her decision does not rationally or reasonably follow from her premise. . . . She would be labeled incompetent."[15(p120)]

The Problem of Religious Beliefs

Consider a different case now, that of a Jehovah's Witness who refuses a lifesaving blood transfusion. Recall that "a person is labeled competent if (1) he or she has an understanding of the situation and the consequences of the decision, and (2) the decision is based upon rational reasons."[15] The application of part 1 of this test is relatively straightforward, even in cases involving religious beliefs. We ask whether the patient understands the situation and the consequences of the decision. If the patient understands that he has a life-threatening bleed and is likely to die without the transfusion, he will have passed the first part of the test of competency. If instead he insists that he will be cured by Jehovah without the need for a blood transfusion, that belief might be treated as a religious delusion and the patient adjudged to be incompetent.[16]

However, what about part 2 of the test for competency? Even the Jehovah's Witness who understands that he has a life-threatening bleed and is likely to die without the transfusion, when asked to give reasons for his refusal, is likely to give religious reasons—such as fear of eternal damnation.[17] The problem, of course, is that religious beliefs, based as they are upon that which cannot be proved, cannot be said to be rational. In the words of Sam Harris in his provocative book *The End of Faith,*

> Is a person really free to believe a proposition for which he has no evidence? No . . . We have names for people who have beliefs for which there is no rational justification. When their beliefs are extremely common we call them "religious"; otherwise, they are likely to be called "mad," "psychotic," or "delusional."[18]

Of course, we do not, as a rule, deem patients to be incompetent merely because the reasons for their refusal are religious.[19] Chell explains that if the reason for a patient's refusal is a religious one, the patient will not be deemed incompetent on that basis so long as the religious beliefs are "held by a sufficient number of persons for a sufficient period of time or [are] sufficiently similar to other orthodox beliefs such that we do not label the beliefs crazy or nonreligious."[15(p123)]

When might a religious belief be considered crazy or nonreligious? Consider, as an example, a patient who claimed to belong to the Church of the Fonz[20] and refused potentially lifesaving treatment because of his interpretation of the teachings of the "sacred texts" of his religion, old *Happy Days* episodes. It is likely that such a patient would be deemed to be incompetent.

Competency and Respect for Autonomy

Deciding whether a patient is competent is an important and unavoidable decision. The choice is unavoidable because the default position is that the patient's choice will be implemented absent some objection on the part of the HCP (the law, after all presumes that all persons are competent absent evidence to the contrary). The choice is important because, in making it, we walk a fine line between Scylla and Charybdis—that is, between the Scylla of erroneously adjudging an autonomous choice to be nonautonomous (and thus wrongfully failing to acknowledge the patient's autonomy) and the Charybdis of erroneously adjudging a nonautonomous choice to be autonomous (and thus wrongfully failing to protect from harm a patient unable to protect himself or herself).

Ultimately, a number of factors will influence an HCP's determination as to whether a particular patient is competent or not. Not surprisingly, one of them is the HCP's degree of certainty that the patient is competent. The more certain I am that a patient has decisional capacity, the more likely I am to honor his or her decision, whether I agree with it or not. A second factor concerns the HCP's medical certainty regarding the facts of the situation and the patient's prognosis. Whether or not I decide to honor the decision of a patient of arguable competency to refuse a lifesaving intervention will depend at least in part on how certain I am that the intervention is in fact lifesaving. Perhaps the patient might survive even without the intervention. To the extent that I as an HCP am uncertain about my prognostication, I will be more likely to err on the side of deciding that the patient's wishes should be honored. A third factor concerns the HCP's assessment of the severity of the situation and the potential outcome of the patient's decision. A patient with a lower extremity venous stasis ulcer who refuses to wear a compressive dressing runs the risk that her wound may not heal or that wound healing will be delayed; a patient with clinical and computed tomographic evidence of acute appendicitis who refuses appendectomy runs the risk of death. It should be clear that, when the decisional capacity of these two patients is in question and all other things are equal, an HCP would be more likely to honor the treatment refusal of the former than the latter.

Case 2-B "When Is Odysseus to Be Believed?"

A fifty-eight-year-old woman with chronic obstructive pulmonary disease (COPD) had, over a period of years, repeatedly expressed a desire not to be endotracheally intubated and mechanically ventilated "unless such an intervention were to be purely temporary."[21(p54)] The patient was brought to the hospital in terminal respiratory failure, and it was the opinion of the medical staff—including a consulting pulmonologist—that if she were placed on a ventilator there was almost no chance of her ever being weaned. When her physician asked her whether she wanted to be intubated, she expressed a wish to be placed on a ventilator "even if she would never again be able to be weaned from it." The physicians caring for her decided that her request to be intubated did not represent an autonomous choice because it was made under the "internal coercion of panic, fear, anoxia [and] hypercarbia," and because it was entirely inconsistent with her repeatedly and emphatically stated prior wishes. The patient was sedated and allowed to die. Do you agree with the decision not to intubate her?

Analysis

As mentioned previously, this case can be analyzed on a number of levels. Because this chapter deals with the principles of biomedical ethics, our analysis will proceed from that level.

The question to be answered is whether the patient should have been intubated. To answer this question, the first issue that needs to be addressed is whether this patient's death-bed consent to intubation was *autonomous*. (Assume that the patient's choice to refuse even life-sustaining treatment, if autonomous, should be respected.) Recall that a choice is autonomous if it is voluntary, informed, and made by an agent with decisional capacity (a competent agent).

In this case it is the decisional capacity or competency of the patient and the voluntariness of her choice that are in question. Thus, there are two questions that must be answered: (1) Did she have decisional capacity or competency? And (2) was her choice voluntary?

First, did she have decisional capacity or competency? Recall that a patient is competent if (1) she has an understanding of the situation and the consequences of her decision, and (2) her decision is based on rational reasons. We are told that she was "slightly 'fuzzy'—albeit grossly oriented," and that the physicians responsible for her care were concerned about her anoxia and hypercarbia. Regarding her anoxia and hypercarbia, was she anoxic and/or hypercarbic enough to be rendered incompetent? We simply do not seem to have enough information to be able to answer this question. Luckily, under the law there is a rebuttable presumption that

(continues)

Case 2-B "When Is Odysseus to Be Believed?" *(continued)*

patients are competent—that is, the burden of persuasion rests with those who would argue that a person lacks decisional capacity or competency. Because of this presumption, we would argue that absent probative evidence to the contrary, the patient was competent to consent to intubation and mechanical ventilation.

Second, was her choice to refuse mechanical ventilation voluntary? As stated earlier, "a person acts voluntarily to the degree that he or she wills the action without being under the control of another's influence." Clearly this patient was not under the control of any other person's influence. Beauchamp and Childress state, however, that conditions such as debilitating disease (among others) can diminish or void voluntariness.[22] In this case, the physicians responsible for her care expressed concern regarding the "internal coercion of panic [and] fear."[23] Were the patient's panic and fear great enough to void voluntariness? We would argue that the same policy considerations that undergird the presumption of competency should undergird a presumption of voluntariness. Who is to say that, faced with the real and immediate specter of one's death, one does not possess a certain insight or clarity lacking in the rest of us? Why should we believe that fear of death precludes the ability to choose autonomously? We believe that her (later) choice to consent to intubation and mechanical ventilation should have been honored and that she should have been intubated.[24]

Nonmaleficence

The Hippocratic imperative to physicians, "Bring benefit and do no harm," expresses the principles of nonmaleficence ("do no harm") and beneficence ("bring benefit").[12(p18)]

The *principle of nonmaleficence* refers to the duty to refrain from causing harm. It underlies the medical maxim *Primum non nocere*: "Above all [or first] do no harm."[11(p113)] The principle of nonmaleficence says, "One ought not to inflict evil or harm,"[11(p116)] where a harm is defined as an adverse effect on one's interests. According to Beauchamp and Childress, the principle of nonmaleficence supports a number of more specific moral rules, including the following:

1. Do not kill.
2. Do not cause pain or suffering.
3. Do not incapacitate.
4. Do not cause offense.
5. Do not deprive others of the goods of life.[11(p117)]

In terms of the moral rules you will learn about in the next chapter, Gert has suggested that the principle of nonmaleficence is

> most reasonably interpreted as . . . summarizing . . . the moral rules "Don't kill," "Don't cause pain," . . . "Don't disable," . . . and probably the rule "Don't deprive of pleasure" as well. Even the rule "Don't deprive of freedom" can be included in

the principle of nonmaleficence, but principlism seems to prefer to include it under the principle of autonomy.[3(p76)]

Harmful acts are generally prima facie[25] wrong, but will not be considered wrong if the harm is justifiable. Harm is justifiable if there is a "just, lawful excuse or reason for the [prima facie harmful] act or [omission]."[5(p599)] For example, killing is prima facie prohibited under the principle of nonmaleficence, but killing in self-defense, although clearly harmful of another, is not wrongful. Likewise, "[s]aving a person's life by a blood transfusion clearly justifies the inflicted harm of venipuncture on the blood donor."[26]

The Rule of the Double Effect

Case 2-C demonstrates the application of the principle of nonmaleficence and introduces the derivative *rule of the double effect (RDE)*.

Case 2-C

A patient with a long smoking history is hospitalized with advanced COPD and lung cancer metastatic to bone.[27] Consider the following scenarios and questions:

1. The patient's wife requests that the physician increase the rate of the morphine infusion to a point adequate to control the patient's pain, irrespective of any effect it might have on his respiratory rate. Should the physician acquiesce?

2. The patient's wife requests that the inevitable be hastened and that sufficient morphine be administered to end the patient's life and hence his suffering. Should the physician acquiesce?

Analysis

The principle of nonmaleficence imposes a prima facie prohibition on the infliction of harm or risk thereof on this patient, and increasing the amount of morphine the patient is receiving will expose the patient to an increased risk of respiratory depression and death. On the other hand, inadequate or suboptimal dosing of this patient's morphine will harm the patient as well by causing pain and suffering. What, therefore, should be done? The answer lies in the RDE, which recognizes that there is a morally relevant difference between the intended effects of an action and its unintended though foreseen effects. Under the RDE, when an action has two inextricably linked foreseen effects (one ethically permissible and the other ethically questionable), the permissible effect may be pursued (even though the questionable or harmful one will follow) provided that all of the following conditions are met.

1. *The nature of the act.* The act must be good, or at least morally neutral (independent of its consequences).

2. *The agent's intention.* The agent intends only the good effect. The bad effect can be foreseen, tolerated and permitted, but it must not be intended.

(continues)

Case 2-C *(continued)*

3. *The distinction between means and effects.* The bad effect must not be a means to the good effect. If the good effect were the direct causal result of the bad effect, the agent would intend the bad effect in pursuit of the good effect.

4. *Proportionality between the good effect and the bad effect.* The good effect must outweigh the bad effect. That is, the bad effect is permissible only if a proportionate reason compensates for permitting the foreseen bad effect.[11(p129)]

In this case, morphine indeed has two inextricably linked effects—one ethically permissible (analgesia) and the other ethically problematic (respiratory depression). The act in question (intravenous administration of a pharmaceutical) is arguably at least a morally neutral act, satisfying condition 1. Condition 2 is satisfied in scenario 1 if the physician titrates the morphine drip only as high as is needed to achieve adequate analgesia. Likewise, condition 3 is satisfied in scenario 1 because respiratory depression is not the means to analgesia. Finally, condition 4 is satisfied in scenario 1 because most people would agree that achieving adequate pain control at the end of life of a terminal cancer patient is worth any foreseeable shortening of the patient's life that might occur as a result of narcotic administration. Therefore, in scenario 1 the RDE applies and the physician's acquiescence does not violate the principle of nonmaleficence.

In scenario 2, on the other hand, condition 2 is not satisfied because the physician intends the bad effect (respiratory depression). Likewise, in scenario 2 the bad effect (respiratory depression) becomes the means to the good effect (analgesia). Thus, a physician who acquiesced under scenario 2 would be violating the principle of nonmaleficence.

Beneficence

The *principle of beneficence* "asserts the duty to help others further their important and legitimate interests."[28] Under the principle of beneficence,

1. One ought to prevent evil or harm.

2. One ought to remove evil or harm.

3. One ought to do or promote good.[11(p115)]

According to Beauchamp and Childress, the principle of beneficence supports a number of more specific rules, including the following:

1. Protect and defend the rights of others.

2. Prevent harm from occurring to others.

3. Remove conditions that will cause harm to others.

4. Help persons with disabilities.

5. Rescue persons in danger.[11(p167)]

Unlike the negative prohibitions of nonmaleficence, beneficence exhorts those to whom it applies to act affirmatively. In other words, one can obey the dictates of *nonmaleficence* by merely refraining from acting; not so in the case of *beneficence*.

Beauchamp and Childress distinguish between specific beneficence and general beneficence. *Specific beneficence* is obligatory beneficence. It refers to those positive obligations (i.e., duties to act) we owe to others to further their important and legitimate interests. We owe a duty of specific beneficence to those others with whom we are in some special relationship. (We shall consider such relationships again in Chapter 15.) Thus, we owe a duty of specific beneficence, for example, to our children, and, as HCPs, to our patients. As HCPs, we are obligated not merely to refrain from harming our patients (under the principle of nonmaleficence), but to act in their best medical interests.

General beneficence "is directed beyond those special relationships to all persons."[11(p169)] For the most part, general beneficence is ideal beneficence—that is, although moral ideals encourage us to act affirmatively so as to help others with whom we do not find ourselves in a special relationship, we are not obliged to do so by the moral rules (see Chapter 3). I say "for the most part" because Beauchamp and Childress argue that, even apart from special relationships, a person X owes an obligatory duty of beneficence toward a person Y if each of the following conditions is true:

1. Y is at risk of significant loss of or damage to life or health or some other major interest.

2. X's action is needed (singly or in concert with others) to prevent this loss or damage.

3. X's action (singly or in concert with others) has a high probability of preventing it.

4. X's action would not present significant risks, costs or burdens to X.

5. The benefit that Y can be expected to gain outweighs any harms, costs, or burdens to X that is likely to occur.[11(p171)]

Case 2-D

A seventy-nine-year-old female patient (Mrs. Y) was admitted to the hospital with an acute, non-Q-wave myocardial infarction.[29] On cardiac catheterization, she was found to have a tapering stenosis of the left anterior descending (LAD) coronary artery, a sixty percent obstruction proximally increasing to a ninety percent obstruction distally. The right and circumflex systems were found to be diffusely but mildly diseased. Her ejection fraction was about forty percent. The patient was evaluated at a medical-surgical conference, and because the nature of the LAD lesion rendered percutaneous transluminal coronary angioplasty (PTCA) difficult, coronary artery bypass grafting (CABG) was considered. Ultimately, however, the recommendation was for medical therapy.

(continues)

Case 2-D (*continued*)

Two days after being discharged from the hospital on medical therapy, the patient was brought to the hospital in cardiac arrest and pulmonary edema. She was resuscitated and found to have suffered no permanent neurologic sequelae, and she was stabilized through the use of an intra-aortic balloon pump (IABP). Myocardial infarction was ruled out. Over the following days, numerous efforts to remove the IABP were unsuccessful; the patient's coronary artery perfusion was dependent on the IABP. Her physicians believed that her only chance for survival was revascularization. Because the facility at which she was hospitalized did not offer cardiac surgery or angioplasty, her physicians contacted cardiothoracic surgeons at a number of regional facilities; all of them refused to accept the patient in transfer because her surgical mortality was felt to be unacceptably high, and it was believed that her (likely) death would adversely affect their mortality statistics, which were being published in the state in which they practiced. By day 9 of hospitalization, her condition had deteriorated further and, believing at this point that it was riskier for the patient to undergo CABG than PTCA, her physicians contacted interventional cardiologists at a number of regional facilities. All refused to accept the patient because she was so high risk. On day 21 of hospitalization, the patient expired. Was the refusal of the subspecialists to accept Mrs. Y in transfer a violation of the principle of beneficence?

Analysis

The issue is whether the subspecialists violated the principle of beneficence. Recall from the previous discussion that there are two categories of beneficence—specific and general. Specific beneficence is the obligatory beneficence that we owe to those others with whom we are in a special relationship. Were any of the subspecialists who were asked to accept Mrs. Y in transfer in a special relationship with her? Probably not. There is no indication in the facts provided that any of them were in a preexisting doctor–patient relationship with her. What about the fact that they were asked by the physicians caring for her to accept her in transfer? Does that create a special relationship? Because, traditionally, physicians have been free to determine which patients they will and will not see, the answer is probably no. (A special relationship might exist if, for example, there was a law in place prohibiting subspecialists from refusing transfers such as the one in question. Alternatively, a special relationship might be found to exist if the referring physicians and the subspecialists were all on the medical staff at the institution where the patient was hospitalized, and there was in place a call schedule for subspecialists.) Therefore, the subspecialists arguably owe no duty of specific beneficence to Mrs. Y.

Do the subspecialists owe an obligatory duty of beneficence to Mrs. Y under the principle of general beneficence? Recall that a person X owes an obligatory duty of beneficence toward a person Y if (1) Y is at risk of significant loss of or damage to life or health or some other major interest; (2) X's action is needed (singly or in concert with others) to prevent this loss or damage; (3) X's action (singly or in concert with others) has a high probability of preventing this loss or damage; (4) X's action would not present significant risks, costs, or burdens to X; and (5) the benefit that Y can be expected to gain outweighs any harms, costs, or burdens to X that are likely to occur. Because strong arguments can be made that each of these conditions apply to the case under discussion, we believe a very strong argument can be made that the subspecialists' refusal constituted a violation of the principle of beneficence—specifically of an obligatory (as opposed to ideal) duty of general beneficence.

Paternalism

Stated simply, *medical paternalism* consists in the judgment that the principle of beneficence trumps the principle of autonomy. Probably most of us have heard the term *paternalism* bandied about pejoratively, though that was not always the case. Historically, beneficence was thought to express the primary obligation of physicians and HCPs; only more recently has the principle of respect for autonomy gained ascendancy.

Beauchamp and Childress define paternalism as "the intentional overriding of one person's known preferences . . . by another person, where the person who overrides justifies the action by the goal of benefiting or avoiding harm to the person whose preferences . . . are overridden."[11(p178)] Further, they distinguish between weak (soft) and strong (hard) paternalism.

> In weak paternalism, an agent intervenes on grounds of beneficence . . . only to prevent *substantially [nonautonomous] conduct*. . . . [Such conduct] include[s] cases of consent or refusal that is not adequately informed, severe depression that precludes rational deliberation, and addiction that prevents free choice and action.
>
> . . .
>
> Strong paternalism, by contrast, involves interventions intended to benefit a person, despite the fact that the person's risky choices . . . are informed, voluntary and autonomous.[11(p181)]

Whether weak paternalism is even a prima facie wrong in need of a defense is arguable,[11(p181)] because if a person's choice is not autonomous, it need not be respected. Strong paternalism is, on the other hand, more controversial. According to Beauchamp and Childress,

> Normally, strong paternalism is appropriate and justified in health care only if the following conditions are satisfied:
>
> 1. A patient is at risk of a serious, preventable harm.
>
> 2. The paternalistic action will probably prevent the harm.
>
> 3. The projected benefits to the patient of the paternalistic action outweigh its risks to the patient.
>
> 4. The least autonomy-restrictive alternative that will secure the benefits and reduce the risks is adopted.[11(p186)]

Justice

The *principle of justice* underlies concerns about how social benefits and burdens should be distributed. For example, is it fair that two patients, otherwise similarly situated, are treated disparately by the health care system because one is affluent and the other is indigent? Between two otherwise similarly situated patients in need of a liver transplant, who should receive the one organ that is available—the recovering alcoholic who has been sober for one year or the patient dying of biliary atresia?[30]

The *principle of formal justice* is common to all theories of justice, and is traditionally attributed to Aristotle. It holds that justice requires that equals be treated equally, and unequals be treated unequally, but in proportion to their relevant inequalities. The question that naturally arises is, When is an inequality a relevant inequality? The various answers to this question constitute the *material principles of distributive justice.* Thus,

> Philosophers . . . have proposed each of the following principles as a valid material principle of distributive justice. . . .
>
> 1. To each person an equal share
>
> 2. To each person according to need
>
> 3. To each person according to effort
>
> 4. To each person according to contribution
>
> 5. To each person according to merit
>
> 6. To each person according to free-market exchanges[11(p228)]

The material principle of justice that one applies will depend on the theory of justice to which one subscribes.

Utilitarian Theories of Justice

Under utilitarian theories (see Chapter 1), "justice is merely the name for the . . . obligation created by the principle of utility,"[11(p231)] under which we should "strive to produce as much overall happiness as possible."[31] Thus, for utilitarians a just distribution of benefits and burdens would be one that produces the most overall happiness. For the utilitarian, "all rules of justice, including equality, can bow to the demands: 'each person maintains that equality is the dictate of justice, except where he thinks that expediency requires inequality.' Whatever does the greatest overall good will be 'just' [internal footnotes omitted]."[32]

Egalitarian Theories of Justice: Rawls

"*Egalitarian* theories of justice hold that persons should receive an equal distribution of certain goods. . . . *Qualified egalitarianism* requires only some basic equalities among individuals and permits inequalities that redound to the benefit of the least advantaged [italics added]."[11(p233)] John Rawls's "justice as fairness," as described in his work *A Theory of Justice,* is probably the foremost modern version of such a qualified egalitarianism. Rawls argues that the principles of justice are those principles that would be chosen by persons behind a metaphorical "veil of ignorance"—that is, persons who "would not know their own race, sex, degree of wealth, or natural abilities."[33] According to Rawls, those principles of justice to which persons would agree would be as follows:

First: each person is to have an equal right to the most extensive basic liberty compatible with a similar liberty for others.

Second: social and economic inequalities are to be arranged so that they are both (a) reasonably expected to be to everyone's advantage, and (b) attached to positions and offices open to all.[33(p450)]

The first principle applies, for example, to the distribution of political liberty and rights such as those protected in the American Bill of Rights. The second principle applies, for example, to the distribution of income and wealth; what the second principle means is that social and economic goods "are to be distributed equally unless an unequal distribution of any, or all, of these values is to everyone's advantage."[33(p451)]

Libertarian Theories of Justice: Nozick

Unlike the theories of justice just discussed, libertarian theories do not focus on maximizing utility or on achieving an equal distribution of goods; rather, libertarian conceptions of justice tend to emphasize the importance of "the unfettered operation of fair procedures."[11(p232)] Robert Nozick developed a libertarian theory of justice—the so-called *entitlement theory*—in his work *Anarchy, State, and Utopia*. Therein, he distinguishes between *historical* principles of justice and *unhistorical* (or end-result) principles of justice (such as utilitarian justice or egalitarian justice), arguing that the justice of any particular distribution of a good among a number of individuals depends not upon how much of the good each individual has, but upon how that distribution came about. Under Nozick's theory,

A distribution is just if it arises from another just distribution by legitimate means. The legitimate means of moving from one distribution to another are specified by the principle of justice in transfer. The legitimate first "moves" are specified by the principle of justice in acquisition. Whatever arises from a just situation by just steps is itself just.[34]

There are three principles of justice under Nozick's theory of justice: (1) the *principle of justice in acquisition*, which deals with the appropriation by persons of previously unheld things; (2) the *principle of justice in transfer*, which deals with the appropriation by persons of holdings from other persons; and (3) the *principle of rectification*, which, as the name suggests, deals with what may be done in order to rectify past injustices that have shaped present holdings.[34(pp150–153)]

The following excerpt illustrates how a person's past actions can influence his or her present entitlements.

Ordinary prudence ... require(s) that a (driver) be prepared to stop short ... if by doing so he can avoid death or injury to another person. Let it be conceded also that a person need not in general take an action sacrificing his own life in order to avert a grave risk to another. Now let us imagine the case where A loads his truck with heavy steel pipe in such a way that if he stops short [the pipe] will shift forward and is very likely to crush him. . . . A, thus laden, sees B drive out of a side road into his path. If A stops short he will avoid hitting and perhaps killing B, but he will also risk being killed by the pipe stacked in his truck. It would seem that A had the right to impose no more than a certain level of risk on others in venturing out on the highway. If he stays within that level and . . . something goes wrong . . . he is not at fault . . . [and] need not sacrifice his life to avoid taking the life of another person who is involved in the encounter. But since [A] ventured out bearing this particularly heavy and dangerous burden he forfeits that right. This argument makes the rightfulness of A's conduct depend on choices made on some distinct, earlier occasion. We can see this if we contrast A's situation with that of C, a hitchhiker who is a passenger [in] A's truck. C is not constrained to risk his life to save B. If A in a fit of cowardice had leapt from the cab leaving C at the controls, we feel that C would be justified in not stopping short. Yet at the moment of the crucial option—to stop or not to stop—the choice of risks presented to A or to C would be exactly the same. This must show that A's prior action in loading the truck in some way obligated him to drive so as to avert danger to persons in B's position, even at the risk of his own life.[35]

This example may help explain our intuition that "it is fairer to give a child dying of biliary atresia an opportunity for a *first* normal liver than it is to give a patient with ARESLD [alcohol-related end-stage liver disease] who was born with a normal liver a *second* one."[30(p1297)]

Absolutely Scarce Resources

As a rule, in medicine we believe that the "health care system should respond based on the actual medical needs of patients" (i.e., that the operative material principle of justice is need) and that "whenever possible all in need should be treated."[36] When all in need cannot be treated, however, then what? If we are dealing with an absolutely scarce resource (such as organs for transplantation), how do we decide who shall receive it when it cannot simply be divided equally between all in need? Generally, some type of selection system must be employed. Such systems include the *chronological system* ("first come, first served"), the *lottery system* (self-explanatory), the *waiting list system* (which differs from the chronological system in that medical criteria are taken into account), and *criteria systems*. Criteria employed in criteria systems include, for example, medical criteria (e.g., how good an HLA "match" exists between the organ donor and the organ recipient) and age (e.g., all other things being equal, it makes more sense to transplant an organ into a child whose life expectancy is, say, seventy years, than into an adult whose life expectancy is twenty-five years).[37]

Critique of Principlism

Although principlism has been the dominant approach to bioethics over the past several decades, Gert and colleagues have criticized it on a number of grounds.[38] We shall examine just a few of those criticisms here.

First, they have argued that, except for the principle of nonmaleficence (see below), the principles of biomedical ethics are flawed because they are not true action guides. Rather, Gert and associates argue, they

> function as checklists, naming issues worth remembering when one is considering a biomedical moral issue. "Consider this . . . consider that . . . remember to look for . . ." is what they tell the agent; they do not embody an articulated, established, and unified moral system capable of providing useful guidance.[3(p75)]

Beauchamp and Childress concede that their "four clusters of principles do not constitute a general moral theory. They provide only a framework for identifying and reflecting on moral problems."[11(p15)]

Second, principlism has been criticized as failing to distinguish between what is morally required (by the moral rules) and what is morally encouraged (by the moral ideals). For example, the principle of respect for autonomy does not distinguish between "Tell the truth" (a moral rule) and "When asked, help others make important decisions" (a moral ideal).[3(p81)]

Third, principlism has been criticized as failing to provide an "agreed-upon method for resolving . . . conflicts" between the principles when in fact they conflict with each other.[3(p87)]

Chapter Summary

Principles, like rules, are action guides, although the guidance they provide is more abstract or general. The principles of biomedical ethics emerged from the 1974 Belmont Report. The principles, as subsequently described by Beauchamp and Childress, include respect for autonomy; nonmaleficence; beneficence; and justice. Under the principle of respect for autonomy, a patient's choice is autonomous if (1) the choice is voluntary (i.e., it is free of controlling constraints by others), (2) the patient is adequately informed, and (3) the patient possesses decision-making capacity or competence. The principle of nonmaleficence refers to the duty to refrain from causing harm. The principle of beneficence asserts the duty to help others and encompasses both specific (obligatory) and general (ideal, and sometimes obligatory) beneficence. Medical paternalism consists in the judgment that the principle of beneficence trumps the principle of autonomy. The principle of formal justice holds that justice requires that equals be treated equally, and unequals be treated unequally, but in proportion to their relevant inequalities. The material principles of distributive justice purport to answer the question, When is an inequality a relevant inequality? Principles that have been proposed as valid material principles of distributive justice include the following: to each person an equal share; to each person according to need; to each person according to effort; to each person according to contribution; to each person according to merit; and to each person according to free-market exchanges.

Review Questions

1. How do the principles of biomedical ethics relate to ethical theory? To the moral rules?

2. List four principles of biomedical ethics.

3. What does the principle of respect for autonomy demand of us?

4. What elements must be present in order for a choice to be autonomous? Why does it matter whether a choice is autonomous?

5. How does one decide whether a patient possesses decisional capacity?

6. How does one decide whether a patient's choice is a voluntary choice?

7. What does the principle of nonmaleficence demand of us?

8. What is the rule of the double effect? What elements must be present in order for it to apply?

9. What does the principle of beneficence demand of us?

10. What is the difference between specific and general beneficence? Between obligatory and ideal beneficence?

11. What is paternalism? Is it ever justified? When?

12. What does the formal principle of justice require?

13. What are the material principles of justice under utilitarian, egalitarian, and libertarian views of justice?

Endnotes

1. Gibson J. Thinking about the "ethics" in bioethics. In: Furrow BR, Greaney TL, Johnson SH, Jost TS, Schwartz RL, eds. *Bioethics: Health Care Law and Ethics.* 5th ed. St. Paul, MN: Thomson, 2001:1–5.

2. *Oxford American Dictionary.* Heald College ed. New York: Avon, 1980:710; italics added.

3. Gert B, Culver CM, Clouser KD. *Bioethics: A Return to Fundamentals.* New York: Oxford University Press, 1997:71–92, p. 75; italics added.

4. In Chapter 1, we learned about a number of ethical theories, as we were introduced to the thinking of Descartes, Aristotle, Aquinas, Kant, and Mill. The theory of *common morality* was not discussed therein, but will be developed in Chapter 3.

5. "Prior cases which are close in facts or legal principles to the case under consideration are called precedents." *Black's Law Dictionary.* Abridged 6th ed. St. Paul, MN: West Publishing, 1991:814.

6. *Roe v. Wade,* 410 U.S. 113 (1973).

7. *Planned Parenthood of Southeastern Pennsylvania v. Casey,* 505 U.S. 833 (1992).

8. Justices Scalia, Thomas, and White, along with Chief Justice Rehnquist, dissented in part. In his dissent, Justice Scalia wrote:

    The authors of the joint opinion, of course, do not squarely contend that *Roe* v. *Wade* was . . . *correct* . . . ; merely that it must be followed, because of *stare decisis.* But in their exhaustive discussion of all the factors that go into the determination of when *stare decisis* should be observed and when disregarded, they never mention "how wrong was the decision on its face?" Surely, if "[t]he Court's power lies . . . in its legitimacy, a product of substance and perception," the "substance" part of the equation demands that plain error be acknowledged and eliminated. *Roe* was plainly wrong—even on the Court's methodology of "reasoned judgment," and even more so (of course) if the proper criteria of text and tradition are applied. (Internal citations omitted)

9. Simmonds NE. Philosophy of law. In: Bunnin N, Tsui-James EP, eds. *The Blackwell Companion to Philosophy*. Oxford, England: Blackwell Publishers, 1996:396.

10. The Belmont Report: ethical principles and guidelines for the protection of human subjects of research. Available at: http://ohsr.od.nih.gov/guidelines/belmont.html. Accessed June 11, 2008.

11. Beauchamp TL, Childress JF. *Principles of Biomedical Ethics*. 5th ed. Oxford: Oxford University Press, 2001.

12. Jonsen AR, Siegler M, Winslade WJ. *Clinical Ethics*. 6th ed. New York: McGraw-Hill, 2006.

13. Some distinguish competency from decisional capacity. Thus, strictly speaking, *incompetency* refers to a formal judicial finding that a person cannot make legally effective decisions regarding his or her own affairs. *Decisional capacity,* on the other hand, refers to a person's ability to make a particular decision and is not dependent on any formal judicial finding. Herein we shall use the two terms interchangeably in the latter sense.

14. Hall MA, Bobinski MA, Orentlicher D. *Health Care Law and Ethics*. 7th ed. Austin, TX: Aspen Publishers, 2006:203–204.

15. Chell B. Competency: what it is, what it isn't, and why it matters. In: Monagle JF, Thomasma DC, eds. *Health Care Ethics: Critical Issues for the 21st Century*. Sudbury, MA: Jones and Bartlett, 2004:117–127.

16. In *In re Milton*, 505 N.E. 2d 255 (Ohio 1987), treatment was allowed despite the patient's religious refusal. The court disregarded the patient's belief that her evangelist husband would heal her as a "religious delusion," characterizing her decision as a nonchoice.

17. Dixon JL. Blood: whose choice and whose conscience? Available at: http://www.watchtower.org/e/hb/index.htm?article=article_07.htm Accessed June 10, 2008. Reprinted there by permission of the *New York State Journal of Medicine*, 1988;88:463–464, copyright by the Medical Society of the State of New York.

18. Harris S. *The End of Faith: Religion, Terror, and the Future of Reason*. New York: W. W. Norton & Company, 2004.

19. Thus, the First Amendment holds that "Congress shall make no law respecting an establishment of religion, or prohibiting the free exercise thereof; or abridging the freedom of speech, or of the press; or the right of the people peaceably to assemble, and to petition the Government for a redress of grievances." State governments are similarly constrained by the Fourteenth Amendment, which makes the First Amendment applicable to them.

20. "The Father, the Son, and the Holy Fonz." Available at: http://en.wikipedia.org/wiki/The_Father,_the_Son,_and_the_Holy_Fonz. "The Father, the Son, and the Holy Fonz" was the eighteenth episode of the fourth season of *Family Guy*.

21. Loewy E. Changing one's mind: when is Odysseus to be believed? *J Gen Intern Med* 1988;3:54–58. See also Paola F. Changing one's mind [letter]. *J Gen Intern Med* 1988;3:416.

22. In the criminal law context, a controlling influence exerted by person A on person B is sometimes referred to as *duress*, and under certain circumstances will cause the law to excuse the

(otherwise criminal) conduct of B; a controlling influence exerted by nonhuman events or circumstances on person B is sometimes referred to as *necessity*. Necessity does not excuse B's conduct, but may be used to argue that what he or she did was justified. See Emanuel S. *Criminal Law*. 2nd ed. Larchmont, NY: Emanuel Law Outlines, 1987:91–101.

23. Recall room 101 in Orwell's *1984*, where Winston Smith finds "the worst thing in the world"—rats—and under the coercion of fear and panic betrays his lover Julia. See Orwell G. *1984*. New York: Signet Classics, 1949.

24. This case illustrates another important point. One should not ask a question unless one is willing to act on the answer one gets. If the patient's request to be intubated was not going to be heeded, why ask?

25. *Prima facie* means "at first sight; . . . a fact presumed to be true unless disproved by some evidence to the contrary." See *Black's Law Dictionary* (abridged 6th ed.), 825.

26. Beauchamp TL, Walters L, Kahn JP, Mastroianni AC. Ethical theory in bioethics. In: Beauchamp TL, Walters L, Kahn JP, Mastroianni AC, eds. *Contemporary Issues in Bioethics*. 7th ed. Belmont, CA: Thomson, 2008:1–34.

27. Adapted from a case in *Clinical Ethics* (6th ed.), pp. 129–130.

28. Beauchamp TL, Childress JF. *Principles of Biomedical Ethics*. 2nd ed. New York: Oxford University Press, 1983.

29. Paola FA, Freeman I. The skilled specialist's ethical duty to treat. *J Clin Ethics* 1994;5(1):16–18.

30. Moss AH, Siegler M. Should alcoholics compete equally for liver transplantation? *JAMA* 1991;265:1295–1298.

31. Mill JS. Utilitarianism. In: Sher G, ed. *Moral Philosophy*. San Diego: Harcourt, Brace, Jovanovich, 1987:369–383, p. 369.

32. Lebacqz K. *Six Theories of Justice*. Minneapolis: Augsburg Publishing House, 1987:21.

33. Rawls J. A theory of justice. In: Sher G, ed. *Moral Philosophy*. New York: Harcourt, Brace, Jovanovich, 1987:453–472, p. 457.

34. Nozick R. *Anarchy, State, and Utopia*. New York: Basic Books, 1974:151.

35. Fried C. Imposing risks upon others. In: Sher G, ed. *Moral Philosophy*. San Diego: Harcourt Brace Jovanovich, 1987:705.

36. Kilner JF. *Who Lives? Who Dies? Ethical Criteria in Patient Selection*. New Haven, CT: Yale University Press, 1992.

37. Leenen HJJ. Selection of patients: an insoluble dilemma. *Med Law* 1988;7:233–245.

38. It should be kept in mind, however, than many of their criticisms of principlism were leveled at its earlier versions, as formulated in earlier editions of the Beauchamp and Childress text *Principles of Biomedical Ethics*. Principlism has evolved over the years.

Chapter 3

The Common Moral System

The utility of moral and civil philosophy is to be estimated, not so much by the commodities we have by knowing these sciences, as by the calamities we receive by not knowing them.

—Hobbes, *De Corpore*

Chapter Learning Objectives
At the conclusion of this chapter the reader will be able to:

1. Define *morality*
2. Explain the relationships among moral value judgments, moral rules or ideals, the principles of biomedical ethics, and ethical theory
3. Apply the procedure discussed herein to distinguish between morally acceptable and morally unacceptable solutions to moral problems
4. Define *impartiality, rationality, reasons,* and the concept of a *public system,* and explain how they relate to common morality
5. Explain the etiology of moral disagreements
6. List the moral rules and explain their significance and those of the moral ideals
7. Explain the determinants of a justified violation of moral rules
8. Define *moral virtue* and explain the relationship existing among the moral virtues

This chapter is an attempt to provide a clear and explicit description of our common morality; it is not an attempt to revise it. Common morality does not provide a unique solution to every moral problem, but it always provides a way of distinguishing between morally acceptable solutions and morally unacceptable solutions; that is, it places significant limits on legitimate moral disagreement. Thus, this chapter will not provide the unique correct solution to every moral problem, but it will provide a clear account of the procedure that one should follow to make sure that the solution that one does put forward is morally acceptable.

One reason for the widely held belief that there is no common morality is that the amount of disagreement in moral judgments is vastly exaggerated. Most people, including most moral philosophers, tend to be interested more in what is unusual than in what is ordinary. It is routine to start with a very prominent example of unresolvable moral disagreement, for example, abortion, and then treat it as if it were typical of the kinds of issues on which one makes moral judgments. It may, in fact, be typical of the kinds of issues on which one makes moral judgments, but this says more about the word *issues* than it does about the phrase *moral judgments*. Generally, the word *issues* is used when talking about controversial matters. More particularly, the phrase *moral issues* is always used to refer to matters of great controversy. Moral judgments, however, are not usually made on moral issues; we condemn murderers and praise heroic rescuers, we reprimand our children or our neighbor's children for taking away the toys of smaller children, and we condemn cheating and praise giving to those in need. None of these are "moral issues," yet they constitute the subject matter of the vast majority of our moral judgments. These moral judgments, usually neglected by both philosophers and others, show how extensive our moral agreement is.

Areas of Moral Agreement

There is general agreement that such actions as killing, causing pain or disability, and depriving people of freedom or pleasure are immoral unless one has an adequate justification. Similarly, there is general agreement that deceiving, breaking a promise, cheating, breaking the law, and neglecting one's duties also need justification in order not to be immoral. There are no real doubts about this. There is some disagreement about what counts as an adequate moral justification for any particular act of killing or deceiving, but there is overwhelming agreement on some features of an adequate justification. There is general agreement that what counts as an adequate justification for one person must be an adequate justification for anyone else in the same situation, that is, when all of the morally relevant features of the two situations are the same. This is part of what is meant by saying that morality requires impartiality.

There is also general agreement that everyone knows what kinds of behavior morality prohibits, requires, discourages, encourages, and allows. Although it is difficult even for philosophers to provide an explicit, clear, and comprehensive account of morality, once all the morally relevant facts are known, most cases are clear enough that almost everyone knows whether or not some particular piece of behavior is morally acceptable. No one engages in a moral discussion of questions such as "Is it morally acceptable to deceive patients in order to get them to participate in an experimental treatment that one wants to test?" because everyone knows that such deception is not justified. The prevalence of hypocrisy shows that people do not always behave in the way that morality requires or encourages, but it also shows that everyone knows what kind of behavior morality *does* require and encourage. This is part of what is meant by saying that morality is a public system.

Finally, there is general agreement that the world would be better if everyone acted morally, and that it gets worse as more people act immorally more often. This explains why it makes sense to try to teach everyone to act morally even though we know that this effort will not be completely successful. In particular cases a person might benefit personally from acting immorally—for example, providing false information in order to get a grant when there is almost no chance of being found out—but in addition to unfairly depriving honest applicants of the possibility of getting a grant, this kind of behavior, if generally practiced, would clearly have bad overall consequences. Further, even in this case it would not be irrational to act morally—namely, not to provide false information even though this will mean that one will not get that grant—because acting to benefit others, even at some cost to oneself, is not acting irrationally. Although acting morally is not always in one's self-interest, it usually is, and it is always in the general interest for people to act morally. Part of what is meant by saying that morality is rational is that morality is the kind of public system that every rational person can support.

Moral Theories

A *moral theory* is an attempt to make explicit, explain, and, if possible, justify morality— that is, the moral system that people use, usually unconsciously, in making their moral judgments and in deciding how to act when confronted with moral problems. It attempts to provide a usable account of our common morality—an account of the moral system that can actually be used by people when they are confronted with new or difficult moral decisions.[1] It must include an accurate account of the concepts of rationality, impartiality, and a public system, not only because these are necessary for providing a justification of morality, but also because they are essential to providing an adequate account of it. Indeed, a moral theory can be thought of as an analysis of the concepts of rationality, impartiality, a public system, and morality itself, showing how these concepts are related to each other. This chapter hopes to use the clear account of morality or the moral system presented by the moral theory to clarify and resolve some of the moral problems that have arisen and will arise in the health care field for health care professionals.

Rationality is the fundamental normative concept. A person seeking to convince people to act in a certain way must try to show that this way of acting is rational, that is, either rationally required or rationally allowed. This chapter uses the term *irrational* in such a way that everyone would admit that if a certain way of acting has been shown to be irrational (i.e., not even rationally allowed), no one ought to act in that way.[2] But that a way of acting is rationally allowed does not mean that everyone agrees that one ought to act in that way. On the contrary, given that it is often not irrational (i.e., rationally allowed) to act immorally, it is clear that many hold that one should not act in some ways that are rationally allowed. However, there is universal agreement that any action that is not rationally allowed ought not be done; that is, no one ever ought to act irrationally. If rationality is to have this kind of force, the account of rationality must make it clear why everyone immediately agrees that no one ever ought to act irrationally.

To say that everyone agrees that they ought never act irrationally is not to say that people never do act irrationally. People sometimes act without considering the harmful consequences of their actions on themselves, and strong emotions sometimes lead people to act irrationally. Regardless of how they actually act, however, people acknowledge that they should not act irrationally. A moral theory must provide an account of rationality such that, even though people do sometimes act irrationally, no one thinks that he or she ought to act irrationally. It must also relate this account of rationality to morality.

Impartiality is universally recognized as an essential feature of morality. Most philosophical accounts of morality fail to recognize the complexity of the concept of impartiality. No one is or should attempt to be impartial in all respects. An adequate account of impartiality requires stating in what respect one is impartial; for example, a teacher should be impartial when grading student papers. A moral theory must make clear why morality requires impartiality when one is considering violating a moral rule (i.e., acting in a kind of way that harms people or increases their probability of suffering harm) but does not require impartiality when acting on a moral ideal (i.e., preventing or relieving harm, such as deciding to which charity to give). Impartiality must also be related to some group; for example, a teacher should be impartial with respect to grading papers with regard to the students in her class. Abortion and the treatment of animals are such difficult problems because people differ in their views concerning who belongs in the group with regard to which morality requires impartiality. Some hold that this group is limited to actual moral agents, some hold that it should include potential moral agents (e.g., fetuses), and still others claim that it includes all sentient beings (e.g., all animals). There are no conclusive arguments for or against any of these views, which is why questions about the scope of moral protection have no unique correct answer.

Most moral theories, unfortunately, present an oversimplified account of morality. Philosophers seem to value simplicity more than adequacy as a feature of their theories. Partly, this is because they do not usually think that their theories have any practical use. Many are more likely to accept theories that lead to obviously counterintuitive moral judgments than to make their theories complex enough to account for many of our actual considered moral judgments. This has led many in applied ethics to claim to be anti–moral theory. They quite rightly regard these very simple kinds of theories as worse than useless. Unfortunately, they seem to accept the false claim of the theorists that all ethical theories must be very simple. Thus they become anti-theory and are forced into accepting the incorrect view that moral reasoning is ad hoc or completely relative to the situation.

The correct Aristotelian middle ground is that moral reasoning is not ad hoc, nor is there any simple account of morality that is adequate to account for our considered moral judgments. Any adequate moral theory must recognize that neither consequences nor moral rules, nor any combination of the two, are the only matters that are relevant when one is deciding how to act in a morally acceptable way or in making moral judgments. Some morally relevant features, such as the relationship between the parties involved, were almost universally ignored until feminist ethical theory emphasized them. When morally relevant features change, they change the kind of action involved and thus may change the moral acceptability of the action under consideration even though the consequences and the moral rules remain the same.

Another reason for the current low esteem in which philosophical accounts of moral-ity are held is that most of these accounts present morality as if it were primarily a per-sonal matter—that is, as if each person decided for herself not only whether she would act morally, but also what counted as acting morally. But this cannot be, for moral judgments are made on all normal adults, and everyone agrees that the moral system must be known to everyone who is judged by it. This means that morality must be a public system, one that is known to all responsible adults; all of these people must know what morality requires of them. In order to justify morality, a moral theory must show that morality is the kind of public system that, given plausible conditions, all impartial rational persons support.

Rationality as Avoiding Harms

Rationality is very intimately related to harms and benefits. Everyone agrees that unless one has an adequate reason for doing so, it would be irrational not to avoid any harm to or to avoid any benefit for oneself or those for whom one is concerned. The present account of rationality, although it accurately describes the way in which the concept of rationality is ordinarily used, differs radically from the accounts normally provided by philosophers in two important ways. First, it starts with irrationality rather than ratio-nality, and second, it defines irrationality by means of a list rather than a formula. The basic definition is as follows: People act irrationally when they act in a way that they know or should know will significantly increase the probability that they, or those they care for, will suffer death, pain, disability, loss of freedom or loss of pleasure, and they do not have an adequate reason for so acting.

The close relationship between irrationality and harm is made explicit by this defini-tion, for this list also defines what counts as a harm or an evil. Everything that anyone counts as an evil or a harm (e.g., diseases, maladies, and punishment) is related to at least one of the items on this list. All of these items are broad categories, so that nothing is ruled out as a harm or evil that is normally regarded as a harm. Although everyone agrees on what the harms are, they do not all agree on the ranking of these harms. Further, pain and disability have degrees, and death occurs at very different ages; thus, there is no uni-versal agreement that any one of these harms is always worse than the others. Some people rank dying several months earlier as worse than a specified amount of pain and suffering, whereas other people rank that same amount of pain and suffering as worse. Thus, for most terminally ill patients, it is rationally allowed either to refuse death-delaying treat-ments or to consent to them.

Most actual moral disagreements, such as whether or not to discontinue the treatment of an incompetent patient, are based on a disagreement on the facts of the case—for example, how painful is the treatment and how long does it relieve the painful symptoms of the patient's disease? Differences in the rankings of the harms account for most of the rest of moral disagreements—for example, how much pain and suffering is it worth to cure some disability? Often the factual disagreements about prognoses are so closely combined with different rankings of the harms involved that they cannot be distinguished. Further complicating the matter, the probability of suffering any of the harms can vary from insignificant to almost certain, and people can differ in the way that they rank a given probability of one harm against a different probability of another harm. Disagreement about involuntary commitment of people with mental disorders that make them dangerous to themselves involves a disagreement both about what percentage of these people would die if not committed and whether a significant probability of death within one week—say, five percent—compensates for a one hundred percent probability of three to five days of a very serious loss of freedom and a thirty percent probability of long-term mental suffering. Actual cases usually involve much more uncertainty about outcomes as well as the rankings of many more harms. Thus, complete agreement on what counts as a harm or evil is compatible with considerable disagreement on what counts as the lesser evil or greater harm in any particular case.

If a person knowingly makes a decision that involves an increase in the probability of his suffering some harm, his decision will be irrational unless he has an adequate reason for that decision. Thus, it is necessary to make clear not only what counts as a reason, but also what makes a reason adequate. A *reason* is a fact or rational belief that one's action will help anyone, not merely oneself or those one cares about, avoid a harm or gain some good, namely, ability, consciousness, freedom, or pleasure. What was said about evils or harms earlier also holds for the goods or benefits mentioned in this definition of a reason. Everything that people count as a benefit or a good (e.g., health, love, and friends) is related to one or more of the items on this list or to the absence of one or more of the items on the list of harms. Complete agreement on what counts as a good is compatible with considerable disagreement on whether one good is better than another, or whether gaining a given good or benefit adequately compensates for suffering a given harm or evil.

A reason is adequate if any significant group of otherwise rational people regard the harm avoided or benefit gained as at least as important as the harm suffered. People are otherwise rational if they do not knowingly suffer any avoidable harm without some reason. No rankings that are held by any significant religious, national, or cultural group are irrational; for example, the ranking by Jehovah's Witnesses of the harms that would be suffered in an afterlife as worse than dying decades earlier than one would if one accepted a transfusion is not an irrational ranking. Similarly, psychiatrists do not regard any beliefs held by any significant religious, national, or cultural group as delusions or irrational beliefs; for example, the belief of Jehovah's Witnesses that accepting blood transfusions will have bad consequences for one's afterlife is not regarded as an irrational belief or delusion. The intent is to count as an adequate reason any relevant fact or rational belief that has any plausibility; the goal is to count as irrational actions only those actions on which there is close to universal agreement that they should not be done.

Any action that is not irrational is rational. This results in two categories of rational actions: those that are rationally required and those that are rationally allowed. Because no action will be irrational if there is a relevant religious or cultural reason for doing it and that reason is taken as adequate by a significant group of people, in what follows we shall ignore particular religious or cultural beliefs by assuming that the persons involved have no beliefs that are not commonly held. Given only commonly held beliefs, an example of a rationally required action (i.e., an action that it would be irrational not to do) would be taking a proven and safe antibiotic for a life-threatening infection. Given the same beliefs, refusing a death-delaying treatment for a painful terminal disease would be a rationally allowed action (i.e., an action that it is rational to do or not to do). The two categories of rationally required and rationally allowed share no common feature except that neither is irrational. This account of rationality has the desired result that everyone who is regarded as rational always wants herself and her friends to act rationally. Certainly, on this account of rationality, people would never want themselves or anyone for whom they are concerned to act irrationally.

Although this account of rationality may sound obvious, it is in conflict with the most common account of rationality, in which rationality is limited to an instrumental role. A rational action is often defined as one that maximizes the satisfaction of all of one's desires, but without putting any limit on the content of those desires. This results in an irrational action being defined as any action that is inconsistent with such maximization. But unless desires for any of the harms on the list are ruled out, it turns out that people would not always want those for whom they are concerned to act rationally. No one would encourage a young patient who, after finding out that he has the gene for Huntington disease, becomes extremely depressed and desires to kill himself now, more than twenty years before he will become symptomatic, to satisfy that desire even if doing so would maximize the satisfaction of his present desires. Rather, everyone concerned with him would encourage him to seek counseling. They would all hope that he would be cured of his depression and then come to see that he has no adequate reason to deprive himself of twenty good years of life.[3] That rationality has a definite content and is not limited to a purely instrumental role—for example, acting so as to maximize the satisfaction of all one's desires conflicts with most accounts of rational actions, both philosophical and in the social sciences.[4]

Scientists may claim that both of these accounts of rationality are misconceived. They may claim that in the basic account of rationality, it is not primarily related to actions at all, but rather that rationality is reasoning correctly. Scientific rationality consists of using those scientific methods best suited for discovering truth. Although this is a plausible account of rationality, it cannot be taken as the fundamental sense of rationality; rather, the account of rationality as avoiding harms is more basic than that of reasoning correctly, or scientific rationality. Scientific rationality cannot explain why it is irrational not to avoid suffering avoidable harms when no one benefits in any way. The avoiding-harm account of rationality does explain why it is rational to reason correctly and to discover new truth, namely, because doing so helps people to avoid harms and to gain benefits.

Rationality, Morality, and Self-Interest

Although morality and self-interest do not usually conflict, the preceding account of rationality makes clear that when they do conflict, it is not irrational to act in either way. Although this means that it is never irrational to act contrary to one's own best interests in order to act morally, it also means that it is never irrational to act in one's own best interest even though this is immoral. Further, it may even be rationally allowed to act contrary both to self-interest and morality, if, for example, friends, family, or colleagues benefit. This is often not realized, and some health care professionals and scientists believe that they cannot be acting immorally if they act contrary to their own self-interest in order to benefit their colleagues. This leads some to immorally cover up the mistakes of their colleagues, believing that they are acting morally because they, themselves, have nothing to gain and are even putting themselves at risk.

Although some philosophers have tried to show that it is irrational to act immorally, this conflicts with the ordinary understanding of the matter. When there is little chance of being found out, it may be rational for a health care professional to deceive a patient about a mistake that he or one of his colleagues has made, even if this is acting immorally. This chapter does not attempt to provide the motivation for one to act morally. That motivation primarily comes from one's concern for others, together with a realization that it would be arrogant to think that morality does not apply to oneself and one's colleagues in the same way that it applies to everyone else. The attempt to provide a useful guide for determining what ways of behaving are morally acceptable presupposes that the readers of this chapter want to act morally.

Impartiality

Impartiality, like simultaneity, is usually taken to be a simpler concept than it really is. Einstein showed that one cannot simply ask whether A and B occurred simultaneously; one must ask whether A and B occurred simultaneously with regard to some particular observer, C. Similarly, one cannot simply ask whether A is impartial; one must ask whether A is impartial with regard to some group in a certain respect. The following analysis of the basic concept of impartiality shows that to fully understand what it means to say that a person is impartial involves knowing both the group with regard to which her impartiality is being judged and the respect in which her actions are supposed to be impartial with regard to that group: A is impartial in respect to R with regard to group G if and only if A's actions in respect to R are not influenced at all by which members of G benefit or are harmed by these actions. Moral impartiality requires not only this basic impartiality, but also not violating a moral rule unless one would be willing for everyone to know that they can violate the rule in a situation with the same morally relevant features.

The minimal group toward which morality requires impartiality consists of all moral agents (those who are held morally responsible for their actions), including oneself, and former moral agents who are still persons (incompetent but not permanently unconscious patients). This group is the minimal group because everyone agrees that the moral rules (e.g., do not kill and do not deceive) require acting impartially with regard to a group including at least all of these people. Further, in the United States and the rest of the industrialized world, almost everyone would include infants and older children who are not yet moral agents in the group toward whom the moral rules require impartiality. However, the claim that moral rules require impartiality with regard to any more inclusive group is controversial. Many hold that this group should not be more inclusive, whereas many others hold that this group should include all potential moral agents, whether sentient or not—for example, a fetus from the time of conception. Still others hold that this group should include all sentient beings (i.e., all beings who can feel pleasure or pain), whether potential moral agents or not—for example, all animals.

The debates about abortion and animal rights are best understood as debates about who should be included in the group toward which the moral rules require impartiality. Because fully informed rational persons can disagree about who is included in the group toward which morality requires impartiality, there is no way to resolve the issue philosophically. Fully informed rational persons who hold that animals are not impartially protected can also disagree about how much they should be protected; that is, they can disagree about how strong a reason one needs in order to kill or cause pain to an animal. This is why discussions of abortion and animal rights are so emotionally charged and often involve violence. Morality, however, does set limits to the morally allowable ways of settling unresolvable moral disagreements. These ways cannot involve violence or other unjustified violations of the moral rules, but must be peaceful. Indeed, one of the proper functions of a democratic government is to settle unresolvable moral disagreements by peaceful means.

Morality requires impartiality toward the minimal group (or arguably some more inclusive group) when one is considering violating a moral rule (e.g., killing or deceiving). Persons are not required to be impartial in following the moral ideals (e.g., relieving pain and suffering). The failure to distinguish between moral rules, which can and should be obeyed impartially with respect to (at least) the minimal group, and moral ideals, which cannot be obeyed impartially even with regard to the minimal group, is the cause of much confusion in discussing the relationship of impartiality to morality. The kind of impartiality required by the moral rules does not allow a violation of a moral rule with regard to one member of the group (e.g., a stranger) unless such a violation would be allowed with regard to everyone else in the group (e.g., friends or relatives). It also does not allow a violation of a moral rule by one member of the group (e.g., oneself) unless everyone else in the group (e.g., a stranger) is allowed to commit such a violation.

Acting in an impartial manner with regard to the moral rules is analogous to a referee impartially officiating a basketball game, except that the referee is not part of the group toward which he is supposed to be impartial. The referee judges all participants impartially if he makes the same decision regardless of which player or team is benefited or harmed by that decision. All impartial referees need not prefer the same style of basket-ball; one referee might prefer a game with less bodily contact, hence calling more fouls, whereas another might prefer a more physical game, hence calling fewer fouls. Impartial-ity allows these differences as long as the referee does not favor any particular team or player over any other. In the same way, moral impartiality allows for differences in the ranking of various harms and benefits as long as these rankings are the ones one would make part of the moral system. Also, one cannot allow anyone to violate a moral rule unless one would be willing for everyone to know that they can violate the rule in a situation with the same morally relevant features.

Public Systems

A *public system* is a system that has the following two characteristics. In normal circum-stances, (1) all persons to whom it applies (i.e., those whose behavior is to be guided and judged by that system) understand it, that is, know what behavior the system prohibits, requires, discourages, encourages, and allows. (2) It is not irrational for any of these persons to accept being guided and judged by that system. The clearest example of a public system is a game, such as poker or basketball. A game has an inherent goal and a set of rules that form a system that is understood by all of the players; that is, they all know what kind of behavior is prohibited, required, discouraged, encouraged, and allowed by the game, and it is not irrational for all players to use the goal and the rules of the game to guide their own behavior and to judge the behavior of other players. Although a game is a public system, it applies only to those playing the game; if one does not want to abide by the rules, one can quit playing the game. Morality is a public system that applies to all moral agents, however, no one can quit being governed by morality. All people who understand morality and can guide their behavior accordingly are subject to moral judgments simply by virtue of being rational persons who are responsible for their actions.

For morality to be known by all rational persons, it cannot be based on any beliefs that are not shared by all rational persons. Those beliefs that are held by all rational persons (rationally required beliefs) include general factual beliefs such as the following: people can be killed, can be caused pain, can be disabled, and can be deprived of freedom or plea-sure. Also included are beliefs that all people have limited knowledge—that is, no one knows everything and everyone is fallible (i.e., everyone makes mistakes). On the other hand, not all rational people share the same scientific and religious beliefs, so that no sci-entific or religious beliefs can form part of the basis of morality itself, although, of course, such beliefs are often relevant to making particular moral judgments. Parallel to the ratio-nally required general beliefs, only personal beliefs that all rational persons have about themselves (e.g., beliefs that they themselves can be killed and suffer pain) can be included as part of the foundation for morality. Also included is the fact that no one wants to be killed, caused pain, and so on, except in special circumstances. All personal beliefs about one's race, sex, religion, and so forth are excluded as part of a foundation for morality because not all rational persons share these same beliefs about themselves.

Although morality itself can be based only on those factual beliefs that are shared by all rational persons, particular moral decisions and judgments obviously depend not only on the moral system but also on factual beliefs about the situation. Most actual moral disagreements are based on a disagreement about the facts of the case, but particular moral decisions and judgments may also depend on the rankings of the harms and benefits. A decision about whether to withhold a patient's prognosis from him involves a belief about the magnitude of the risk (e.g., what the probability is of the information causing him to suffer a major depression or leading him to kill himself) and the ranking of that degree of risk of depression or death against the certain loss of freedom (to act on the information) that results from withholding that information. Equally informed impartial rational persons may differ not only in their beliefs about the degree of risk but also in their rankings of the harms involved, and either of these differences may result in their disagreeing on what morally ought to be done.

Morality or the Moral System

Although morality is a public system that is known by all those who are held responsible for their actions (all moral agents), it is not a simple system. A useful analogy is the grammatical system used by all competent speakers of a language. Few competent speakers can explicitly describe this system, yet they all know it in the sense that they use it when speaking and in interpreting the speech of others. If presented with an explicit account of the grammatical system, competent speakers have the final word on its accuracy. They should not accept any description of the grammatical system if it rules out speaking in a way that they regard as acceptable or allows speaking in a way that they regard as completely unacceptable.

In a similar fashion, a description of morality or the moral system that conflicts with one's own considered moral judgments normally should not be accepted. However, an explicit account of the systematic character of morality may make apparent some inconsistencies in one's own moral judgments. Moral problems cannot be adequately discussed as if they were isolated problems whose solution does not have implications for all other moral problems. Fortunately, everyone has a sufficient number of moral judgments that they know to be both correct and consistent so that they are able to judge whether a proposed moral theory provides an accurate account of morality. Although few, if any, people consciously hold the moral system described in this chapter, I believe that this moral system is used by most people when they think seriously about how to act when confronting a moral problem themselves, or in making moral judgments about others.

Providing an explicit account of morality may reveal that some of one's moral judgments are inconsistent with the vast majority of one's other judgments. Thus one may come to see that what one accepted as a correct moral judgment is in fact mistaken.

Particular moral judgments, even of competent people, may sometimes be shown to be mistaken, especially when those judgments are based on long accepted but unchallenged ways of thinking. In these situations, one may come to see that one was misled by superficial similarities and differences and so was led into acting or making judgments that are inconsistent with the vast majority of one's other moral judgments. For example, today, most doctors in the United States regard the moral judgments that were made by most doctors in the United States in the 1950s about the moral acceptability of withholding information from their cancer patients as inconsistent with the vast majority of their other moral judgments. However, before concluding that some particular moral judgment is mistaken, it is necessary to show how this particular judgment is inconsistent with most of one's more basic moral judgments. These basic moral judgments are not personal idiosyncratic judgments but are shared by all who accept our common moral system—for example, that it is wrong to kill and cause pain to others simply because one feels like doing so.

Morality has the inherent goal of lessening the amount of harm suffered by those included in the protected group, either the minimal group or a more inclusive group. It contains rules that prohibit some kinds of actions, such as killing, and require other kinds, such as keeping promises, and moral ideals that encourage certain kinds of actions, such as relieving pain. It also contains a procedure for determining when it is justified to violate a moral rule, for example, when a moral rule and a moral ideal conflict. Morality does not provide unique answers to every question; rather, it sets the limits to legitimate moral disagreement. One of the tasks of a moral theory is to explain why, even when there is complete agreement on the facts, genuine moral disagreement cannot be eliminated, but it must also explain why this disagreement has legitimate limits. It is very important to realize that unresolvable moral disagreement on some important issues (e.g., abortion) is compatible with total agreement in the overwhelming number of cases where moral judgments are made.

One of the proper functions of a democratic government is to choose among the morally acceptable alternatives when faced with an unresolvable moral issue. One important task of this chapter is to show how to determine those morally acceptable alternatives, in order to make clear the limits of acceptable moral disagreement. Within these limits, it may also be important to show that different rankings of harms and benefits have implications for choosing among alternatives. If one justifies refusing to allow job discrimination on the basis of race or gender because one ranks the loss of the opportunity to work as more significant than the loss of the freedom to choose whom one will employ, impartiality may require one to refuse to allow job discrimination against those having disabilities when they are capable of doing the work.

Moral disagreement not only results from factual disagreement and different rankings of the harms and benefits but also from disagreement about the scope of morality, that is, who is protected by morality. This disagreement is closely related to the disagreement about who should be included in the group toward which morality requires impartiality.

Some maintain that morality is only, or primarily, concerned with the suffering of harm by moral agents, whereas others maintain that the death and pain of those who are not moral agents are as important, or almost so, as the harms suffered by moral agents. Abortion and the treatment of animals are currently among the most controversial topics that result from this unresolvable disagreement concerning the scope of morality. Some interpret the moral rule "Do not kill" as prohibiting killing fetuses and some do not. Some interpret the moral rule "Do not kill" as prohibiting killing animals and some do not. But even if one regards fetuses and animals as not included in the group impartially protected by morality, this does not mean that one need hold they should receive no protection.

There is a wide range of morally acceptable options concerning the amount of protection that should be provided to those who are not included in the group toward which morality requires impartiality. Many hold that although the reasons that are adequate to justify killing or causing pain to animals do not have to be as strong as the reasons that are adequate to justify killing or causing pain to moral agents, some reasons are needed. Few hold that it is morally justifiable to cause pain to animals just because one feels like doing so. Many states have laws prohibiting cruelty to animals to enforce this moral opinion. Yet many hold it is justifiable to use animals in medical experiments that will help provide treatments for important human maladies. Many hold that it is justifiable to kill animals for food, even when vegetarian alternatives are available. Many hold that it is justifiable to deprive animals of their freedom so that people can enjoy seeing them in zoos, but it is now felt that they should be placed in larger, more comfortable surroundings than the small cages in which they used to be placed.

Another source of legitimate moral disagreement is the interpretation of moral rules. This category of disagreements based on interpretations of the rules is limited to different interpretations when the rule involves only moral agents. Even when there is no question that all involved are impartially protected by the moral rules, there is sometimes disagreement on what counts as breaking the rule—for example, what counts as killing or deceiving. People sometimes disagree on when not feeding, or discontinuing other life-sustaining treatment, counts as killing. There is also disagreement about when not telling counts as deceiving, or whether dyeing one's hair ever counts as breaking that rule. Some of these disagreements can be resolved, but some cannot, and often some institution will have to make a decision that settles the matter for the people governed by that institution. States may adopt rules determining when it is allowed to discontinue life-sustaining treatments, and health care professionals following such rules are not regarded as having killed patients but only as having allowed them to die.

Although there is some disagreement regarding the interpretation of moral rules (i.e., determining what behavior in what circumstances counts as violating the rule), most cases are clear and there is complete agreement that the behavior counts as a violation of a moral rule and thus needs to be justified. All impartial rational persons agree on the kinds of actions that need justification (e.g., killing and deceiving) and the kinds that are praiseworthy (e.g., relieving pain and suffering). Even though there is sometimes disagreement about the interpretation of a moral rule, all agree on what moral rules they would include in a public system that applies to all moral agents. They also usually agree on what moral ideals can justify violations of these moral rules. These rules and ideals are part of our common morality; they are not the invention of some moral theory. On the contrary, any adequate moral theory must explain and, if possible, justify these rules and ideals as part of our common morality. However, most moral theories do not do this; rather, they put forward some substitute for our common morality.

In addition to disagreements about the facts, and to the previous three sources of legitimate moral disagreement, there is a source of disagreement that seems like a disagreement about the facts but is really a disagreement of ideology, or views about human nature. This is a disagreement about what the consequences of everyone knowing that they were allowed to break the rule in certain circumstances would be. For example, some people hold that when asked whether one likes someone's clothes or hair, it is justifiable to deceive that individual in order to avoid hurting his or her feelings. They would publicly allow deception in this kind of situation because they believe that everyone knowing that this kind of violation is allowed would result in significant harm being avoided with only a minimal loss of trust. Others would not publicly allow deception in this kind of situation because they believe that the loss of trust would be significant and would outweigh the amount of harm avoided.

With regard to (at least) the minimal group, there are certain kinds of actions that everyone regards as being immoral unless one has an adequate justification for doing them. Among these kinds of actions are killing, causing pain, deceiving, and breaking promises. Anyone who kills people, causes them pain, deceives them, or breaks a promise, and does so without an adequate justification, is universally regarded as acting immorally. Saying that there is a moral rule prohibiting a kind of act is simply another way of saying that a certain kind of act is immoral unless it is justified. Saying that breaking a moral rule is justified in a particular situation—for example, breaking a promise in order to save a life—is another way of saying that a kind of act that would be immoral if not justified is justified in this kind of situation. When no moral rule is being violated, saying that someone is following a moral ideal (e.g., relieving pain) is another way of saying that he or she is doing a kind of action regarded as morally good. Using the terminology of moral rules and moral ideals and justified and unjustified violations allows us to formulate a precise account of morality, showing how its various component parts are related. Such an account may be helpful to those who must confront the often unfamiliar problems raised by the practice of medicine, by helping them to see how these problems are similar to those that are more familiar.

A Justified Moral System

A moral system that all impartial rational persons could accept as a public system that applies to all moral agents is a justified moral system. Like all justified moral systems, the goal of our common morality is to lessen the amount of harm suffered by those protected by it; it is constrained by the fallibility and limited knowledge of people and by the need for the system to be understood by everyone to whom it applies. It includes rules prohibiting causing each of the five harms that all rational persons want to avoid and ideals encouraging the prevention of each of these harms.

Moral Rules

Each of the first five rules prohibits directly causing one of the five harms or evils.

- Do not kill (could include causing permanent loss of consciousness).
- Do not cause pain (including mental suffering, e.g., sadness and anxiety).
- Do not disable (including loss of physical, mental, or volitional abilities).
- Do not deprive of freedom (including opportunities and freedom from being acted on).
- Do not deprive of pleasure (including future as well as present pleasure).

The second five rules are those that when not followed in particular cases usually cause harm, and general disobedience of which always results in more harm being suffered.

- Do not deceive (includes more than lying).
- Keep your promises. (Do not break your promises.)
- Do not cheat. (Do not violate rules of a voluntary activity in which you are participating.)
- Obey the law. (Do not break the law.)
- Do your duty. (Do not neglect your duty.) The term *duty* is being used in its everyday sense to refer to what is required by special circumstances or one's role in society.

Two moral rules can conflict—for example, doing one's duty may require causing pain—so it is clear that it is a mistake to conclude that one must always avoid breaking a moral rule. Sometimes breaking one of these rules is so strongly justified that not only is there nothing immoral about breaking it, but also it would be immoral not to break the rule. A health care professional who, with the rational, informed consent of a competent patient, performs some painful procedure in order to prevent much more serious pain or death breaks the moral rule against causing pain, but is not doing anything that is immoral in the slightest. In fact, refusing to do the necessary painful procedure, given the conditions specified, would itself be a violation of one's duty as a health professional and thus would need justification in order not to be immoral. It is clear, therefore, that saying that someone has broken a moral rule does not necessarily mean that someone has done anything wrong—it is only saying that some justification is needed.

What Counts as a Violation of a Moral Rule?

As mentioned earlier, people often disagree about what counts as violating a moral rule. Sometimes people will disagree about whether to consider an action as a justified violation of a moral rule, as described previously, or as an action that is not even a violation of a rule. Not every action that results in someone suffering a harm or an evil counts as breaking one of the first five rules. A scientist who finds out that another scientist's important new discovery is, in fact, false, may know that publishing her finding will result in the second scientist feeling bad. But publishing her finding is not a justified violation of the rule against causing pain: most would say it is not a violation of that rule at all. Determining whether it is depends on the practices and conventions of the society.

Often these situations are not clear. For example, if a physician responds to a couple's question and informs them that their fetus has some serious genetic problem, such as trisomy 18, he may know that this will result in their suffering considerable grief. However, if he has verified the information and told them in the appropriately considerate way, then many would say that he did not break the rule against causing pain and that his action requires no justification. Indeed, not responding truthfully to their question would be an unjustified violation of the rule against deception. This interpretation is taking the physician to be acting like the scientist reporting a mistake by another scientist. Others might take the physician to be acting like a health care professional justifiably breaking the rule against causing pain because he is doing so with the consent of the couple and for their benefit. In either case, it is at least a moral ideal to be as kind and gentle in telling that truth as one can. Indeed, many would claim it is a duty of health care professionals to minimize the suffering caused by providing information about serious medical problems.

Lying—making a false statement with the intent to deceive—clearly counts as violating the rule prohibiting deception, as does any other action that is intentionally done in order to deceive others. But it is not always clear when withholding information counts as deception. Thus, it not always clear that a health care professional needs a justification for withholding some information—for example, that the husband of the woman whose fetus is being tested did not father that fetus. In scientific research, what counts as deceptive is determined in large part by the conventions and practices of the field or area of research. If it is a standard scientific practice not to report unsuccessful experiments, then doing so is not deceptive, even if some people are deceived. However, a practice that results in a significant number of people being deceived is a deceptive practice even if it is a common practice within the field or area—for example, releasing to the press a premature and overly optimistic account of some medical discovery, thereby creating false hope for those suffering from the related malady. Recognition that one's action is deceptive is important, for then one realizes that one needs a justification for it or else one is acting immorally.

Justifying Violations of the Moral Rules

Almost everyone agrees that the moral rules are not absolute, that they have justified exceptions; most agree that even killing is justified in self-defense. Further, there is widespread agreement on several features that all justified exceptions possess. The first of these involves impartiality. There is general agreement that all justified violations of the rules are such that if they are justified for any person, they are justified for every person when all of the morally relevant features are the same. The major, and probably only, value of simple slogans such as the Golden Rule, "Do unto others as you would have them do unto you," and Kant's categorical imperative, "Act only on that maxim that you would will to be a universal law," is as a device to persuade people to act impartially when they are contemplating violating a moral rule. However, given that these slogans are often misleading, when trying to decide what to do in difficult cases, it would be better to consider whether an impartial rational person could publicly allow that kind of violation.

There is complete agreement that for a violation to be justified it has to be rational to favor everyone being allowed to violate the rule in the same circumstances. Suppose that someone suffering from a mental disorder wants both to inflict pain on others and wants to have pain inflicted on himself. He favors allowing any person who wants others to cause him or her pain to cause pain to others, whether or not those others want pain inflicted on them. Whether this person is acting in accord with the Golden Rule or the categorical imperative, it is not sufficient to justify that kind of violation. No impartial rational person would favor allowing those who want pain caused to themselves to cause pain to everyone else whether or not those others want pain caused to them. The result of allowing that kind of violation would be an increase in the amount of pain suffered with almost no compensating benefit, which is clearly irrational.

Finally, there is general agreement that a violation is justified only if it is rational to favor that violation even if everyone knows that this kind of violation is allowed; that is, it is rational to publicly allow the violation. A violation is not justified simply if it would be rational to favor allowing everyone to violate the rule in the same circumstances, but only if almost no one knows that it is allowable to violate the rule in those circumstances. For example, when almost no one knows that such deception is allowed, it might be rational to favor allowing a health care professional to deceive a patient about his diagnosis if that patient were likely to be upset by knowing the truth. But that would not make deception in these circumstances justified. It has to be rational to favor allowing this kind of deception when everyone knows that one is allowed to deceive in these circumstances. One must be prepared to publicly defend this kind of deception if it were discovered. Only the requirement that the violation be publicly allowed guarantees the kind of impartiality required by morality.

Not everyone agrees on which violations satisfy these three conditions, but there is general agreement that no violation is justified unless it satisfies all three of these conditions. Allowing for some disagreement while acknowledging the significant agreement concerning justified violations of the moral rules results in the following formulation of the appropriate moral attitude toward violations of the moral rules: Everyone is always to obey the rule unless an impartial rational person can publicly allow violating it. Anyone who violates the rule when no impartial rational person can publicly allow such a violation may be punished. (The "unless" clause only means that when an impartial rational person can publicly allow such a violation, impartial rational persons may disagree on whether or not one should obey the rule. It does not mean that they agree one should not obey the rule.)

Morally Relevant Features

When deciding whether an impartial rational person can publicly allow a violation of a moral rule, the kind of violation must be described using only morally relevant features. Because morally relevant features are part of the moral system, they must be such that all moral agents can understand them. This means that any appropriate description of the violation, for the purposes of determining whether an impartial rational person can publicly allow it, must be such that it can be reformulated in a way such that all moral agents can understand it. Limiting the way in which a violation can be described makes it easier for people to discover that their decision or judgment is biased by some considerations that are not morally relevant. If a consideration cannot be reformulated as an instance of some morally relevant feature, then that consideration should not be used when determining whether a violation is justified.

The discovery of a morally relevant feature (e.g., whether the situation is an emergency) comes from finding that the application of the moral system to a situation results in a conflict with one's moral intuitions that can be eliminated by adding that feature. Because morally relevant features must be such that they can be understood by all moral agents and can be used by them in describing a situation, this procedure does not provide an opportunity to introduce one's biases into the moral system. Of course, in any actual situation, it is the particular facts of the situation that determine the answers to these questions, but all of these particular facts must be able to be redescribed in a way that can be understood by all moral agents. The answers to the following ten questions are the morally relevant features that have been discovered so far.

1. What moral rules are being violated?

2. What harms are being (a) avoided (not caused), (b) prevented, or (c) caused?

3. What are the relevant beliefs and desires of the people toward whom the rule is being violated? (This explains why it is important to provide patients with adequate information and why patients' consent to treatment is so important.)

4. Does one have a relationship with the person(s) toward whom the rule is being violated such that, even without consent, one sometimes has a duty to violate

moral rules with regard to the person(s)? (This explains why a parent or guardian is allowed to make decisions about treatment that cannot be made by the health care team.)

5. What benefits are being promoted?

6. Is an unjustified or weakly justified violation of a moral rule being prevented?

7. Is an unjustified or weakly justified violation of a moral rule being punished?

8. Are there any alternative actions that would be preferable?[5]

9. Is the violation being done intentionally or only knowingly?[6]

10. Is it an emergency situation that people do not believe that they will be in?[7]

When considering the harms being avoided (not caused), prevented, or caused and the benefits being promoted, one must consider not only the kind of benefits or harms involved but also their seriousness, duration, and probability. If more than one person is affected, one must consider not only how many people will be affected but also the distribution of the harms and benefits. If two violations are the same in all of their morally relevant features, then they count as the same kind of violation. Anyone who claims to be acting or judging as an impartial rational person who holds that one of these violations should be publicly allowed must hold that the other also be publicly allowed. This follows from the kind of impartiality required by morality. However, this does not mean that two people, both impartial and rational, who agree that two actions count as the same kind of violation must always agree on whether to publicly allow this kind of violation. Impartial rational persons may differ in their estimate of the consequences of publicly allowing this kind of violation, or they may rank the benefits and harms involved differently. The moral system allows for such legitimate moral disagreement.

An impartial rational person decides whether to publicly allow a violation by estimating what effect this kind of violation, if publicly allowed, would have. If all informed impartial rational persons would estimate that less harm would be suffered if this kind of violation were publicly allowed, then all impartial rational persons would publicly allow this kind of violation and the violation is strongly justified; if all informed impartial rational persons would estimate that more harm would be suffered, then no impartial rational person would publicly allow this kind of violation and the violation is unjustified. However, impartial rational persons, even if equally informed, may disagree in their estimate of whether more or less harm will result from this kind of violation being publicly allowed. Sometimes, primarily when considering the actions of governments, it is also appropriate to consider not only the harms but also the benefits that would result from this kind of violation being publicly allowed. When equally informed impartial rational persons disagree on whether to publicly allow this kind of violation, the violation counts as weakly justified. Most controversial moral questions involve weakly justified violations.

Disagreements in the estimates of whether a given kind of violation being publicly allowed will result in more or less harm may stem from two distinct sources. The first is a difference in the rankings of the various kinds of harms. If someone ranks a specified amount of pain and suffering as worse than a specified amount of loss of freedom, and someone else ranks them in the opposite way, then although they agree that a given action is the same kind of violation, they may disagree on whether to publicly allow this kind of violation. The second is a difference in estimates of how much harm would result from publicly allowing a given kind of violation, even when there seems to be no difference in the rankings of the different kinds of harms. These differences may stem from differences in beliefs about human nature or about the nature of human societies. Insofar as these differences cannot be settled by any universally agreed upon empirical method, such differences are best regarded as ideological. The disagreement about the acceptability of voluntary active euthanasia of patients with terminal illnesses is an example of such a dispute. People disagree on whether publicly allowing voluntary active euthanasia will result in various bad consequences, including significantly more people dying sooner than they really want. However, it is quite likely that most ideological differences also involve differences in the rankings of different kinds of harms; for example, does the suffering prevented by voluntary active euthanasia rank higher or lower than the earlier deaths that might be caused? But sometimes there seems to be an unresolvable difference when a careful examination of the issue shows that there is actually a correct answer.

Applying the Moral System to a Particular Case

Suppose a physician claims that deception about a diagnosis (e.g., of Huntington disease in a young adult) to avoid causing a specified degree of anxiety and other mental suffering is justified. She may claim that withholding unpleasant findings in this case will result in less overall harm being suffered than if deception were not practiced. She may hold that it is likely that this patient will be extremely upset with the bad news and is very unlikely to find out about the deception for very many years. Thus she may claim that this kind of deception actually results in this patient suffering less overall harm than if he were told the truth now. However, another physician may claim that deception—no matter how difficult it will be for the patient to accept the facts or how confident the physician is that the deception will not be discovered for a long time—is not justified. The latter may hold that this deception will actually increase the amount of harm suffered because the patient will be deprived of the opportunity to make decisions based on the facts and that if he does find out about the deception he will have less faith in statements made by physicians, thus increasing the amount of anxiety and suffering. Thus there is a genuine empirical dispute about whether withholding bad news from this patient is likely to increase or decrease the amount of harm suffered.

Which of these hypotheses about the actual effects of deception in this particular case is correct I do not know, but if one is concerned with the moral justifiability of such deception, it does not matter. The morally decisive question is not "What are the consequences of this particular act of deception?" but rather "What would be the consequences if this kind of deception were publicly allowed?" Neither physician has taken into account that a justifiable violation against deception must be one that can be publicly allowed, that is, one that everyone knows is allowed. Once one realizes that in making a moral decision one must consider the consequences if everyone knows that it is allowable to deceive in certain circumstances—for example, to withhold bad news in order to avoid anxiety and other mental suffering—then the loss of trust involved will obviously have worse consequences than if everyone knew that such deception was not allowed. And this loss of trust clearly results in worse consequences than the consequences of everyone knowing that this kind of violation is not publicly allowed. Publicly allowing this kind of violation means allowing everyone, not only health care professionals but also patients, to know that deception is allowed in this kind of case. This cannot help but increase the anxiety suffered even by patients who are not deceived.

It is only by concentrating on the results of one's own deception without recognizing that morally allowed violations for oneself must be such that everyone knows that they are morally allowed for everyone that one could be led to think that such deception was justified. Consciously holding that it is morally allowable for oneself to deceive others in this way although one would not want everyone to know that everyone is morally allowed to deceive others in the same circumstances is exactly what is meant by arrogance, namely, the arrogating of exceptions to the moral rules for oneself that one would not want everyone to know are allowed for all. This arrogance is clearly incompatible with the kind of impartiality that morality requires with regard to obeying the moral rules.

Contrasts with Other Systems for Guiding Conduct

For those who are concerned with the philosophical foundations of bioethics, it may clarify this account of our common moral system to compare it with the views put forward by many contemporary followers of Immanuel Kant (1724–1804) and John Stuart Mill (1806–1873). The Kantian categorical imperative, "Act only on that maxim whereby you can at the same time will that it be a universal law of nature," and Mill's utilitarian greatest happiness principle, "Act so as to bring about the greatest happiness for the greatest number," are two of the most popular and influential moral philosophical slogans. But these slogans, though often cited, are inadequate, by themselves, to provide a useful moral guide to conduct. It is not fair to Kant and Mill or their contemporary followers to compare these slogans with the account of the moral system sketched in this chapter, because Kant and Mill and their contemporary followers have far more to say than simply working out the consequences of these slogans. However, these slogans, especially in medical contexts, are often put forward in a simplified way. Further, neither Kant nor Mill nor their contemporary followers provide a list of morally relevant features; that is, there is little effort devoted to providing plausible accounts of how one determines whether two violations count as violations of the same kind for the purpose of moral evaluation.

On a popular interpretation of a Kantian deontological system, one should never act in any way that one could not will to be a universal law. If it would be impossible for everyone always to do a specific kind of action, then everyone is prohibited from doing that kind of action. For example, that it is impossible for everyone always to make lying promises (for then there could be no practice of promising) is what makes it morally prohibited to make lying promises. In the common moral system described in this chapter, one is prohibited from doing a kind of action only if, given the morally relevant facts, no impartial rational person would publicly allow that kind of action. A Kantian system seems to rule out ever making lying promises, whereas our common morality allows the making of lying promises in some circumstances, for example, when it is necessary to make the lying promise to prevent a harm sufficiently great that less overall harm would be suffered even if everyone knew such lying promises were allowed.

On a popular interpretation of a utilitarian or consequentialist system (such as that of Bentham and Mill), one not only may but also should violate any rule if the foreseeable consequences of that particular violation, including the effects on future obedience to the rule, are better than the consequences of not violating the rule. A consequentialist system is concerned only with the foreseeable consequences of the particular violation, not with the foreseeable consequences of that kind of violation being publicly allowed. But on the common moral system, it is precisely the foreseeable consequences of that kind of violation being publicly allowed that are decisive in determining whether it is morally allowed. The consequences of the particular act are important only in determining the kind of violation under consideration. A consequentialist system favors cheating on an exam if one were certain that one would not get caught and no harm would result from that particular violation of the rule against cheating. Assuming that exams serve a useful function, our moral system would not allow this kind of violation of the rule against cheating, for if this kind of violation were publicly allowed, it would be pointless to have exams.

According to consequentialism, the only morally relevant features of an act are its consequences. It is, paradoxically, the kind of moral theory usually held by people who claim that they have no moral theory. Their view is often expressed in phrases like the following: "It is all right to do anything as long as no one gets hurt," "It is the actual consequences that count, not some silly rules," or "What is important is that things turn out for the best, not how one goes about making that happen." According to classic utilitarianism (Bentham and Mill), the only relevant consequences are pleasure and pain. That act is considered morally best which produces the greatest balance of pleasure over pain. In our common moral system, pleasure and pain are not the only consequences that count, and it is not the consequences of the particular violation that are decisive in determining its justifiability, but rather the consequences of such a violation being publicly allowed.

Our moral system differs from a Kantian system and resembles a consequentialist system in that it has a purpose, and consequences are explicitly taken into consideration.

It resembles a Kantian system and differs from a consequentialist system in that common morality is a public system in which rules are essential. The role of impartiality also differs. The Kantian system requires all of one's actions to be impartial, and consequentialist systems require one to regard the interests of everyone impartially. Common morality does not require impartiality with regard to all of one's actions; it requires impartiality only with respect to violation of a moral rule. Nor does morality require one to regard the interests of everyone impartially; it only requires that one act impartially when considering whether to violate a moral rule. Indeed, when concerned with all those in the minimal group, it is humanly impossible to regard the interests of everyone impartially. Impartiality with respect to the moral ideals (Kant and Mill would call these duties of imperfect obligation) is also humanly impossible.

Common morality also differs from the systems resulting from the theories of Kant and Mill, as well as almost all other moral theories, in that it does not require all moral questions to have unique answers, but explicitly allows for a limited area of disagreement among equally informed impartial rational persons. That all of the moral rules are or can be taken as prohibitions is what makes it humanly possible for them to be followed impartially. The public nature of morality and the limited knowledge of rational persons help to explain why achieving the point of morality—lessening the suffering of harm—requires impartial obedience to the moral rules but does not require, or even encourage, that moral ideals be followed impartially.

Moral Ideals

In contrast with the moral rules, which prohibit doing those kinds of actions that cause people to suffer some harm or increase the risk of their suffering some harm, the moral ideals encourage one to do those kinds of actions that lessen the amount of harm suffered (including providing goods for those who are deprived) or decrease the risk of people suffering harm. As long as one avoids violating a moral rule, following any moral ideal is encouraged. In particular circumstances, it may be worthwhile to talk of specific moral ideals; for example, one can claim that there are five specific moral ideals involved in preventing harm, one for each of the five kinds of harms. People often become health care professionals because they are motivated to act on the moral ideals of preventing death, pain, and disability. But when they become health care professionals they may come to have duties to prevent death, pain, and disability with respect to their patients, and so acting in those ways toward those patients is no longer merely acting on moral ideals. One can also specify particular moral ideals that involve preventing unjustified violations of each of the moral rules. Insofar as a misunderstanding of morality may lead to unjustified violations of the moral rules, providing a proper understanding of morality may also be following a moral ideal.

Although it is not important to list all of the specific moral ideals, it is important to distinguish moral ideals from other ideals, because only moral ideals can justify violating a moral rule with regard to someone without his or her consent. I call ideals that involve promoting goods (e.g., abilities and pleasure) for those who are not deprived *utilitarian ideals.* Those who train athletes or who create delicious new recipes are following utilitarian ideals. *Religious ideals* involve promoting activities, traits of character, and so forth, that are idiosyncratic to a particular religion or group of religions. *Personal ideals* involve promoting some activities, traits of character, and so forth, that are idiosyncratic to particular persons (e.g., ambition), about which there is not universal agreement. All of these ideals may be well worth following, but unlike moral ideals, none of them can justify breaking a moral rule with regard to a person without his or her consent. All impartial rational persons would sometimes favor breaking a moral rule in order to follow a moral ideal—for example, breaking a promise to meet someone for dinner in order to aid an accident victim, even when one has no duty to aid.

One of the most important differences between the moral rules and the moral ideals is that moral rules can be impartially obeyed all of the time. That is why impartial rational persons favor people always following the moral rules unless they have an adequate justification for not doing so. People do not favor people following the moral ideals all of the time because it is humanly impossible to do so. The moral rules set constraints on one's behavior regardless of what one's goals are. The moral ideals provide goals for one's behavior. This account of moral rules and ideals should not be surprising at all. Claiming that certain rules are moral rules is only claiming what everyone agrees, namely, that certain kinds of actions (e.g., killing, causing pain, deceiving, and breaking promises) are immoral unless one has an adequate justification for doing these kinds of acts. Claiming that certain ideals are moral ideals is only claiming what no one doubts, namely, that acting to relieve pain and suffering is encouraged by morality. Moral ideals express the point of morality more directly than moral rules, because following them is directly acting to achieve the goal of morality, which is the lessening of suffering harm by all those protected by morality.

Moral Ideals and Moral Worth

Following the moral ideals by providing clarification of morality or even by preaching that everyone adopt the moral attitude toward the moral rules does not usually have moral worth when doing so requires no sacrifice or risk, as in writing this chapter. However, there are occasions on which preaching morality does have significant moral worth. Someone who speaks out openly against the immoral action of some powerful person or group of persons is following a moral ideal in a significant way. Someone who urges his country to stop acting in an immoral fashion often undergoes significant risk in so doing, and his action deserves moral praise. Even someone who does not undergo any risk but merely devotes a great deal of time and effort to encouraging people to act morally may deserve moral praise. Of course, much depends on the motive for the action, but this will not be discussed here.

The moral worth of an action is determined not by the amount of evil prevented or relieved, but by how much it counts in judging the moral character of the person acting. A billionaire who gives a hundred dollars to a worthy charity prevents or relieves more evil than a person with an income only slightly above the poverty level who gives only one percent of that. However, the act of the poorer person has more moral worth. Indeed, when the cost to the individual in obeying a moral rule is very large, simply obeying that moral rule when it would be unjustified to violate it may have more moral worth than most instances of following moral ideals. In such a case obeying the moral rule indicates more about the moral character of the person than most cases of following a moral ideal. The relationship between moral ideals and moral worth is not a simple one, and some following of a moral ideal may even have negative moral worth, such as a very wealthy person giving much too small a donation.

Moral Virtues and Vices

Moral philosophy used to be primarily concerned not with particular acts, but with those traits of character that were virtues and vices. Hobbes says, "The science of virtue and vice, is moral philosophy."[8] However, I have described morality without even mentioning virtue or vice. Nonetheless, I realize that no account of morality is complete without an account of virtue and vice. Moreover, as a practical matter, children should be taught morality by means of the moral virtues. It is only in theoretical contexts that the moral virtues are derived from more basic concepts, although this theoretical understanding is helpful in teaching the virtues.

Teaching children to be virtuous involves not only training them to act virtuously but also to enjoy acting in that way. Children who are taught and trained in the appropriate way will usually not only come to have a disposition to act virtuously but also will come to enjoy acting in that way. The kinds of punishments and rewards that are most effective in affecting the way children feel about acting in a way that exemplifies character traits are often very mild, often only a frown or a smile. A child who is praised for responding to the suffering of others by trying to help is more likely to come to enjoy responding in that way, and hence to develop the virtue of kindness. Simply expressing approval to a child who tells the truth when there is a temptation to lie and expressing disapproval when she lies may result in her coming to view unjustified deception as not even an option. Training to develop virtuous character traits should always involve training a person to come to enjoy acting in that way. Children should be raised to enjoy acting morally, not only because it increases the likelihood of their acting in this way but also because the children will feel better when acting morally. Aristotle would not even consider a person to have a virtuous character trait unless he or she enjoyed exercising that trait, for Aristotle held that virtues must contribute to a person's flourishing.[9]

A clear account of the moral system is necessary for a proper understanding of the moral virtues and vices. A particular moral virtue involves following some part of the moral system significantly more often than most people, that is, justifiably following a moral rule or ideal significantly more often than most people in the same situation. A particular moral vice involves acting contrary to some part of the guide provided by morality significantly more often than most people, that is, unjustifiably violating a moral rule or failing to justifiably follow a moral ideal significantly more often than most people in the same situation. Although it is not discussed in most philosophical accounts of the virtues and vices, the same person may have some moral virtues and some moral vices. What this shows is that character traits are not always, probably not even primarily, formed on the basis of rational deliberation. If they were, all of the moral virtues would go together, because the reasoning that is persuasive with regard to one moral virtue should be persuasive with regard to them all. For most people, heredity and early training explain their particular moral virtues and vices. Understanding the relationship between the moral virtues and vices and the moral system is neither necessary nor sufficient for developing the virtues; however, it is necessary for properly understanding them.

The moral virtues and vices involve free, intentional, voluntary actions related to the moral rules and ideals. Associated with each of the second five moral rules is a moral vice, that is, a disposition to respond to a conflict between a moral rule and one's inclinations, interests, or goals in a way that involves unjustifiable violation of that rule. Associated with the rule concerning deception is deceitfulness; with promises, untrustworthiness; with cheating, unfairness; with obeying the law, dishonesty; and with doing one's duty, undependability. The linking of a particular moral vice with a specific moral rule is somewhat arbitrary; however, this pairing makes discussion easier and does not distort the understanding of the vices.

All the moral vices connected with the second five rules have corresponding virtues. In fact, except for truthfulness, which corresponds to the vice of deceitfulness, the names of all of these other virtues can be derived from those of the corresponding vices simply by removing the prefix. Because these moral virtues involve dispositions not to unjustifiably violate the moral rules, all impartial rational persons favor everyone having these moral virtues. The account of morality makes it obvious why the moral virtues connected with the second five rules—truthfulness, trustworthiness, fairness, honesty, and dependability—are those traits of character that all rational people want others to have and at least pretend to have themselves. Rational persons favor others acquiring the moral virtues in order to lessen their own risk of suffering harm. However, because they know that other rational persons also want them to act morally, they must at least pretend to cultivate these virtues in themselves. This explains the truth of La Rochefoucauld's saying "Hypocrisy is the homage that vice pays to virtue."

The moral virtues and vices connected with the second five moral rules lie on a single scale. As a person becomes less truthful, he or she becomes more deceitful, less trustworthy, more untrustworthy, and so on. A person may be completely dependable, generally dependable, fairly dependable, somewhat dependable or undependable, fairly undependable, generally undependable, or completely undependable. The virtue and the vice are such that as a person moves away from one end of the scale, he or she necessarily moves toward the other. But most people are somewhere in the middle, and it would be incorrect to claim that they have either the virtue or the vice. A person has a particular moral virtue or vice only if, given similar circumstances, the frequency with which he or she unjustifiably breaks the corresponding moral rule is significantly less than others or significantly greater. In fact, the second five moral rules can be restated in terms of either the virtues or the vices. The rules might be either "Be truthful, trustworthy, fair, honest, and dependable" or "Do not be deceitful, untrustworthy, unfair, dishonest, or undependable." This close association between the second five rules and the moral virtues and vices becomes important when discussing the question "Why be moral?"

Although most of what are normally listed as the moral virtues and vices are related to the second five moral rules, some moral virtues and vices are not. Cruelty is a moral vice that is related to the first five rules. It is most obviously related to the rule prohibiting the causing of pain, but it does not seem restricted to this rule. Rather, cruelty can manifest itself in unjustifiable violations of any of the first five rules, that is, any unjustifiable infliction of harm on someone. Of course, some people are crueler than others; whereas some people kill and torture unjustifiably, others may only deprive of pleasure unjustifiably. There do not seem to be distinct vices related to each of the first five moral rules; there are only degrees and kinds of cruelty.

Unlike the moral vices connected to the second five moral rules, a decrease in cruelty does not necessarily lead to an increase in what might be taken as the corresponding moral virtue, kindness. Between kindness and cruelty sits indifference. Unlike the moral virtues connected to the second five rules—honesty, fairness, and so on—kindness does not consist in a disposition to obey the moral rules. Rather, kindness is a disposition to follow the direct moral ideals, to act so as to relieve the harm suffered by others when this does not involve unjustifiably violating a moral rule. This explains the presence of indifference. Kindness is not simply lack of cruelty, as honesty is lack of dishonesty. Nor is cruelty simply lack of kindness, as dishonesty is lack of honesty. Lack of kindness is indifference; when regarded as a moral vice, it is known as callousness and is regarded as close to cruelty. There are no moral virtues related to the first five rules, for no one is thought to deserve praise simply for not unjustifiably causing harm to others. Indeed, if a person never unjustifiably causes harm but also never acts to prevent or relieve it when he or she has an opportunity to do so, that person may be regarded as callous.

Although this list of six moral virtues and seven moral vices is not complete, it is sufficient to confirm a general description of the moral virtues and vices. A moral vice must be a character trait that involves unjustifiably violating the moral rules or that involves failing to follow the moral ideals when this can be done justifiably. A moral virtue must be a character trait that involves justifiably obeying the moral rules or justifiably following the moral ideals. Moral virtues and vices can perhaps be best defined in terms of the attitudes of all impartial rational persons without mentioning the moral rules or ideals. A moral virtue is any trait of character that all impartial rational persons favor all persons possessing.[10] A moral vice is any trait of character that all impartial rational persons favor no person possessing. Regardless of how the moral virtues and vices are defined, however, they all have a direct conceptual relationship to moral rules and moral ideals.

Chapter Summary

A clear account of our common morality shows that there is far more agreement on moral matters than is usually assumed. Everyone agrees that killing, causing pain, disabling, depriving of freedom, depriving of pleasure, deceiving, breaking promises, cheating, breaking the law, and neglecting one's duties are not morally allowed unless one has an adequate justification. Everyone also agrees that preventing and relieving pain, helping the needy, discouraging immoral behavior, and encouraging moral behavior are morally good ways to behave. Finally, there is complete agreement that truthfulness, trustworthiness, fairness, and kindness are moral virtues and that deceitfulness, cruelty, and callousness are moral vices. This chapter, which provides a detailed analysis of the common moral system, including the role of rationality and impartiality, is intended to provide a better understanding of the moral rules, the moral ideals, and the moral virtues. It also is intended to make explicit the procedure that is used for determining what counts as an adequate justification of a moral rule and to make clear not only why some moral disagreements are legitimate but also why there are limits to legitimate moral disagreement.

Review Questions

1. What is the goal of morality?

2. Does common morality provide a unique solution to every moral problem? If not, what does it provide?

3. What does it mean when we say that morality requires impartiality? That morality is rational? That morality is a public system?

4. What are some of the sources of moral disagreements?

5. How are rationality, morality, and self-interest related? As explained in this chapter, what does it mean to say that a person is acting irrationally? Is it irrational to act contrary to one's own best interests in order to act morally? Is it irrational to act in one's own best interest even though this is immoral?

6. List the moral rules. How do the first five differ from the second five?

7. Is it the case that one should always avoid breaking a moral rule? Can two moral rules conflict?

8. How do the moral ideals differ from the moral rules?

9. What is a virtue? A moral virtue? How are virtues related to personality traits? To character traits? How are the moral virtues related to the moral rules?

Endnotes

1. A more extended account of morality and of the moral theory that justifies it are presented in my books: Gert B. *Morality: Its Nature and Justification.* Rev. ed. New York: Oxford University Press, 2005, and *Common Morality: Deciding What to Do.* Rev. ed. New York: Oxford University Press, 2007. The application of this account of morality to problems in medicine is presented in Gert B, Culver CM, Danner Clouser K. *Bioethics: A Systematic Approach.* New York: Oxford University Press, 2006.

2. I am aware that the terms *rational* and *irrational* are used in many different ways; for example, *rational* can mean calculating. However, I think that the basic normative concept of rationality is the one that I am describing.

3. See Gert B. Irrationality and the DSM-III-R definition of mental disorder. *Analyze Kritik* 1990;12(1):34–46.

4. See Gert B. Rationality, human nature, and lists. *Ethics,* 1990;100(2):279–300, and Gert B. Defending irrationality and lists. *Ethics,* 1993;103(2):329–336.

5. This involves trying to find out whether there are any alternative actions such that they would either not involve a violation of a moral rule or that the violations would differ in some morally relevant features (e.g., less evil caused, or more evil avoided or prevented).

6. There are many other questions (e.g., "Is the violation being done freely or because of coercion?") whose answers will affect the moral judgment that some people will make. However, the point in listing morally relevant features is to help those who are deciding whether to commit a given kind of violation. Features that are solely of value in judging violations that have already been committed cannot be used in deciding how to act. Although one does not usually decide whether or not to commit a violation intentionally or only knowingly, sometimes that is possible. Some might publicly allow a kind of violation if it is done only knowingly, but might not publicly allow a violation that differed only in that it is done intentionally. For example, many people would publicly allow nurses, and many nurses would be willing, to administer morphine to terminally ill patients in order to relieve pain even though everyone knows it will hasten the death of the patient, but, with no other morally relevant changes in the situation, they would not allow nurses, nor would nurses be willing, to administer morphine in order to hasten the death of the patient. This distinction explains what seems correct in the views of those who endorse the doctrine of double effect. Such a distinction may also account for what many regard as a morally significant difference between lying and other forms of deception, especially withholding information, because lying is always intentionally deceiving. Nonetheless, it is important to remember that many, perhaps most, violations that are morally unacceptable when done intentionally are also morally unacceptable when done only knowingly.

7. This kind of emergency situation is sufficiently rare that people are not likely to think that they will ever be in it. This feature is necessary to account for the fact that certain kinds of emergency situations seem to change the moral decisions and judgments that many would make even when all of the other morally relevant features are the same. For example, in an emergency when large numbers of people have been seriously injured, health care professionals are morally allowed to abandon patients who have a very small chance of survival in order to take care of those with a better chance, in order that more people will survive. However, in the ordinary practice of medicine, health care professionals are not morally allowed to abandon patients with poor prognoses in order to treat those with better prognoses, even if doing so would result in more people surviving.

8. *Leviathan*, chap. 15, para. 40. However, Hobbes, unlike most other philosophers, clearly distinguishes between moral virtues such as justice and charity, and personal virtues, such as courage, prudence, and temperance. See *De Homine*, chap. 3, sec. 32 in *Man and Citizen* (Indianapolis, IN: Hackett Publishing, 1991).

9. Following Aristotle, many virtue theorists take contributing to flourishing to be an essential feature of virtues. This standard view is the result of the failure to distinguish clearly between moral virtues and personal virtues.

10. Because having either a moral virtue or vice requires acting either significantly better or significantly worse than it is reasonable to expect with respect to following a moral rule or moral ideal, it may seem impossible to favor everyone having a moral virtue or no one having a moral vice. What impartial rational persons favor is everyone having a character trait that now corresponds to a moral virtue, although if everyone had it, it might not be called a virtue any more.

Chapter 4

Case-Based Decision Making in Ethics

Our discussion will be adequate if it has as much clearness as the subject-matter admits of, for precision is not to be sought for alike in all discussions, any more than in all the products of the crafts. ... In the same spirit, therefore, should each type of statement be received; for it is the mark of an educated man to look for precision in each class of things just so far as the nature of the subject admits; it is evidently equally foolish to accept probable reasoning from a mathematician and to demand from a rhetorician scientific proofs.

—Aristotle, *Nichomachean Ethics*

Chapter Learning Objectives
At the conclusion of this chapter the reader will be able to:

1. Understand the four-topics method of case-based decision making

2. Understand the relationship of each of the four topic areas to ethical principles

3. Learn to apply the four-topics method to actual cases

4. Understand the clinical casuistry method and its components—grounds, warrants, provisional conclusions, and rebuttals

5. Recognize the difference in approach between a top-down theoretical argument schema and a bottom-up practical reasoning schema

6. Learn to apply the clinical casuistry method to actual cases

7. Understand key facts and issues in the Terri Schiavo case

8. Understand the combined use of the four-topics method and the clinical casuistry method as applied to complex cases such as the Schiavo case

Previous chapters have addressed the ethical principles that undergird the ethical practice of medicine, as well as the moral rules that are often brought to bear in ethical reasoning. This chapter concerns itself with an actual process of ethical decision making that is case based. The rationale for this is that ethical problems always first appear as a practical difficulty or, in some cases, as a bona fide dilemma. Cases always involve situations where options exist—where decisions of one sort or another must be made. In medicine, it is often the case that indecision and consequent failure to act forces the decision in a particular direction. For example, consider a case in which a patient has indicated a desire not to be resuscitated, but no do-not-resuscitate (DNR) order has yet been written. When a health care professional (HCP) later responds to the patient's sudden and unexpected cardiopulmonary arrest, questions about what to do suddenly arise in the HCP's mind: "Should I honor the patient's wish, or should I go against it because there is no DNR order on the chart?" In other words, the problem lies in choosing between doing what the health care professional knows the patient wants (not performing resuscitative measures) and doing what hospital policy requires (any patient without a DNR order should receive an attempt at resuscitation). In this instance, any delay has the practical effect of deciding against resuscitation, because as time passes the chance of a successful resuscitation dwindles. This means that in some cases indecision is itself a default decision.

Cases like the one just presented do not allow time for deliberation and careful choice. The HCP can only react. If there has been no thought beforehand about how the HCP might respond in such an event, then both the decision-making process and the decision itself are likely to be suboptimal. There is a class of cases, then, that must be considered in advance, because the nature of the cases will not allow time for thought. Thinking ahead about such possibilities allows HCPs to anticipate problems and make decisions appropriately. This has been labeled *preventive ethics*.[1] Had the HCP considered the possibility of an unexpected arrest after it became known that the patient did not want resuscitative measures, a DNR could have been written. Alternatively, a discussion could have been held with the patient to clarify goals and explore the reasons behind the request to not be resuscitated. In any case, once the HCP was clear on the decision, appropriate action could have been taken at the appropriate time. Through preventive ethics, one can avoid common pitfalls that have ethical ramifications.

At the other extreme are those cases in which time is plentiful, but the decision is still hard. In these cases, there is ample time to consider options and weigh them carefully before proceeding. The classic example of this sort of case is the patient in a permanent vegetative state, where the decision is whether to discontinue the patient's artificial nutrition and hydration (ANH). Many famous ethics cases have involved just such a scenario, such as the cases of Karen Ann Quinlan,[2] Nancy Cruzan,[3] and, most recently, Terri Schiavo.[4] Let's look briefly at the Schiavo case.

Terri Schiavo was twenty-seven years old when she suffered a cardiopulmonary arrest in February of 1990. She was resuscitated and placed on a mechanical ventilator. Once she regained the ability to breathe without the ventilator, it was discontinued. During this time, Schiavo was placed on ANH. Despite all efforts to help her, including the placement of a thalamic implant, Schiavo did not improve. After several years with no change in Schiavo's status, a disagreement developed between Schiavo's husband and her parents over whether ANH should be discontinued. Schiavo's husband believed that his wife would not want to continue ANH once it became clear that there was no realistic hope of her improving. Her parents disagreed. As a result, Schiavo's husband turned to the courts to settle the dispute. The court's role was to function as Schiavo's surrogate decision maker in order to make the decision that, based on the available evidence, Schiavo would likely have made for herself. What followed was the most prolonged and contentious right to refuse treatment case in American history.

The core ethical question in the Schiavo case was whether it would be ethical to discontinue ANH. The case evolved over many years and gained such momentum in the media that nearly everyone had an opinion on the case.[5] The Schiavo case involved the court system at the highest levels. It also involved the Florida legislature, the governor of Florida, the U.S. Congress, and the president of the United States. Because the Schiavos were Catholic, Pope John Paul II used the public interest in the case as an opportunity to write about ANH from a Catholic perspective.[6] The media attention was unprecedented and extended beyond the United States to Europe and other parts of the world. In contrast to the Schiavo case, most such cases are handled privately between the involved parties, typically family members and HCPs involved in the direct care of the patient. In hospital settings, one may consult with the hospital's institutional ethics committee. One of the laments of the Schiavo case is that because she was in a long-term care facility when the dispute over her care arose, there was no institutional ethics committee to help the family members work through their differences. The Schiavo case also points out the truth that although the courts ultimately will settle disputes and decide difficult cases, the process can be lengthy.

In sum, whether the time course of a case is so compressed that it requires that it be considered prospectively or whether, like the Schiavo case, there is much time to deliberate before acting, we must have a consistent and informed approach to addressing ethical questions in clinical practice. Most cases fall between the two extremes mentioned thus far. In most cases there is time to decide the best course, to address conflict, and to communicate adequately with persons affected by the decision. In some cases, time remains a factor: we may have hours to days before a decision needs to be made. In other cases, we may have weeks to years.

Approaches to Case-Based Ethical Decision Making

Although there have been many approaches to case-based decision making, two of the most useful are the four-topics method pioneered by Mark Siegler[7] and the clinical casuistry model presented by Albert Jonsen and Stephen Toulmin.[8] These two approaches are especially useful when combined. Both approaches and their combined use are described here.

The Four-Topics Method

The four-topics approach to case-based ethical decision making was first put forth by Mark Siegler in an article entitled "Decision-Making Strategy for Clinical-Ethical Problems in Medicine."[9] This strategy is a way of organizing key information into four domains, or topics. It does not directly guide decision making by providing a reasoning process; rather, it organizes information and key considerations so that they can be usefully thought about.

This approach is analogous to the standard history and physical exam (H&P) in clinical medicine. In the H&P, information and key considerations are organized into domains such as (1) the chief complaint; (2) the history of present illness, which explores the chief complaint in terms of onset, duration, aggravating and alleviating factors, and so on; (3) past medical history; (4) social history; (5) family history; (6) review of systems, which is a standard review of body systems in terms of common symptoms or conditions; (7) physical examination; (8) laboratory data, results of other studies, and review of records; (9) assessment, which is the HCP's conclusions about the patient's problem(s); and (10) plan, which is the HCP's decisions about how to address the patient's problem(s). Notice that all of the categories consist of gathering information except for categories 9 and 10—the assessment and plan. These last two domains document the result of the HCP's thought processes in terms of (a) conclusions about the nature of the patient's problem(s), in the "assessment," and (b) conclusions about what actions to take next, in the "plan." The H&P doesn't tell the health care professional how to think; it organizes complete and accurate information so that he or she can think with an appropriate and complete set of data.

In like fashion, the four-topics method organizes information into domains that are relevant to ethical decision making just as the H&P is relative to medical decision making. The four topics are (1) medical indications, (2) patient preferences, (3) quality of life, and (4) external factors. The last category has been changed in recent years to "contextual features."[10] This system is given full treatment in the book *Clinical Ethics: A Practical Approach to Ethical Decisions in Clinical Medicine*.[7] Table 4-1 summarizes the system, and a brief description of the system follows.

The person analyzing the case collects and organizes information based on the questions in each quadrant of the grid shown in Table 4-1. For each quadrant or cell, the analyst notes the topic heading, followed by the ethical principle or principles typically involved, followed by specific questions that are designed to collect basic information related to each topic. The medical indications topic deals primarily with getting the facts of the case clear, considering the goals of treatment, estimating the chance of success of treatment, making alternate plans in case treatment fails, and estimating potential harm that might result from attempts to treat. The patient preferences quadrant contains questions about the patient's ability to make decisions, identifying a surrogate decision maker in the case of an incapacitated patient, assessing current preferences for patients with capacity and past preferences of patients who lack capacity, inquiring about the existence of advance directives, ensuring that the process of informed consent is carried out to the extent possible, and ensuring that the patient's rights are respected.

Many ethical issues can be decided on the basis of information collected in these two cells alone. For example, if a diabetic patient with a gangrenous limb refuses surgery to amputate the limb, ethical conflict is created because according to medical indications, amputation would be the treatment of choice and withholding that treatment might well result in the patient's death. When the questions under "patient preferences" are asked and it is deter-

TABLE 4-1   The Four-Topics Method

Medical Indications

The Principles of Beneficence and Nonmaleficence

1. What is the patient's medical problem?
2. Is the problem acute? Chronic? Critical? Emergent? Reversible?
3. What are the goals of treatment?
4. What are the possibilities of success?
5. What are the plans in case of therapeutic failure?
6. In sum, how can this patient be benefited by medical and nursing care, and how can harm be avoided?

Patient Preferences

The Principle of Respect for Autonomy

1. Is the patient mentally capable and legally competent? Is there evidence of incapacity?
2. If competent, what is the patient stating about preferences for treatment?
3. Has the patient been informed of the benefits and risks, understood this information, and given consent?
4. If incapacitated, who is the appropriate surrogate? Is the surrogate using appropriate standards of decision making?
5. Has the patient expressed prior preferences (e.g., advance directives)?
6. Is the patient unwilling or unable to cooperate with medical treatment? If so, why?
7. In sum, is the patient's right to choose being respected to the extent possible in ethics and law?

Quality of Life

The Principles of Beneficence and Nonmaleficence and Respect for Autonomy

1. What are the prospects, with and without treatment, for a return to normal life?
2. What physical, mental, and social deficits is the patient likely to experience if treatment succeeds?
3. Are there biases that might prejudice the provider's evaluation of the patient's quality of life?
4. Is the patient's present or future condition such that his or her continued life might be judged undesirable?
5. Is there any plan and rationale to forgo treatment?
6. Are there plans for comfort and palliative care?

Contextual Features

The Principles of Loyalty and Fairness

1. Are there family issues that might influence treatment decisions?
2. Are there provider (physicians and nurses) issues that might influence treatment decisions?
3. Are there financial and economic factors?
4. Are there religious or cultural factors?
5. Are there limits on confidentiality?
6. Are there problems of allocation of resources?
7. How does the law affect treatment decisions?
8. Is clinical research or teaching involved?
9. Is there any conflict of interest on the part of the providers or the institution?

Source: Jonsen AR, Siegler M, Winslade WJ. *Clinical Ethics: A Practical Approach to Ethical Decisions in Clinical Medicine.* 5th ed. © McGraw-Hill 2002. Reprinted with permission.

mined that the patient has mental capacity, that the patient states clear preferences for not undergoing amputation, and that the patient has understood the benefits and risks and has refused to consent to surgery, then we have enough information to conclude that out of respect for the patient's autonomy we should honor the patient's refusal. The actual reasoning behind this is examined later, when we discuss the clinical casuistry model.

The "quality of life" cell of the four-topics method grid addresses topics that often arise when the patient is unable to participate in decisions and has left no clear advance treatment preferences. The questions involve the prognosis of returning to normal life; deficits in physical, mental, and social domains; third-party judgments of patient quality of life; plans to forgo treatment; and plans for comfort care or palliative care. When a competent patient can make contemporaneous choices, or an incapacitated patient has made them in advance, the principle of respect for autonomy comes into play. When the patient is incapacitated and has left no wishes, we default to the principles of beneficence and nonmaleficence because no autonomous choices are known.

Finally, in the "contextual features" cell, the questions address family issues, provider issues, financial conflicts, and religious or cultural issues that can affect decision making. In addition, these questions consider limits on confidentiality, allocation of resources, legal concerns, research and teaching issues, and conflicts of interest. When all of these questions are considered and answered, what emerges is a focused picture of key case data, organized by topic and in relation to the core ethical principles. This arrangement allows the important considerations of the case to be viewed at a glance and thereby facilitates decision making.

One advantage of this approach is that it looks at things from the bottom up rather than the top down. It mirrors the way things work in clinical medicine. Health care professionals don't approach diagnosis from the top down by first considering pathophysiologic principles, even though they are important and vitally inform the HCP's understanding. Instead, HCPs approach diagnosis from the bottom up by first listening to the patient's history of the problem, asking pertinent questions to gain more information, and then reasoning about the collected information in order to arrive at a diagnosis or at least a diagnostic plan. Once the four-topics method has helped us focus our case material, we next turn to a process for practical reasoning that will help us to draw conclusions about the case at hand.

The Clinical Casuistry Model

The clinical casuistry model was described at length by Albert Jonsen and Stephen Toulmin in their book *The Abuse of Casuistry: A History of Moral Reasoning.*[8] Their hope was to reexamine the process by which cases of conscience were resolved by thinkers of the past and to give an account of how that method might be usefully applied to current cases, especially cases involving ethical choices in medicine. Like the four-topics method, this is a bottom-up approach to reasoning about moral problems; thus, it is entirely complementary to the approach taken in the four-topics method. Jonsen and Toulmin contrast their approach with the top-down approach that can be taken when one uses principles or maxims as the starting point.

Let's take as an example the case of an adult man, Mr. Smith, who is refusing blood transfusions even though he has been informed that without the transfusion he will die. The treating physician is uneasy about this because he knows he could save this patient. Is it right for the physician to just stand by and allow Mr. Smith to die for want of readily available treatment?

In approaching this case, the physician recalls learning in ethics class that health care professionals should honor refusals of treatment when they are made by competent patients. Before we use this statement as a starting point for reasoning about the case, let's look at the classic top-down reasoning approach used in formal arguments (Figure 4-1). In this approach, one starts by stating a universal major premise such as the one given: "Health care professionals should honor refusals of treatment when they are made by competent patients." It is then followed by a particular minor premise that describes the current situation; for example, this particular patient, Mr. Smith, is a competent patient who is refusing a lifesaving blood transfusion. The argument produces the necessary conclusion that the physician should honor Mr. Smith's refusal of lifesaving blood transfusion (Figure 4-2).

The problem with this approach is that it is not sufficiently attentive to the level of detail and the complexity of considerations that we typically find in clinical ethics cases.

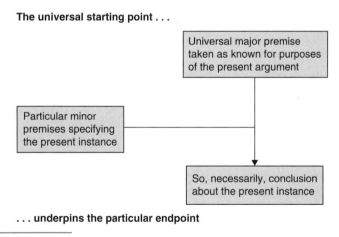

The universal starting point . . .

> Universal major premise taken as known for purposes of the present argument

> Particular minor premises specifying the present instance

> So, necessarily, conclusion about the present instance

. . . underpins the particular endpoint

Figure 4-1 Theoretical top-down argument.

From *Abuse of Casuistry: A History of Moral Reasoning.* Albert R. Jonsen, Stephen Edelston Toulmin. © 1990, the University of California Press. Reprinted with permission.

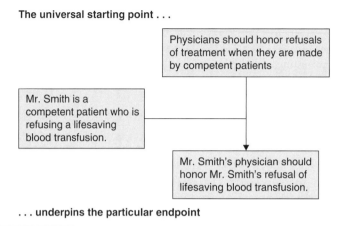

The universal starting point . . .

Physicians should honor refusals of treatment when they are made by competent patients

Mr. Smith is a competent patient who is refusing a lifesaving blood transfusion.

Mr. Smith's physician should honor Mr. Smith's refusal of lifesaving blood transfusion.

. . . underpins the particular endpoint

Figure 4-2 Top-down argument applied to an actual case.

By contrast, the clinical casuistry method does not start from universal maxims, however they might be derived. Instead, it begins with the facts of the case, and then applies considerations that have proven important in previous similar cases in order to reach a provisional conclusion about the case at hand. These considerations from prior cases are called *warrants*, and often resemble or duplicate the maxims that are commonly used in thinking about cases such as the one just presented. The prior cases are called *paradigms*. These can be thought of as classic cases. We have, for example, a number of classic types of treatment refusal cases that present themselves over and over again. We have cases involving competent patients, cases involving incompetent patients, and cases involving patients who were formerly competent but have lost capacity. The final category of cases contains subgroups: those who have made their wishes known before losing capacity, and those who have not. In addition to the cases already described, there are cases involving patients who were never competent, such as adults with congenital mental disability. There are also cases involving children, many of whom are too young to have decision-making capacity, and others who are older and might be regarded as mature minors.

Thus, any situation with which the ethicist might be confronted can be thought of as belonging to a specific category of cases that has its own set of classic cases that can be regarded as paradigms. One of the most important aspects of the clinical casuistry method is that one needs skill in judgment to pick the correct paradigmatic case that the case at hand most closely resembles. If the match is a clear fit, then the case can usually be easily handled. If the degree of fit for the paradigm is not very tight, then applying the paradigm is more likely to lead to erroneous results. Finally, the provisional conclusion reached by this method can be rebutted if it can be established that there are exceptional circumstances that are sufficient to override the conclusion to which the paradigmatic

The outcomes of experience . . .

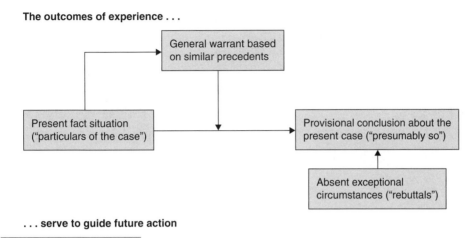

. . . serve to guide future action

Figure 4-3   Practical reasoning: the clinical casuistry method.

From *Abuse of Casuistry: A History of Moral Reasoning.* Albert R. Jonsen, Stephen Edelston Toulmin. © 1990, the University of California Press. Reprinted with permission.

case would ordinarily lead us. Figure 4-3 illustrates this method graphically, and Figure 4-4 uses this method to look at the case of Mr. Smith's refusal of a transfusion.

The first question is, Where do we get our paradigms, or classic cases, from? Many of these come from cases that have been tried in the courts. Because similar cases have been tried in numerous states over the past forty years, with the different courts reaching similar conclusions in the vast majority of instances, these legal cases can serve as paradigms for clinical ethical decision making. Because clinical decisions must comply with the law, a knowledge of key legal cases can be very helpful in working toward the resolution of an ethics problem that arises in clinical practice. Many books on ethics also feature classic cases and problems. *Clinical Ethics: A Practical Approach to Ethical Decisions in Clinical Medicine*, by Jonsen, Siegler, and Winslade, has a wealth of classic cases that can serve as paradigms.[7]

In Figure 4-4, we should note that if there are no exceptional circumstances that make the case significantly different from the paradigmatic case from which we derived our warrant, then the conclusion stands. Mr. Smith's doctor should honor his refusal even if Mr. Smith will die as a result. This, of course, assumes that we have chosen the right paradigm in the first place, and that the degree of fit between the paradigm and the present case is good.

When we examine the case further and obtain more information, we learn that Mr. Smith's wife died a year ago, and that he subsequently became a member of the Jehovah's

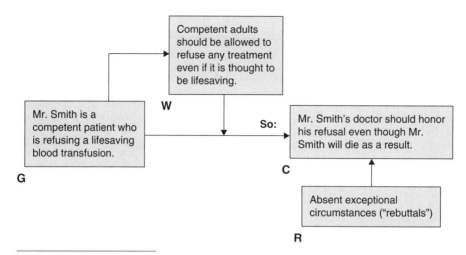

Figure 4-4 Actual case: refusal of blood transfusion, without rebuttal.
G, grounds—the core situation that creates a difficulty that requires resolution;
W, warrant—consideration(s) from prior paradigmatic cases, stated as a maxim;
C, conclusion—provisional conclusion reached by applying warrants to present case; R,
rebuttal—exceptional circumstances sufficient to override the provisional conclusions.

Witnesses. He is the sole caretaker for her three minor children, aged three, five, and eight.
If Mr. Smith dies for want of a transfusion, his three children will end up as wards of the
state. In looking at this new information, there might be several exceptional circumstances
or "rebuttals" one could posit. Figure 4-5 shows one rebuttal in graphical form.

In verbal form, the argument reads as follows. Several possible rebuttals have been
added.

(G) Mr. Smith is a competent patient who is refusing a lifesaving blood transfusion.

(W) Competent adults should be allowed to refuse any treatment even if it is thought
to be lifesaving.

So:

(C) Mr. Smith's doctor should honor his refusal even though Mr. Smith will die as a
result.

   (R₁) Except that his three children will end up as wards of the state.

   (R₂) Except that the reason for refusing is based on a religious belief that is not
   shared by most people in our society.

   (R₃) Except that he joined the Jehovah's Witnesses less than a year ago, and so
   may not be as firm on refusing transfusion as someone who has been in the
   faith for a longer period of time.

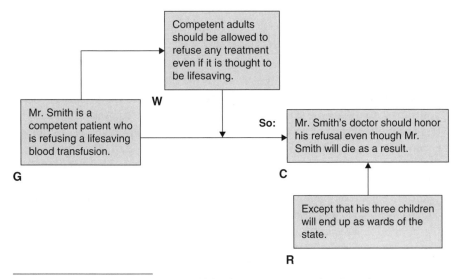

Figure 4-5 Actual case: refusal of blood transfusion, with rebuttal.

(R₄) Except that the treating physician believes it is wrong to allow a patient to die for lack of a transfusion.

Are any of the exceptional circumstances listed significant enough to rebut the provisional conclusion? This is ultimately a matter of judgment, but one that needs to be adequately informed. Our next step, then, is to look to see whether these issues have been addressed in the courts, the clinical ethics literature, the medical literature, and so forth. It turns out that there are court cases that have addressed these and other exceptions.[11,12] Thus these exception-based cases themselves form paradigms for common proposed rebuttals for cases involving a competent patient who is refusing a lifesaving blood transfusion.

When one studies the court cases and the literature on cases involving Jehovah's Witnesses, one finds that only the first exception (R₁) has been found sufficient to override the conclusion. There have indeed been a small number of cases of court-ordered transfusion of adults to prevent their minor children from being left as orphans and wards of the state.[13] This leads, therefore, to the next step of petitioning the appropriate court for an order to transfuse. Upon review, the court will either issue or deny the order based on relevant state law.

The fact that Jehovah's Witnesses have beliefs about blood that are not shared by most people in our society is not sufficient to rebut the provisional conclusion. What matters is the choice of a competent adult, not the basis, religious or otherwise, upon which that choice is made. Similarly, the short duration of Mr. Smith's membership in the fellowship of Jehovah's Witnesses does not devalue his decision in any way. Again, if this is the choice of a competent adult, then that fact alone will usually outweigh any other consideration. If the physician is concerned the patient may be ambivalent about refusing transfusion, he or she can approach the patient directly about this rather than overriding Mr. Smith's refusal because of an unverified concern.

Finally, although the physician may disagree with the patient's decision and morally object to it, believing it wrong, this nevertheless does not override the provisional conclusion. Physicians who disagree with patient refusals are not free to override them. The proper course of action for the physician is to withdraw appropriately from the case, allowing another physician without the same reservations to assist the patient in his medical care. This way, no one's autonomy, the patient's or the physician's, is compromised.

As you can see, it is possible for the student of clinical ethics to build up a taxonomy of cases of certain types, complete with subsets of these cases that deal with common exceptions. One could have categories such as those shown in Table 4-2.

As one learns about classic cases and their variants, one is better positioned to resolve ethical issues from an informed perspective. This lessens the risk that one will reinvent the wheel with his or her own cases. Armed with a sufficient knowledge of case paradigms, the information-gathering potential of the four-topics method combined with the practical reasoning approach of the clinical casuistry method will yield the best results. The tools of ethics are not as sharp as those of science, and the conclusions of ethics are impre-

---

TABLE 4-2   Taxonomy Structure for Paradigmatic Cases

Treatment refusal
Adults
  Competent
    Mechanical ventilation
    Artificial nutrition and hydration
    Blood transfusion (Jehovah's Witness)
      With minor children
      With concern regarding religious basis
      With concern regarding sincerity of belief
      With moral objection by physician
    Dialysis
  Incompetent
    With living will or health surrogate
    With oral past wishes only
    With no past wishes
Minors
  Mature minor with assent

cise because of the messy nature of ethical disputes. Nevertheless, these disputes are some of the most engaging in medicine, and their questions are some of the most in need of answers.

Using the Combined Approach for Case-Based Decision Making

Although a number of simple cases could be provided to further illustrate the use of the four-topics method in combination with the clinical casuistry method, let us instead consider a complex case—that of Terri Schiavo (Case 4-A), which we briefly considered earlier.[4] The simple ethics cases have been called "thin" cases because of their lack of detail. "Thick" cases, on the other hand, are rich in detail and more likely to be what we encounter in clinical life. It is in the details that we often find fine, but important, distinctions that can turn the case in one direction or another. It should also be pointed out that as cases evolve, the tools for analyzing and deciding about cases must be able to negotiate changes as they occur and to respond appropriately to new information.

Case 4-A   Terri Schiavo

Cardiac Arrest and Persistent Vegetative State

On February 25, 1990, twenty-seven-year-old Terri Schiavo suffered a cardiac arrest as a result of a low blood potassium level. Her husband of five years, Michael Schiavo, called 911. When emergency medical services arrived, they resuscitated Mrs. Schiavo and rushed her to the hospital. From the time of her collapse until the time she was resuscitated, Mrs. Schiavo's brain was without blood flow and oxygen. This resulted in devastating and permanent brain damage.

Mrs. Schiavo was comatose when she arrived at the hospital. She initially required mechanical ventilation and ultimately a tracheostomy tube; however, the ventilator and tracheostomy tube were withdrawn after Mrs. Schiavo regained the ability to breathe on her own. Mrs. Schiavo also required a surgical procedure to insert a gastrostomy tube (g-tube) into her stomach through her abdominal wall. This allowed Mrs. Schiavo to receive artificial nutrition and hydration (ANH). Eventually Mrs. Schiavo awoke from her coma, but she never regained consciousness.

After two and a half months, Mrs. Schiavo was discharged to a long-term care facility. Later that year, her husband was granted an appointment to serve as his wife's legal guardian. Mrs. Schiavo remained in a persistent vegetative state, completely bed-bound and in need of total care. Despite vigorous attempts at rehabilitation, including being taken by her husband to California to receive surgical implantation of an experimental thalamic stimulator, Mrs. Schiavo's condition did not improve.

(continues)

Case 4-A Terri Schiavo (*continued*)

The Malpractice Award

In November 1992, Mrs. Schiavo and her husband were awarded $1,000,000 in a medical malpractice lawsuit that linked Mrs. Schiavo's cardiac arrest to her fertility specialist's failure to diagnose a potassium deficit. Some suspect that Mrs. Schiavo's low potassium level may have been a result of excess fluid intake and weight loss caused by an eating disorder. The bulk of the malpractice award ($700,000) went into a trust fund to pay for Mrs. Schiavo's perpetual care. The rest went to her husband for loss of consortium.

The relationship between Mrs. Schiavo's husband and her parents, the Schindlers, was initially a good one, but it began to deteriorate in the immediate aftermath of the malpractice trial. In July of the following year, Mrs. Schiavo's parents fought unsuccessfully to have their son-in-law removed as their daughter's sole guardian. This was the first step in what became a truly unprecedented legal fight that made the Terri Schiavo case the most intensely litigated case in U.S. history.

The Artificial Nutrition and Hydration Case

By mid-1996, six years after Mrs. Schiavo's cardiac arrest, she remained unchanged. A computed tomographic scan of her brain showed a severely abnormal structure. Much of her cerebral cortex was absent, having been replaced by cerebral spinal fluid. Her uncontested diagnosis at the time was persistent vegetative state. During this period Mrs. Schiavo's husband gradually came to accept that his wife had no realistic hope of improvement, and that in such a circumstance she would not want interventions that would only maintain her in her current condition.

Even though Mrs. Schiavo's husband was the legal guardian and could have authorized his wife's physician to discontinue the g-tube, he chose to ask a judge to decide because there was strong disagreement between himself and his in-laws over what to do, as well as suspicion on both sides about monetary motives. In May 1998, eight years after Mrs. Schiavo's heart attack, Judge George Greer of the Pinellas-Pasco County Circuit Court began to hear the case, serving as Mrs. Schiavo's surrogate decision maker. As surrogate, the judge's purpose was to make the decision that, based on available evidence, Mrs. Schiavo would likely have made for herself.

The judge heard from both sides regarding Mrs. Schiavo's wishes. Like many young people without children, Mrs. Schiavo had not prepared a will, much less a living will. She had been raised in the Catholic faith, but did not regularly attend Mass or have a religious advisor. Her statements to her friends and family about the dying process were few and were oral rather than written. At the trial, Mrs. Schiavo's husband and two of his relatives who were close to Mrs. Schiavo testified that, prior to her heart attack, Mrs. Schiavo spoke of not wanting to be kept alive should she ever become incapacitated with no realistic medical hope of recovery. Mrs. Schiavo's parents and a friend from Mrs. Schiavo's high school days also testified, recounting statements that suggested Mrs. Schiavo might want to continue living.

Case 4-A   Terri Schiavo (*continued*)

Judge Greer also heard testimony about Mrs. Schiavo's condition. The physician in the case testified that Mrs. Schiavo's cerebral cortex had been virtually destroyed and that any reactions she appeared to have were purely reflexive. However, Mrs. Schiavo was clearly not brain dead. Her parents believed their daughter's expressions and sounds were not reflexes, but real responses. Mrs. Schiavo's parents also expressed hope that their daughter might one day improve, just as coma patients have been known to improve after years and even decades of illness.

Judge Greer finally made the decision he believed was in accord with Mrs. Schiavo's wishes and her rights under the law. He found that there was clear and convincing evidence that Mrs. Schiavo was in a persistent vegetative state, from which there was no reason to believe she would ever emerge. He also found that there was clear and convincing evidence regarding Mrs. Schiavo's previously expressed wishes—namely, that she would not want to be maintained in a persistent vegetative state by receiving ANH via a g-tube. Accordingly, on February 11, 2000, he ruled that the ANH should be discontinued. Mrs. Schiavo's parents appealed. Almost a year later, the Second District Court of Appeals ruled in agreement with Judge Greer's decision.

Mrs. Schiavo's parents appealed to the Florida State Supreme Court, but the court declined to review the case. A subsequent appeal to the U.S. Supreme Court was also denied hearing. Mrs. Schiavo's g-tube was finally clamped shut on April 24, 2001.

The Artificial Nutrition and Hydration Case Revisited

Soon after Mrs. Schiavo's g-tube was clamped, her parents learned that an ex-girlfriend of her husband had been interviewed on a local radio station and disputed the fact that Mrs. Schiavo's husband had evidence of his wife's wishes. She claimed he told her he had no idea what Mrs. Schiavo would have wanted. Allegations also surfaced, based on an old bone scan report, that Mrs. Schiavo had been physically abused by her husband. Mrs. Schiavo's parents filed an emergency motion to resume the ANH and asked that the case be reopened in light of this new evidence. They also initiated a civil suit against their son-in-law, alleging "fraud and perjury." The judge assigned to this new civil suit, not Judge Greer, ordered that Mrs. Schiavo's g-tube be unclamped and that ANH be resumed. This took place two days after the g-tube had been clamped.

Mrs. Schiavo's husband immediately went to the Second District Court of Appeals, filing a motion to block the new judge's order. The court denied this motion and instead instructed Judge Greer to rehear the case. After doing so, he again found that Mrs. Schiavo would not have wanted to continue the ANH. Mrs. Schiavo's parents again appealed, disputing the claim that Mrs. Schiavo would have wanted her g-tube clamped. They also presented statements from physicians questioning the diagnosis of persistent vegetative state. One of these statements suggested that Mrs. Schiavo could be improved with treatment.

(continues)

Case 4-A Terri Schiavo (*continued*)

Reexamining the Evidence

On review, the Second District Court of Appeals found no basis for reversing Judge Greer's conclusion that Mrs. Schiavo's wishes were clear and convincing. However, the appeals court did agree with Mrs. Schiavo's parents that there should be a reexamination of the evidence regarding Mrs. Schiavo's diagnosis and possible treatments. The court stipulated that five physicians should independently review Mrs. Schiavo's medical data and examine her. Two physicians would be chosen by each side, with a fifth physician being chosen by mutual agreement or by the court, should the two parties fail to agree on the fifth physician. Testimony would be heard on two issues: (1) Mrs. Schiavo's diagnosis; and (2) the evidence for any new treatments, their likelihood of success, and their acceptability within the scientific community. What was not in dispute was the court's earlier finding that there was clear and convincing evidence Mrs. Schiavo would not want to be maintained in a persistent vegetative state by receiving ANH via a g-tube.

On November 22, 2002, after an exhaustive reconsideration of the evidence in Mrs. Schiavo's case, Judge Greer ruled that Mrs. Schiavo was indeed in a persistent vegetative state and that there was no effective treatment for this condition. He therefore ordered that the provision of ANH be discontinued in accordance with Mrs. Schiavo's wishes. When Mrs. Schiavo's parents appealed, the Second District Court of Appeals affirmed Judge Greer's ruling. Mrs. Schiavo's parents next appealed to the Florida State Supreme Court and then the U.S. Supreme Court, both of which declined to hear the case. In desperation, Mrs. Schiavo's parents attempted to have the case introduced into the federal court system, but federal judge Richard Lazzara ruled that he lacked jurisdiction to hear the case. Mrs. Schiavo's parents also requested the personal intervention of Jeb Bush, governor of Florida.

The Legislature and Governor Intervene

Mrs. Schiavo's g-tube was finally removed on October 15, 2003. In the days that followed, there was intense media attention and also enormous public pressure on lawmakers, largely from a telephone and e-mail campaign orchestrated through a foundation created by Mrs. Schiavo's parents to help publicize and fund their legal fight. Five days after Mrs. Schiavo's g-tube was removed, the Florida legislature hastily passed a bill giving the governor the authority to issue a stay of the court's ruling and authorize the reinsertion of Mrs. Schiavo's g-tube. The bill, named "Terri's Law," was signed the following day by Governor Bush, who also issued an executive order for surgical reinsertion of a g-tube into Mrs. Schiavo.[14] He also requested that an independent guardian be appointed to review the case. Jay Wolfson, of the University of South Florida Health Sciences Center, was given this task.

Immediately after the passage of Terri's Law, her husband requested an injunction to prevent the reinsertion of the tube and filed suit against Governor Bush in state court, arguing that Terri's Law was unconstitutional. On May 6, 2004, the Pinellas Circuit Court judge handling the case regarding Terri's Law (not Judge Greer, but Judge W. Douglas Baird) ruled that the law was indeed unconstitutional. Governor Bush immediately appealed. The attorney for

Case 4-A Terri Schiavo (*continued*)

Mrs. Schiavo's husband asked the appeals court to defer hearing the case and instead send it straight to the Florida State Supreme Court. They did so. On September 23, 2004, the Florida Supreme Court unanimously found Terri's Law to be unconstitutional.[15] Governor Bush subsequently appealed to the U.S. Supreme Court, but the case was denied hearing.

Mrs. Schiavo's Final Months

With the stay of Terri's Law no longer in effect, Judge Greer's earlier decision to stop the g-tube remained in force. A date was eventually set for the removal of the g-tube. The last months of Mrs. Schiavo's life were marked by a flurry of legal, political, and media activity involving Florida's governor, the Florida legislature, Florida's Department of Children and Families, the U.S. Senate and House of Representatives, various state and federal courts, the Florida State Supreme Court, the United States Supreme Court, the president of the United States, Pope John Paul II, Randall Terry of Operation Rescue, and Jesse Jackson, among others.

Mrs. Schiavo's ANH was stopped for the third and final time on March 18, 2005. She died on March 31, 2005, amid great public and political rancor, thirteen days after her g-tube was removed. An autopsy revealed that Terri Schiavo was cortically blind, that there was no evidence that she had ever been abused, and that her severe and irreversible brain damage was consistent with the diagnosis of persistent vegetative state.

The Schiavo case is immensely complicated. The details are numerous and well known. One of the challenges in dealing with real-world ethics cases is getting enough detail to characterize the problem accurately and then to decide about it, knowing that all relevant considerations have been addressed. In the Schiavo case our difficulty is in the opposite direction: it is to sort through the questions, speculations, and accusations to get to the essence of the case. In the Schiavo case the set of people looking at it and proffering opinions about it expanded to people across the world. With so many voices, it was hard to know what to think, much less what to do. By contrast, the easiest clinical situation is small scale, and has at its center a patient and family who are in agreement about the facts of the case and about the choices that are to be made. If the set of people is small, limited to a handful of relatives, then there is some real potential for education, understanding, and ultimately consensus about the right thing to do. When the case is being followed and commented on by a worldwide set of people, there is little chance that consensus will be achieved. In reality, it is far better to resolve these questions early on in the process before intransigent conflict emerges. Further, once the case gets into the legal system, matters become even more prolonged. The unusual thing about the Schiavo case was that it became a media event or, more accurately, a media drama that unfolded with each legal twist and turn.

Some of the questions in this case include the following: Who should make decisions in the case—the husband or the parents? Is administering ANH via a g-tube a form of medical treatment or a form of basic care? If the g-tube is clamped or removed, will the patient starve to death? If a doctor clamps or removes the tube, is the doctor thereby killing the patient or allowing her to die a natural death? Should patients in a persistent vegetative state be given unproven treatments? Rather than trying to address these questions in general, the purpose of case-based decision making is to render a decision in the particular case.

To get to the essence of the case, we will need to employ both the four-topics method and the clinical casuistry method. Let's start by looking at the case as it stood just before Terri Schiavo died. We'll start first with organizing basic information using the four-topics method, which helps us distill the case down to its essence (Table 4-3). The "medical

TABLE 4-3   The Four-Topics Method: The Terri Schiavo Case

Medical Indications	Patient Preferences
The Principles of Beneficence and Nonmaleficence	The Principle of Respect for Autonomy
1. What is the patient's medical problem? —*Persistent vegetative state due to anoxic brain injury.*	1. Is the patient mentally capable and legally competent? Is there evidence of incapacity? —*No; there is clear evidence of incapacity.*
2. Is the problem acute? Chronic? Critical? Emergent? Reversible? —*Chronic.*	2. If competent, what is the patient stating about preferences for treatment? —*N/A*
3. What are the goals of treatment? —*To maintain the patient in her current condition, her treatment consists of basic nursing care and the provision of ANH via g-tube.*	3. Has the patient been informed of the benefits and risks, understood this information, and given consent? —*N/A*
4. What are the possibilities of success? —*As long as the patient remains in her current care setting with her current treatment plan, she could be maintained for many years to come.*	4. If incapacitated, who is the appropriate surrogate? Is the surrogate using appropriate standards of decision making? —*The appropriate surrogate would be the patient's husband; however, he has asked the court to serve as surrogate for his wife because of a disagreement with his in-laws regarding his wife's care, particularly over the issue of discontinuing ANH.*
5. What are the plans in case of therapeutic failure? —*There are no plans in case the current plan of care fails.*	5. Has the patient expressed prior preferences (e.g., advance directives)?
6. In sum, how can this patient be benefited by medical and nursing care, and how can harm be avoided?	

TABLE 4-3   The Four-Topics Method: The Terri Schiavo Case *(continued)*

Medical Indications	Patient Preferences
—*The patient can be benefited insofar as she is maintained in her current condition. Harm can be avoided by managing side effects associated with ANH administration via g-tube; harm can also be avoided by providing diligent nursing care to minimize skin breakdown problems and aspiration of stomach contents.*	—*No; the patient does not have an advance directive, but she did make statements in other situations involving care of relatives at the end of life. The court has ruled that these statements constitute clear and convincing evidence the patient would not want to continue to receive ANH in the context of persistent vegetative state.*

6. Is the patient unwilling or unable to cooperate with medical treatment? If so, why?
   —*The patient is unable to cooperate with medical treatment because she is in a persistent vegetative state.*
7. In sum, is the patient's right to choose being respected to the extent possible in ethics and law?
   —*Because medical ethics upholds patient autonomy, the patient's right to choose how to be cared for is paramount and should be decisive. Her right to choose is being respected in the decisions of the courts; however, it is not being respected in a practical sense because the patient is still connected to an intervention the court has ruled she would not want. Her right to choose has yet to be upheld because of the efforts of the patient's parents and others who have joined their cause to prevent the carrying out of what the court has found to be the patient's choice*

Quality of Life	Contextual Features
The Principles of Beneficence and Nonmaleficence and Respect for Autonomy	The Principles of Loyalty and Fairness
1. What are the prospects, with and without treatment, for a return to normal life? —*There are no prospects, irrespective of treatment, for the patient to return to a normal life.*	1. Are there family issues that might influence treatment decisions? —*Yes; there is major conflict in the family, notably between the patient's husband and his in-laws.*

(continues)

TABLE 4-3   The Four-Topics Method: The Terri Schiavo Case (*continued*)

Quality of Life	Contextual Features
2. What physical, mental, and social deficits is the patient likely to experience if treatment succeeds? —*The physical deficits associated with her current treatment are related to ANH via g-tube. She is at risk of aspiration of stomach contents into her lungs with resulting aspiration pneumonia and possibly death. She is also at risk of diarrhea from concentrated nutritional preparations; the risk of skin breakdown and infection and possible sepsis will increase if any diarrhea is not quickly controlled.*	2. Are there provider (physicians and nurses) issues that might influence treatment decisions? —*None identified.* 3. Are there financial and economic factors? —*None identified. Although there have been disputes over the proper use of money awarded to the patient in a malpractice suit, currently there are no financial issues affecting care.*
3. Are there biases that might prejudice the provider's evaluation of the patient's quality of life? —*None are known.*	4. Are there religious or cultural factors? —*Yes; although the entire family is Catholic, the patient's father claims that stopping ANH is not consistent with the beliefs of his religious faith.*
4. Is the patient's present or future condition such that his or her continued life might be judged undesirable? —*Yes; her current condition, persistent vegetative state, is such that many would judge living in it to be undesirable.*	5. Are there limits on confidentiality? —*No; there is no condition that would limit the patient's physician from keeping full confidentiality.*
5. Is there any plan and rationale to forgo treatment? —*Yes. The courts have ruled that her current treatment be stopped—that she stop receiving ANH; however, the court's ruling is being challenged on many fronts.*	6. Are there problems of allocation of resources? —*Not at present.* 7. How does the law affect treatment decisions? —*The law addresses the issue of ANH, regarding it as a treatment that can be forgone when that is the wish of the patient; in this unusual case, the law has yet to be effective in carrying out the patient's wishes because of constant legal challenges.*
6. Are there plans for comfort and palliative care? —*Yes; the patient is currently a resident at a local hospice.*	8. Is clinical research or teaching involved? —*No.* 9. Is there any conflict of interest on the part of the providers or the institution? —*There does not appear to be any conflict of interest.*

ANH, artificial nutrition and hydration; g-tube, gastrostomy tube; N/A, not applicable.

indications" questions establish that the patient is in a persistent vegetative state and that the only reasonable medical goal is to maintain the patient in that state. The "patient preferences" questions establish that Terri Schiavo would not want to accept continued treatment with ANH. The court heard testimony from both sides about statements Mrs. Schiavo made to other adults in serious situations such as attending a funeral or visiting a sick loved one in the hospital. Her recounted statements from several persons were found to constitute clear and convincing evidence that Terri Schiavo would not want to accept continued treatment with ANH. When the patient's treatment preferences are known, either directly or by inductive inference from clear past statements, the ethical course of action is to honor the patient's choice about his or her own care. Although others might wish to treat the patient differently, the principle of respect for autonomy mandates that the patient's choice be the one that is honored. It should be noted that the lower court's hearing regarding Mrs. Schiavo's treatment preferences was reviewed and ratified by Florida's Second District Court of Appeals. This conclusion was never challenged afterward, as were other conclusions, such as the existence of viable treatment for Mrs. Schiavo and the diagnosis of persistent vegetative state, both of which where reheard in court and reaffirmed.

The "quality of life" questions affirm that regardless of treatment, there is no prospect of the patient returning to a normal life. The "contextual features" questions highlight the intense family conflict that exists. The questions also indicate that religious ideas regarding ANH may be playing a role in the conflict. Most important, the questions highlight the legal understanding of ANH—that it is a medical treatment pure and simple, and that, as such, it can be forgone like any other medical treatment, if that is the wish of the patient. In the case of Terri Schiavo, we already know from the "patient preferences" section that her wish is exactly that—to forgo ANH.

The four-topics method has helped us to focus and distill a large amount of information down to its essential core, which we can then reason about using the clinical casuistry method. The essential problem in the Schiavo case is that she is a permanently incapacitated patient who would not want to accept continued treatment with ANH. The problem is that she is receiving the very thing that the court has established she would not want. What is more, there is heated conflict over what to do. The parents want to treat their daughter based on their desires for her. The husband claims that he only wants to treat his wife the way she would have wanted to be treated.

Figure 4-6 looks at the argument in graphical form. In verbal form, the argument reads as follows. Several possible rebuttals have been added.

(G) Mrs. Schiavo is a permanently incapacitated patient who would not want to accept continued treatment with ANH.

(W) Patient preferences regarding nonacceptance of treatment should be honored.

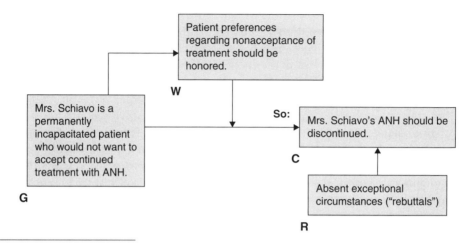

Figure 4-6 Terri Schiavo case: nonacceptance of artificial nutrition and hydration.

So:

   (C) Mrs. Schiavo's ANH should be discontinued.

     (R_1) Except that her parents disagree with the decision.

     (R_2) Except some people do not believe that ANH is a treatment.

     (R_3) Except that she did not have a living will.

     (R_4) Except some people do not believe she is in a persistent vegetative state.

     (R_5) Except that some people do not trust the legal process.

     (R_6) Except that some people think she is being denied treatment.

     (R_7) Except that some people think she is being discriminated against because she is profoundly disabled.

     (R_8) Except that she will suffer greatly in the process because she will starve to death.

     (R_9) Except that some people are suspicious of the motives of her husband.

     (R_{10}) And so on.

Just as we did in the transfusion case, we should examine whether any of the exceptional circumstances listed are significant enough to rebut the provisional conclusion. We should look to see whether these issues have been addressed in the courts, the clinical ethics literature, the medical literature, and so on, to see whether paradigms exist for the exceptions.

With regard to R$_1$, "except that her parents disagree with the decision": Courts and legislatures have consistently affirmed that the wishes of an adult patient should control care, not the interests of others, such as parents. Indeed, in cases where a surrogate does not follow the incapacitated patient's known wishes, the surrogate can be removed from the case.

With regard to R$_2$, "except some people do not believe that ANH is a treatment": Courts across the country, and many legislatures, have stated consistently that ANH, in the eyes of the law at least, is a medical treatment. As such, it can be refused by a competent adult either contemporaneously or in advance of incapacity via an advance directive or via past statements to others.

With regard to R$_3$, "except that she did not have a living will": It is well established that the right to refuse or forgo unwanted medical intervention is not contingent on having a living will. Living wills can be useful, but they are by no means required.

With regard to R$_4$, "except some people do not believe she is in a persistent vegetative state": Whether members of the public question the diagnosis of persistent vegetative state is not relevant to rebutting the conclusion. As for medical opinion, more than one hearing was devoted to this issue, with the conclusion being that she was in fact in a persistent vegetative state. Even if she was not, the decision would not be affected. Being in a persistent vegetative state is not a precondition to have one's right to be free of unwanted intervention honored.

With regard to R$_5$, "except that some people do not trust the legal process": Distrust of the legal system on the part of some is not sufficient to rebut the conclusion that ANH should be discontinued. Further, an independent guardian was appointed by the Florida governor, who himself did not agree with the ruling of the courts, to look at the legal handling of this case, and other matters. With regard to the legal issues, the guardian found the judge's treatment of the matter to be exemplary.[16]

With regard to R$_6$, "except that some people think she is being denied treatment": There was testimony from two physicians who said they wanted to treat Mrs. Schiavo, one with hyperbaric treatments and the other with vasodilation treatments. The merits of these two approaches were weighed by the court and found wanting. The physicians provided no scientific basis for the use of their proposed treatments in patients in persistent vegetative state. These two approaches were thus found by the court to have no evidence in their favor.

With regard to R$_7$, "except that some people think she is being discriminated against because she is profoundly disabled": The basis for the court's conclusion was grounded in the wishes of Mrs. Schiavo. There was clear and convincing evidence that she would not want ANH continued in the setting of permanent mental and physical incapacity. The court decisions were not based on any consideration of disability. It is interesting to note that in the latter years of the case, opponents of the courts' decisions made an attempt to reframe the case from the paradigm of treatment refusal to one of discrimination against the disabled.

With regard to R_8, "except that she will suffer greatly in the process because she will starve to death": People in a persistent vegetative state have no capacity to perceive suffering, and so cannot suffer from starvation.

With regard to R_9, "except that some people are suspicious of the motives of her husband": Such suspicion does not rebut the conclusion in the case, because the husband removed himself from the decision-making process by asking an impartial court to review the matter and settle the issue in terms of existing law. The court is a neutral third party whose only interest is in deciding the matter based on the facts and making sure that Mrs. Schiavo's rights under the law are upheld. In taking a neutral surrogate role, the court sought to make the decision that, based on all available evidence, would be the decision Mrs. Schiavo would make for herself if she were able.

As we can see, the clinical casuistry method places concerns about the case in the form of rebuttals to the central conclusion of the case, testing them against that conclusion to see if any concerns are sufficient to rebut the conclusion. If not, the conclusion stands. This approach is different from raising questions and concerns and discussing them apart from their specific connection to the central conclusion in the case. The method allows us to stay focused on the conclusion of the matter and to weigh concerns in light of that conclusion.

Although the Schiavo case is exceedingly complicated and unusual, and our treatment of it brief, it is at least sufficient to show that the combination of the four-topics method and the clinical casuistry method is up to the task of taking complex situations and rendering an analysis that is focused and clinically relevant, concrete rather than abstract, and above all, useful. Familiarity and facility with the combined use of these methods will lead to decisions that are well informed and well reasoned.

Chapter Summary

Case-based decision making in ethics is a clinical activity that consists of a practical approach to collecting and analyzing information about the case at hand and then using that information in a process of practical reasoning that results in particular conclusions about what action to take. This chapter described two approaches and then combined the two to produce a complete and functional model for case-based decision making. The first approach is the four-topics method, which serves to collect key case information based on questions that are grouped under four topics: medical indications, patient preferences, quality of life, and contextual features. Each of these topics, in turn, is related to one or more of the standard ethical principles: beneficence, nonmaleficence, respect for autonomy, and loyalty and fairness (justice). This method helps to focus and organize the case material, relate it to principles, and emphasize the considerations that should drive the decisions that are made.

The clinical casuistry method is a structured process of practical reasoning. It takes the basic issue or problem, as defined by the four-topics method, and puts it into an argument form that leads to decisions. It does so chiefly by applying conclusions or maxims from paradigmatic cases to the case at hand to yield a provisional conclusion. If there are no exceptions that are significant enough to rebut or overturn the provisional conclusion, then the conclusion will stand. If the provisional conclusion is rebutted, then a different conclusion will be reached.

The combination of the four-topics method and the clinical casuistry method is a powerful and flexible approach that can accommodate a high level of detail and a large number of concerns or issues that commonly arise in real clinical ethics cases. It has the benefit of distilling the case down to a central issue and providing a well-reasoned basis for resolving the issue in terms of a next action.

Review Questions

1. Describe the four-topics method.
2. List the ethical principles associated with each topic.
3. Describe the clinical casuistry method.
4. Describe the difference between a theoretical argument and practical reasoning.
5. What is a warrant?
6. What is a paradigmatic case?
7. Explain the advantage of the combined use of the four-topics method and the clinical casuistry method.
8. Describe the central ethical problem in the Schiavo case.

Endnotes

1. Forrow L, Arnold RM, Parker LS. Preventive ethics: expanding the horizons of clinical ethics. *J Clin Ethics* 1993;4:287–294.
2. *In re Quinlan*, 70 NJ 10 (1976).
3. *Cruzan v Director, Missouri Department of Health*, 110 S Ct 2841 (1990).
4. Cerminara KL, Goodman KW. Key events in the case of Theresa Marie Schiavo. Available at: http://www.miami.edu/ethics/schiavo/timeline.htm. Accessed June 17, 2008.
5. Walker RM, Black J. Should news practices trump legal and medical practices? The Terri Schiavo case. *Media Ethics* 2006;17:1–13.
6. Pope John Paul II. Care for patients in a "permanent vegetative state." *Origins* 2004;33(43):737, 739–740. Also available at: http://www.vatican.va/holy_father/john_paul_ii/speeches/2004/march/documents/hf_jp-ii_spe_20040320_congress-fiamc_en.html. Accessed June 17, 2008.
7. Jonsen AR, Siegler M, Winslade WJ. *Clinical Ethics: A Practical Approach to Ethical Decisions in Clinical Medicine.* 5th ed. New York: McGraw-Hill, 2002.
8. Jonsen AR, Toulmin S. *The Abuse of Casuistry: A History of Moral Reasoning.* Berkeley, CA: University of California Press, 1988.

9. Siegler M. Decision-making strategy for clinical-ethical problems in medicine. *Arch Intern Med* 1982;142:2178–2179.

10. Walker RM, Miles SH, Stocking CB, Siegler M. Physicians' and nurses' perceptions of ethics problems on general medical services. *J Gen Intern Med* 1991;6:424–429.

11. *Matter of Dubreuil,* 629 So.2d 819 (Fla., 1993).

12. Cantor NL. *Legal Frontiers of Death and Dying.* Bloomington, IN: Indiana University Press, 1987.

13. See, for example, *Application of the President & Directors of Georgetown College,* 331 F.2d 1000 (D.C. Cir. 1964).

14. Senate amendment, bill no. HB 35-E. Available at: http://www.miami.edu/ethics2/schiavo/102003_HB35-E.pdf. Accessed June 17, 2008.

15. Supreme Court of Florida, no. SC04-925: corrected opinion. September 23, 2004. Available at: http://www.floridasupremecourt.org/decisions/2004/ops/sc04-925.pdf. Accessed June 17, 2008.

16. Wolfson J. A report to Governor Jeb Bush in the matter of Theresa Marie Schiavo, December 1, 2003. Available at: http://www.miami.edu/ethics2/schiavo/wolfson%27s%20report.pdf. Accessed June 17, 2008.

Chapter 5

Professionalism and the Internal Morality of Medicine

> **More.** *You want me to swear to the Act of Succession?*
>
> **Margaret.** *"God more regards the thoughts of the heart than the words of the mouth." Or so you've always told me.*
>
> **More.** *Yes.*
>
> **Margaret.** *Then say the words of the oath and in your heart think otherwise.*
>
> **More.** *What is an oath then but words we say to God?*
>
> **Margaret.** *That's very neat.*
>
> **More.** *Do you mean it isn't true?*
>
> **Margaret.** *No, it's true.*
>
> **More.** *Then it's a poor argument to call it "neat," Meg. When a man takes an oath, Meg, he's holding his own self in his own hands. Like water. [He cups his hands.] And if he opens his fingers <u>then</u>—he needn't hope to find himself again.*
>
> —Robert Bolt, *A Man for All Seasons*

Chapter Learning Objectives

At the conclusion of this chapter the reader will be able to:

1. Understand the concept of the internal morality of medicine and its relationship to the moral rules

2. List the goals of medicine

3. Understand what is meant by the means of medicine

4. Apply the concepts of goal illegitimacy, means illegitimacy, and means–ends disjunction

5. Define *medical futility* and distinguish among the various subtypes of medical futility

6. Define *profession* and *professionalism*

7. List, recognize, distinguish, and apply the tenets of professionalism

Chapter 3 discussed the moral rules. This chapter begins to explore in greater depth the last of the listed rules—"do not neglect your duty"—as it pertains to medicine and the

121

allied health professions.[1] More specifically, this chapter considers two related questions: What is the scope of a health care professional's duty? and What does it mean to say that medicine is a profession? A subsequent chapter (Chapter 15) reconsiders the moral rule prohibiting neglect of duty in the context of medical malpractice.

Medical Futility

Oddly enough, we begin our discussion with medical futility, for reasons that will become apparent later on. The concept of medical futility has received much attention in the literature of bioethics and medicine over the past seventeen years,[2] although the concept is not a new one. "In the Hippocratic writing entitled *The Art,* the physician is advised to . . . 'refuse to treat those who are overmastered by their diseases, recognizing that in such cases medicine is powerless.' "[3]

Something is said to be futile if it is "ineffective" or "incapable of producing any result."[4] Consider, for example, the fate of the mythological Sisyphus.

> For a crime against the gods . . . he was condemned to an eternity at hard labor. And frustrating labor at that. For his assignment was to roll a great boulder to the top of a hill. Only every time Sisyphus, by the greatest of exertion and toil, attained the summit, the darn thing rolled back down again.[5]

Consider alternatively the plight of the mythological Tantalus, from whom the word *tantalize* derives:

> Tantalus . . . so offended the gods that he was condemned in the afterlife to an eternity of hunger and thirst. He was made to stand in a pool in Tartarus, the Underworld zone of punishment. Each time he reached down for the water that beckoned to his parched lips, it drained away. Overhanging the pool were boughs laden with luscious fruit. But each time Tantalus stretched to pluck this juicy sustenance, the boughs receded from his grasp.[6]

Sisyphus's attempt to push the rock to the top of the mountain is futile because it cannot achieve its intended goal. The same may be said of Tantalus's attempts to eat and drink. These allusions to mythology illustrate an important concept regarding futility—specifically, the idea that futility must be defined with reference to a specific goal. For example, the acts of Sisyphus and Tantalus would not be futile if their goals were to "get some exercise" or "pass the time" (assuming such a thing is even possible in eternity).

Interventions are said to be *medically* futile if they "have no realistic chance of achieving the goals of medicine."[7] We shall have more to say about the goals of medicine later in this chapter. For now, understand that characterizing an intervention as medically futile is of importance because health care professionals (HCPs) are generally under no obligation to provide medically futile treatments.[8-11] Jecker and Schneiderman have made the even stronger argument that HCPs are professionally obligated to resist demands for futile treatment.[12] As such, medical futility arguably delimits the sphere of proper unilateral decision making by HCPs.

Medical futility has been divided into three subtypes: physiologic, qualitative, and quantitative.

Physiologic Futility

An act is *physiologically futile* if it is clearly futile in achieving its physiologic objective and thus offers no physiologic benefit to the patient. Such acts are sometimes described as being "medically futile because ineffective." An example of a physiologically futile act would be the use of CPR on a patient in whom rigor mortis has set in or on a patient decapitated in a freak accident in the hospital cafeteria. CPR in these patients simply cannot achieve its intended goal—the restoration of cardiopulmonary function. This is the least controversial type of medical futility, because it appears not to involve any value judgment.

Qualitative Futility

An act is *qualitatively futile* if it has important physiologic effects that medical judgment concludes are nonbeneficial to the patient as a person. Such acts are sometimes described as being "medically futile because nonbeneficial." An example of a qualitatively futile act would be the use of artificial feeding and hydration in patients in a permanent vegetative state (e.g., the Terry Schiavo case). Because these patients lack conscious awareness, such treatment arguably does not benefit them as persons, despite the fact that it is effective physiologically in meeting their nutritional and fluid requirements. This is a more controversial type of medical futility, because it incorporates a value judgment of sorts—specifically, the judgment that consciousness is a sine qua non of personhood. Stated otherwise, it incorporates the value judgment that a human life divorced from consciousness is not the proper object of medicine.

Quantitative Futility (Probabilistic Futility)

An act is *quantitatively futile* if it is very unlikely to produce either a desired physiologic effect or a personal benefit. Such acts are sometimes described as being "medically futile because improbable." How unlikely or improbable must an effect be to render an act quantitatively medically futile? Well, Schneiderman and associates have, for example, proposed that "when physicians conclude (either through personal experience, experiences shared with colleagues, or consideration of reported empiric data) that in the last 100 cases, a medical treatment has been useless, they should regard that treatment as futile."[13] Of course, any such numeric cutoff will be arbitrary and controversial.

The Wanglie Case

Helga Wanglie was an eighty-six-year-old, ventilator-dependent woman in permanent vegetative state (PVS).[14] In November 1990, her physicians informed the Wanglie family that continued mechanical ventilation was nonbeneficial to her as a person and that it should be discontinued.

Mrs. Wanglie's husband (an attorney), daughter, and son rejected the idea of withdrawing ventilator support, insisting that Mrs. Wanglie would not be better off dead than in PVS and that, in any event, a miracle could occur. Although Mr. Wanglie allegedly originally reported that his wife had never stated her preferences concerning life-sustaining treatment in PVS, he later insisted that his wife had consistently said that she wanted such treatment even in the face of such a condition.

The hospital asked the court to appoint an independent conservator to decide whether the continued use of the ventilator was beneficial to Mrs. Wanglie; in the event the conservator found its use nonbeneficial, the hospital asked that a second hearing be held on the question of whether it was legally obliged to provide the respirator.

On July 1, 1991, the court appointed Mr. Wanglie his wife's conservator and, noting that the hospital had not yet made any request for permission to stop the ventilator, declined to address the merits of the case. The hospital announced that it would not discontinue ventilator support. Three days later, Mrs. Wanglie died of sepsis-induced multisystem organ failure.

The Baby K Case

Baby K was a female anencephalic infant born in October 1992 in Virginia.[15] Because of perinatal respiratory distress, she was intubated and mechanically ventilated. Baby K's mother, Mrs. H, was told that no treatment existed for anencephaly and that no therapeutic or palliative purpose was served by continued mechanical ventilation. Nevertheless, she refused to consent to a do-not-resuscitate (DNR) order.

The treating physicians consulted the institutional ethics committee, which concluded that ventilator support was futile and should be stopped after allowing Mrs. H a "reasonable time." Mrs. H rejected the committee's recommendation, and rather than pursuing legal action, the hospital took advantage of a window of opportunity—a period during which Baby K was not ventilator dependent—to transfer Baby K to a nursing home in November 1992.

Unfortunately, Baby K required readmission to the hospital in January and again in March 1993. Because it was expected that she would continue to experience episodes of respiratory distress requiring admission, intubation, and mechanical ventilation, the hospital finally commenced legal action, and a guardian was appointed to represent Baby K. The guardian agreed that ventilator support should be withheld from Baby K when she experienced respiratory distress. The hospital requested a declaratory judgment that the withholding of ventilator support would not be illegal.

In July 1993, the U.S. District Court for the Eastern District of Virginia held that under the federal antidumping law (the Emergency Medical Treatment and Active Labor Act, or EMTALA), "the hospital would be liable . . . if Baby K arrived there in respiratory distress . . . and the hospital failed to provide [the] mechanical ventilation . . . necessary to stabilize her acute medical condition."

EMTALA requires that hospitals provide stabilizing treatment to any person who comes to an emergency department in an "emergency medical condition," where "emergency medical condition" is defined as "acute symptoms of sufficient severity . . . such that the absence of immediate medical attention could reasonably be expected to result in . . . serious impairment to bodily functions, or serious dysfunction of any bodily organ or part."[16] EMTALA, the court wrote, "does not admit of any 'futility' . . . exceptions."[15]

Interestingly, the district court seemed to adopt the definition of medical futility equating it to physiologic futility when it wrote, "Even if EMTALA contained [a futility exception, it] . . . would not apply here. The use of a mechanical ventilator to assist breathing is not 'futile' . . . in relieving the acute symptoms of respiratory difficulty which is the emergency medical condition that must be treated under EMTALA."[15]

The Gilgunn Case

Catherine Gilgunn was a seventy-one-year-old woman with Parkinson disease, diabetes, and heart disease, and was one year status-post cerebrovascular accident and a mastectomy for breast cancer.[17,18] She was admitted to the Massachusetts General Hospital (MGH) in June 1989 for surgery to repair a hip fracture, and while there developed extensive and irreversible brain damage secondary to status epilepticus, resulting in a coma.

> [The patient's daughter] Joan, who was the surrogate, informed the physicians . . . that Catherine always said she "wanted everything done" that was medically possible. With the encouragement of the hospital's Optimum Care Committee (OCC), Mrs. Gilgunn's attending physician wrote a DNR order on July 5th, despite these expressed wishes. Dr. Ned Cassem, the Chair of that committee and acting as the consultant, took the view that the family's opinion was not relevant, since CPR was not a "genuine therapeutic option." The social worker's notes concurred that the family's inability to prepare for the inevitable did not "justify mistreating the patient." Because of his inability to argue strongly on medical grounds against Joan and her family's beliefs, the doctor revoked the DNR order two days later.
>
> The following month a new attending physician, Dr. William Dec, took over the case. The new attending physician couldn't convince Joan of the inappropriateness of CPR for her mother. Dr. Dec asked the OCC to review the case again. Dr. Cassem, still acting as a consultant on behalf of the committee, once again endorsed a DNR order because CPR would be "medically contraindicated, inhumane, and unethical." Dr. Dec, with the approval of the MGH legal counsel, wrote

the DNR order. He also began to wean Catherine from the ventilator, since he regarded her as imminently dying. Her blood gases were not monitored during the weaning, because Dr. Dec did not expect her to survive on her own. Three days later, on August 10, 1989, Catherine Gilgunn died.[19]

Joan Gilgunn sued the hospital and the physicians for intentional infliction of emotional distress. In a jury trial before the Suffolk County Superior Court, the hospital and the physicians were found not guilty of negligently imposing emotional distress on the patient's daughter. The judge had asked the jury to consider whether the patient, had she been able to, would have requested CPR and continued mechanical ventilation. The jury answered yes to both questions, but agreed with the defendants that such treatment would have been futile.

The Scope of the Health Care Professional's Duty

This is all very interesting, but why, you might well ask, is medical futility being discussed in this chapter? What does medical futility have to do with professional duty as it pertains to physicians and other health care professionals?

You will recall from the material discussed earlier that characterizing an intervention as medically futile is of importance because HCPs are generally under no obligation to provide medically futile treatments. Recall, too, that some have made the even stronger argument that HCPs are professionally obligated to resist demands for futile treatment. Of course, saying that an HCP has no obligation to provide a particular treatment means that he or she has no duty to do so; saying that an HCP is obligated to resist demands for a particular treatment means that he or she has a duty not to provide that treatment. Thus, medical futility is all about professional duty.

The converse is not true, however. Professional duty is not all about medical futility. Medically futile acts represent but a proper subset of those acts (acts falling outside the scope or limits of medicine), demands for which HCPs are arguably professionally obligated to resist. Consider, for example, a case pulled from an article in the Washington post in 1994: a young woman wishes to undergo breast augmentation to size 56 FF so that she can embark on a career as an exotic dancer.[20] Should a physician accommodate her wishes in this regard?

Whatever concerns one might have about the appropriateness of a physician accommodating the wishes of the young woman, such accommodation does not implicate the concept of medical futility. Clearly, breast augmentation surgery almost uniformly achieves its intended goal. If, therefore, we believe that there is something wrong about a physician being involved in such a case, the wrongness lies elsewhere.

Compare the question actually posed—Should a *physician* accommodate her wishes in this regard?—with the following question: Should a *nonphysician licensed to practice cosmetic surgery*[21] accommodate her wishes in this regard? It should be apparent that these two questions differ, and that the difference revolves around the moral rule prohibiting neglect of duty—in this case, the physician's duty versus the duty of the nonphysician licensed to practice cosmetic surgery. We simply cannot answer the question as it pertains to a physician without knowing something about the physician's duty, for to answer the question we must first determine whether accommodating the young woman's wishes would be consistent or inconsistent with that duty. As we begin to formulate an approach to these questions of duty, let's consider something called the *internal morality of medicine*.[22]

The Internal Morality of Medicine

Building on the work of John Ladd,[23] Brody and Miller argued that the "goals and means of medicine constitute an internal morality" and that the "professional integrity of physicians is constituted by allegiance to this internal morality."[22] Along with others,[24-27] they have argued that the goals of medicine derive from the nature of medical practice. Thus, acts promoting no medical goal violate the internal morality of medicine or at best constitute what they refer to as "borderline medical activities." Further, Brody and Miller have pointed out that an act might promote the legitimate goals of medicine and yet, because of the unacceptability of the means being employed, violate the internal morality of medicine. They use the example of a physician treating members of his or her own family to illustrate such a (means) violation.

The Goals of Medicine

Although some bioethicists deny the very existence of goals of medicine, "the majority position [is] that there are goals that mark the profession and that these goals are normative."[28] A number of formulations of the goals of medicine have been proffered.[28-31] For example, in the Hastings Center's Goals of Medicine Project, representatives from fourteen countries proposed four goals of medicine: (1) the prevention of disease and injury and the promotion and maintenance of health; (2) the relief of pain and suffering caused by maladies; (3) the care and cure of those with a malady, and the care of those who cannot be cured; and (4) the avoidance of premature death and the pursuit of a peaceful death.[32] Brody and Miller proffered a formulation of the goals of medicine that made the important contribution of pointing out that the goals must include the threshold goals of "diagnosing the disease or injury" (because appropriate treatment depends on proper diagnosis) and of "reassuring the 'worried well' who have no disease or injury."[22]

It is important to mention here that the relevant goal or end is the one actually *intended* by the HCP. In cases where an HCP's action has more than one effect, the principle of the double effect may be applicable.[3(pp129-130)] For example, it has been reported that patients receiving Botox injections to smooth forehead wrinkles experienced relief from chronic headaches as an unanticipated side effect.[33] Assuming a restrictive formulation of the goals of medicine (one that excludes reversal of the signs of aging as a goal), one could argue that the medical legitimacy of the procedure—that is, its consistency with the internal morality of medicine—depends on whether the HCP's intended goal was one of headache relief (legitimate) or cosmetic enhancement (illegitimate).

Let us return momentarily to the case of the young woman who would be a 56 FF. We might conclude that breast augmentation in her case violates the internal morality of medicine because it advances no legitimate medical goal. Although this terminology is somewhat cumbersome, it is more specific and informative than saying that the procedure is not medically indicated.

The Means of Medicine

As noted earlier, an act might promote the legitimate goals of medicine and yet, because of the unacceptability of the means being employed, violate the internal morality of medicine. Brody and Miller suggested four standards limiting the morally acceptable means physicians (and by extension other health care professionals) may use to promote legitimate goals:[22,34]

1. The physician must employ technical competence in practice.

2. The physician must honestly portray medical knowledge and skill to the patient and to the general public, and avoid any sort of fraud or misrepresentation.

3. The physician must avoid harming the patient in any way that is out of proportion to expected benefit, and must seek to minimize the indignity and the invasion of privacy involved in medical examinations and procedures.

4. The physician must maintain fidelity to the interests of the individual patient.

These standards relate to limitations upon the means of medicine rather than to the means themselves. They do not answer the question that concerns us here: "When is a means a medical means?"

Insight into the nature of medical means is provided by American medical malpractice case law. Thus, in *Pike v. Honsiger*, 155 N.Y. 201 (1898), the court described the standard of care in the following way: "The physician is under an obligation to exercise the same degree of knowledge, skill, diligence and care that the ordinary competent practitioner would exercise under the same or similar circumstances. The physician is under the further obligation to use his best judgment in exercising his skill and applying his knowledge."

Knowledge refers to "an organized body of information."[35] *Medical* knowledge, then, refers specifically to the organized body of *medical* information. Such medical information includes, for example, the basic sciences of anatomy, embryology, physiology, biochemistry and molecular biology, histology, microbiology, pathology, and genetics. Medical information also includes clinical sciences such as internal medicine, surgery, obstetrics and gynecology, pediatrics, and psychiatry. *Skill*, on the other hand, refers to "the ability to *do* something well."[35] In the context of the present discussion, it refers to the ability to do something *medical* well. That something medical might be a particular procedure, such as inserting a central venous catheter, performing a lumbar puncture, or removing an appendix.

Something done *diligently* refers to something done with care and effort; and *care*, in turn, refers to "serious attention and thought," or "caution to avoid damage or loss."[35] Although there may be differences of degree between the diligence and care employed in a medical context and those employed in other contexts (given what is at stake), we do not believe there are qualitative differences.

Thus, a health care professional employs medical means when he or she exercises medical knowledge or skill in the pursuit of some goal.

The Means–End Fit

In their excellent discussion of the internal morality of medicine, Brody and Miller discuss goals (ends) and means, but do not explicitly discuss the relationship between the two—what we refer to here as the means–end fit. However, the idea that the tightness of the fit between the ends being pursued and the means being employed is important is implicit in the third of their proposed standards limiting the means that physicians may use in pursuing legitimate medical goals: "The physician must avoid harming the patient in any way that is out of proportion to expected benefit, and must seek to minimize the indignity and the invasion of privacy involved in medical examinations and procedures."[22]

Precedent for applying a means–end fit test can be found in the analyses employed by American courts in reviewing the legitimacy of governmental acts. Regulations affecting fundamental rights are reviewed under a "strict scrutiny" standard: they are struck down unless necessary to achieve a compelling government purpose. In contrast, regulations affecting rights deemed not fundamental are reviewed under a "rational basis" standard: they are upheld if reasonably related to any legitimate government purpose.[36] Thus, in the context of due process analysis, a sliding scale exists: the more intrusive the governmental act being reviewed, the tighter the means–end nexus must be in order for that act to pass review.

Employing the Internal Morality of Medicine Analysis

The previous discussion suggests a possible approach to thinking about whether a particular act is consistent with a health care professional's duty as a health care professional—that is, consistent with the internal morality of medicine. Such an approach, analogous to the approach employed by American courts in deciding whether a particular legislative act exceeds constitutional authority, would involve consideration of the following three questions:

1. Is a legitimate medical goal being pursued?
2. Are the means being employed legitimate medical means?
3. Are the goals and the means appropriately related?

Accordingly, an HCP acts in conformity with the internal morality of medicine when he or she employs legitimate and appropriate medical means in the pursuit of a legitimate medical end. In contrast, either when the ends being pursued or the means being employed by the HCP are not legitimately medical, or when the means and the ends are not appropriately related, the act is beyond the HCP's authority and consequently inconsistent with the internal morality of medicine.

Categorizing Violations of the Internal Morality of Medicine

Acts violating the internal morality of medicine may be further subclassified depending on which prong of the trident discussed earlier is defective. When the goal (or end) of the act, though achievable, is not a legitimate medical goal, the act may be said to be a violation of the internal morality of medicine because of goal illegitimacy. When the means being employed are not legitimate medical means, the act may be said to be a violation of the internal morality of medicine because of means illegitimacy. When the means and the ends are not appropriately related—in other words, when the means–end fit is not sufficiently tight—the act may be said to be a violation of the internal morality of medicine because of means–ends disjunction.[37]

Medical futility, with which we opened this chapter, represents a paradigmatic example, albeit an extreme form, of a means–ends disjunction. A medically futile act is one that is incapable of achieving its desired medical goal. Consider, for example, a patient with metastatic cancer, bilateral pneumonia, and overwhelming sepsis who develops progressive hypoxia despite mechanical ventilation with 100 percent oxygen. Resuscitation of such a patient in the event of a cardiac arrest resulting from progressive hypoxia would be medically futile because none of the goals of medicine are achievable. If resuscitation is a violation of the internal morality of medicine in this case (as we believe it is), what makes it so is neither goal illegitimacy nor means illegitimacy, but rather a weakness of the nexus between a legitimate medical goal (prolongation of life) and a legitimate medical means (advanced cardiac life support). Medical futility represents an extreme form of means–ends disjunction, one in which the disconnectedness between goals and means is complete.

Cases 5-A through 5-D illustrate each of these principles in action.

Case 5-A

A plastic surgeon performs a breast augmentation on a young woman of average height (preprocedure breast size of 34C, postprocedure size 56 FF) who wishes to embark on a career as an exotic dancer. Would breast augmentation be consistent with the internal morality of medicine?

Case 5-A (*continued*)

Analysis

Recall that the goals of medicine as enumerated earlier included (1) the prevention of disease and injury and the promotion and maintenance of health; (2) the relief of pain and suffering caused by maladies; (3) the care and cure of those with a malady, and the care of those who cannot be cured; and (4) the avoidance of premature death and the pursuit of a peaceful death.[32] There is, however, nothing in the facts of this case to suggest that the woman in question is afflicted by any disease or malady because, as defined by Clouser, Culver and Gert, "a person has a malady if and only if he has a condition, other than his rational beliefs and desires, such that he is suffering, or is at increased risk of suffering, a harm or an evil (death, pain, disability, loss of freedom or opportunity, loss of pleasure) in the absence of a distinct sustaining cause."[38] The pursuit of any of the first three goals requires that a malady be present. Nor can we seriously argue that the fourth goal is being pursued here. Consequently, the act of augmenting her breasts surgically advances no legitimate medical goal (i.e., is goal illegitimate) and is therefore a violation of the internal morality of medicine.

Case 5-B

A retired military officer with pain secondary to incurable metastatic cancer asks his physician to shoot him in order to put an end to his pain because, in the words of his hero George S. Patton, "There's only one proper way for a professional soldier to die: the last bullet of the last battle of the last war."[39] Would shooting this patient be consistent with the internal morality of medicine?

Analysis

The act under consideration furthers the goal of relieving pain and suffering caused by maladies (goal 2) and might arguably result in a peaceful death (goal 4), and therefore is goal legitimate. The means under consideration, however, are nonmedical; thus, the act in question employs an illegitimate means (i.e., is means illegitimate) and would therefore be a violation of the internal morality of medicine.

Case 5-C

A patient with a thin (<0.76 mm) melanoma on his left leg undergoes an appropriate surgical excision. He subsequently requests that his surgeon amputate his entire limb "just to be sure." Would such an amputation be consistent with the internal morality of medicine?

(continues)

Case 5-C (continued)

Analysis

Patients with such lesions treated as the patient has already been treated enjoy virtually a 100 percent cure rate. Although the goals being pursued (cure of disease and prevention of premature death) and the means employed (amputation) here are legitimate, in this case the connection or nexus between them is too loose. The standard of care demands the less extensive surgery that the patient has already undergone because the performance of the more extensive surgery that he is requesting will neither increase the likelihood that he will be cured nor decrease the likelihood of premature death. Amputation of the limb would be a violation of the internal morality of medicine because of means–ends disjunction.

Case 5-D

In November 2004, Kentucky governor Ernie Fletcher, a former family physician, signed the death warrant for fifty-one-year-old convicted killer Thomas Clyde Bowling.[40] Did Governor Fletcher's act violate the internal morality of medicine and, if so, how?

Analysis

We submit that the act described in this case is unambiguously nonmedical. The authority involved in this case was Fletcher's legal authority, not his expert authority as a physician. The signing of the death warrant did not take place within the context of a doctor–patient relationship. Fletcher employed no medical means in signing the death warrant, nor did he pursue any medical ends. In short, Fletcher was acting as the chief executive of a state, not as a physician. Consequently, Fletcher's act, while provoking no small measure of controversy,[41] triggers no internal morality of medicine analysis or inquiry and thus cannot be said to violate the internal morality of medicine. Indeed, the Kentucky Board of Medical Licensure ruled that there was no merit to the complaint that Governor Fletcher had violated any tenets of medical ethics when he signed the death warrant.[42]

   In contrast, consider another case in which the Georgia Board of Medicine ruled that Dr. H. V. Sanjeeva Rao did not violate the state's medical practice act when he inserted a catheter into a prisoner to start a lethal injection. Dr. Rao employed medical means in placing the intravenous catheter, thus triggering the internal morality of medicine inquiry, but was arguably engaged in the pursuit of no legitimate medical goals. We believe, therefore, that Dr. Rao's act was arguably a violation of the internal morality of medicine.

Professionalism

A *profession* is "a vocation or occupation requiring special, usually advanced, education, knowledge, and skill."[43] Originally the term applied to theology (or divinity), law, and medicine. Herein, of course, we concern ourselves with the latter.

" 'Professionalism' has come to be accepted as a watchword for those qualities and modes of conduct proper to professions."[44] One way to think about professionalism is as the virtue-based analogue (see Chapters 1 and 3) of the duties we referred to earlier in discussing the internal morality of medicine. In other words, just as virtue ethics focuses on the character of the agent or actor in its examination of morality (as opposed to the rightness or wrongness of particular acts or their consequences), so too medical professionalism focuses on the character of medical professionals. Because, as we shall see, medical professionals invite patients to trust them, they should aspire to make themselves into the kinds of people who will be trusted and who will be trustworthy. More broadly, they should aspire to make themselves into the kind of people who will be good medical professionals.

> The good physician will be one who exhibits those character traits which most effectively achieve and indeed are indispensable for attainment of the ends of medicine . . . [, including]
>
> - Fidelity to trust . . .
> - Benevolence . . .
> - Intellectual honesty . . .
> - Courage . . .
> - Compassion . . .
> - Truthfulness[44]

Latham has written that, although the Parsonian model that follows may fail "as a factual description of medical professionalism in America, [there is] much to recommend it as a normative description of what American medical professionalism ought to look like."[45] Under that model, the elements of medical professionalism include (1) the expert authority of the medical profession, (2) medical professionals as mediators between individuals and society, (3) the medical professionals' motivations, and (4) acts of profession.

The Authority of the Medical Professional

Authority, according to sociologist Max Weber, is "essentially the probability that one's commands [will] be obeyed."[45] According to Arendt, the hallmark of authority is obedience without either coercion or persuasion.[46] Thus, as regards the authority of the medical professional, "[my] physician does not need to persuade me to take my medicine; and he is not at liberty to force me to take it. He tells me to take it . . . and I do. . . . [A] professional's authority allows her to secure our actions or beliefs without use of coercion, and without persuasion."[45]

But how does authority secure obedience absent coercion or persuasion? Weber identified and explained three types of legitimate authority:

Legal authority, in which people obey your commands because they recognize the legal legitimacy of your having issued them; *traditional authority,* in which people obey your commands because they have always done so; and *charismatic authority,* in which people obey your commands because something in your personality emotionally compels their obedience.

Parsons ... felt that Weber had missed a fourth ... variety of legitimate authority. This was *expert authority:* people obey your commands because they believe you know something they don't know.[45] (Internal footnotes omitted)

It was this last type of authority—expert authority—that Parsons associated with professionals. According to Parsons, "the authority of [medical] professionals is grounded in their [medical] knowledge and expertise."

Medical Professionals as Mediators Between Individuals and Society

One might ask, on whose behalf does the medical professional exercise expert authority? The obvious answer is on the patient's behalf; although this is true, it is only partly true. Sometimes, Parsons believed, professionals exercise expert authority on society's behalf.

Under normal circumstances, the patient's goals and society's goals are the same. The patient is sick and wants to get well. Society, too, wants him or her to get well for any number of reasons—because we care about him or her, because we want the individual to return to being a productive member of society, because we want the patient to cease being a drain on societal resources, or because of public health concerns. The patient's goals and society's goals are sometimes inconsistent with each other. In such cases, the medical professional acts as a mediator between individuals and society. "Part of the time, they [use] their authority to curb their own [patient's] deviance—to align their [patient's] interests and actions with broad social norms."[45] Consider, for example, the physician who properly refuses to write a sick note for a well patient who is looking for an excuse to avoid work. "In [such a] case, the 'deviant' ... is 'mainstreamed' through the intercession of the professional. On the other hand, professional authority is sometimes used to create safety zones for individuals against the demands of social norms."[45] Consider, for example, the physician who properly excuses his or her sick patient from having to go to work, or the psychiatrist who testifies as an expert that the defendant in a criminal case was insane at the time he or she committed a criminal act and therefore is not guilty by reason of insanity.

Case 5-E

A forty-three-year-old prisoner on death row for stabbing a woman to death during a robbery twenty-four years earlier is diagnosed as suffering from paranoid schizophrenia.[47] His execution is stayed under guidelines formulated by the U.S. Supreme Court case of *Ford v Wainwright,*

Case 5-E (*continued*)

477 US 399 (1986), which held that the Eighth Amendment's prohibition of cruel and unusual punishment prevents the state from executing an insane prisoner. The state of Arkansas wants the patient medicated involuntarily with antipsychotics so that he can be restored to competency and executed. Should psychiatrists medicate the prisoner?

Analysis

Clearly this case revolves around the question of whether medicating the prisoner is an appropriate exercise of the physician's professional role in mediating between the individual (here, the prisoner-patient) and society. Remembering that professionalism and the internal morality of medicine are two sides of the same coin, we begin by asking whether a legitimate medical goal is being pursued in treating the prisoner. Were this patient not on death row, involuntary treatment would almost certainly be justified under the third of the goals of medicine discussed earlier (the care and cure of those with a malady, and the care of those who cannot be cured) and possibly under the second (the relief of pain and suffering caused by maladies, if indeed the prisoner was suffering mentally).[48]

Alas, the patient is on death row, and the psychiatrist knows that as a consequence of his treatment the prisoner's mental disturbance will be corrected and he will surely die. Would we ever seriously consider the involuntary use in an otherwise healthy forty-four-year-old man of an antipsychotic that, though effective, had a one-year mortality rate of 100 percent? Clearly we would not, if other safer treatment choices were available. But what if no safer alternatives were available? What if the stark choice were between effective treatment followed by death within one year versus withholding treatment and allowing the profoundly psychotic patient to continue to suffer?

The principle of respect for autonomy normally dictates that, when possible, the person who should make the choice is the competent patient. If we could be certain that the state would not take the opportunity to promptly execute the prisoner as soon as his psychosis was successfully controlled, it would be consistent with the internal morality of medicine to treat the patient in order to restore his decisional capacity so that he could make the choice—successful control of his psychosis followed by execution within the year versus nontreatment of his psychosis—for himself. In the absence of such certainty, powerful arguments can surely be made against involuntarily medicating this patient.

The Medical Professional's Motivations

The third element of the Parsonian model of medical professionalism concerns the motivations of medical professionals.

> Professionals, Parsons thought, must not be too strongly motivated by the desire for power, lest they attempt to achieve it by promoting social norms at the expense of individual liberty. On the other hand, they must not be too strongly

motivated by profit, lest they allow their authority to be bought out by wealthy private [patients] seeking exemption from social norms. Instead, Parsons concluded, the professional project is successful only because professionals are motivated primarily by the desire for status and reputation—both among their peers and in society at large—rather than by the desire for money or power.[45]

Closely related to their role as mediators and to the motivations of medical professionals is their right of self-regulation. Thus, their interest in status and reputation as opposed to wealth

afffords a crucial counterbalance to the professionals' right of self-regulation: for while the right of *self-regulation* implies that professionals could not be induced by regulators into favoring the public interest over that of their private [patients], the non-pecuniary character of professionals' . . . interests helps guarantee that they could not be induced to favor private, moneyed interests over the interests of the public. . . . Parsons was adamant that professional *self-regulation* can work . . . even if physicians are . . . self-interested. What is required is only that their self-interest be non-pecuniary in character.[45] (Italics added)

Acts of Profession

As the name implies, the professions are characterized as well by acts of profession. To profess something means to declare it aloud, or to proclaim it publicly. According to Pellegrino, in the medical context such acts of profession occur in two ways.

One is the public profession—the solemn proclamation on graduation from medical school when the "Oath" is taken. This is the moment when the newly graduated physician enters the profession, not when she receives her degree. The degree is simply evidence of completion of the academic requirements for the degree "doctor of medicine." It says nothing of the commitment to the way the acquired knowledge and skill are to be used. Without the Oath the doctor is a skilled technician or laborer whose knowledge fits him for an occupation but not a profession. When the Oath is proclaimed, if it is taken seriously as a binding commitment to place one's special knowledge and skill at the service of the sick, the graduate has then made his "profession." He or she enters the company of others with similar commitments. At this moment, one enters a moral community whose defining purpose is to respond to and to advance the welfare of patients—those who are ill, who are in need of help, healing, or relief of suffering, pain or disability. The second way the profession is "declared" is in the daily encounter with patients. Every time a physician sees a patient and asks "What can I do for you, what is wrong, what is the problem?" he or she is professing (committing oneself) to two things: one is competence (i.e., having the knowledge and skill to help) and the other is to use that competence in the best interests of the patient. This "profession" or commitment, by its very declaration, invites trust. The doctor voluntarily promises that he can be trusted and incurs the moral obligations of that promise.[44]

The oldest of these public oaths is the Hippocratic Oath:

I will apply dietetic measures for the benefit of the sick according to my ability and judgment; I will keep them from harm and injustice. [beneficence, nonmaleficence]

I will neither give a deadly drug to anybody who asked for it, nor will I make a suggestion to this effect. [prohibition of physician-assisted suicide, euthanasia]

Similarly I will not give to a woman an abortive remedy. [prohibition of abortion]

Whatever houses I may visit, I will come for the benefit of the sick, remaining free of all intentional injustice, of all mischief and in particular of sexual relations with both female and male persons . . . [prohibition of sexual relations with patients]

What I may see or hear in the course of the treatment or even outside of the treatment in regard to the life of men, which on no account one must spread abroad, I will keep to myself. [confidentiality][49]

In 2002, ostensibly because "[c]hanges in the health care delivery systems in countries throughout the industrialized world threaten the values of professionalism,"[50] leaders of the American Board of Internal Medicine (ABIM) Foundation, the American College of Physicians-American Society of Internal Medicine (ACP-ASIM) Foundation, and the European Federation of Internal Medicine met as the Medical Professionalism Project and drafted the so-called Charter on Medical Professionalism. This document was published simultaneously in the *Annals of Internal Medicine*[50] and *Lancet*. The charter consisted of three "fundamental principles"—primacy of patient welfare, patient autonomy, and social justice—and ten "professional commitments":

- Professional competence
- Honesty with patients
- Confidentiality
- Maintaining appropriate relations with patients
- Improving quality of care
- Improving access to care
- Just distribution of finite resources
- Scientific knowledge
- Maintaining trust/managing conflicts of interest
- Professional responsibilities

In their summary, the Project's authors wrote:

> To maintain the fidelity of medicine's social contract during this turbulent time, we believe that physicians must reaffirm their active dedication to the principles of professionalism. . . . This Charter on Medical Professionalism is intended to encourage such dedication and to promote an action agenda for the profession of medicine that is universal in scope and purpose.[50]

An interesting point to consider is that the charter, unlike the Hippocratic Oath, makes no mention of abortion or euthanasia.

Chapter Summary

An intervention is said to be medically futile if it has no realistic chance of achieving any legitimate medical goal. An intervention that is medically futile may be subclassified as being physiologically futile, qualitatively futile (medically futile because nonbeneficial) or quantitatively futile (probabilistically futile). Health care professionals are generally under no obligation to provide medically futile treatments.

The goals and means of medicine constitute an internal morality of medicine, and the professional integrity of health care professionals is constituted by allegiance to this internal morality. When the goal (or end) of an act, though achievable, is not a legitimate medical goal, the act violates the internal morality of medicine because of goal illegitimacy. When the means employed are not legitimate medical means, the act violates the internal morality of medicine because of means illegitimacy. When the means and the ends are not appropriately related—in other words, when the means–end fit is not sufficiently tight—the act violates the internal morality of medicine because of means–ends disjunction. Medical futility represents an extreme form of means–ends disjunction, one in which the disconnectedness between goals and means is complete.

Just as virtue ethics focuses on the character of moral agents as opposed to the rightness or wrongness of particular acts, medical professionalism focuses on the character of medical professionals. The Parsonian model of professionalism is characterized by the following elements: (1) the expert authority of the professional, (2) the professional as a mediator between individuals and society, (3) professional motivations, and (4) acts of profession.

Review Questions

1. Define *medical futility*.

2. List and explain each of the various types of medical futility. How do they differ? Give examples of each.

3. Who were Helga Wanglie, Baby K, and Catherine Gilgunn?

4. List the goals of medicine as formulated by the Hastings Center Goals of Medicine Project.

5. What three questions should be considered in asking whether an act violates the internal morality of medicine?

6. Explain the relationship between medical futility and the internal morality of medicine.

7. Explain the relationship between medical professionalism and the virtues.

8. According to Parsons, what elements characterize—or should characterize—a profession?

Endnotes

1. Much of this chapter dealing with the internal morality of medicine is substantially reproduced from Paola F, Nixon L, Walker R. Beyond medical futility: a proposed taxonomy of ultra vires acts in medicine. *Intern Emerg Med* 2006;1(4):267–272.

2. From 1966 through the week of August 3, 2006, there were 681 bibliographic records in Medline listed under the focused MeSH heading of medical futility—all between 1989 and 2005. None were listed from 1966 through 1988.

3. Jonsen AR, Siegler M, Winslade WJ. *Clinical Ethics.* 6th ed. New York: McGraw-Hill, 2006:28.

4. Dictionary.com. Available at: http://dictionary.reference.com/browse/futile. Accessed December 21, 2007.

5. Encyclopedia of Greek Mythology. Available at: http://www.mythweb.com/encyc/entries/sisyphus.html. Accessed December 21, 2007.

6. Mythweb. Available at: http://www.mythweb.com/encyc/entries/tantalus.html. Accessed December 21, 2007.

7. Schneiderman LJ, Jecker NS, Jonsen AR. Medical futility: response to critiques. *Ann Intern Med* 1996;125:669–674.

8. Brett AS, McCullough LB. When patients request specific interventions: defining the limits of the physician's obligation. *N Engl J Med* 1986;315:1347–1351.

9. Blackhall LJ. Must we always use CPR? *N Engl J Med* 1987;317:1281–1285.

10. Paris JJ, Crone RK, Reardon F. Physician's refusal of requested treatment. The case of Baby L. *N Engl J Med* 1990;322:1012–1015.

11. McCormick RA. To save or let die. The dilemma of modern medicine. *JAMA* 1974;229:172–176.

12. Jecker NS, Schneiderman LJ. Medical futility: the duty not to treat. *Camb Q Healthc Ethics* 1993;2:151–159.

13. Schneiderman LJ, Jecker NS, Jonsen AR. Medical futility: its meaning and ethical implications. *Ann Intern Med* 1990;112:949–954.

14. *In re Helga Wanglie,* Fourth Judicial District (Dist. Ct., Probate Div.) PX-91-283. Minnesota, Hennepin County.

15. *In the Matter of Baby K,* 832 F.Supp. 1022 (U.S. District Court, Eastern District Virginia, 1993).

16. 42 U.S.C.A. § 1395dd (1995).

17. Super. Ct. Civ. Action No. 924820, Suffolk Co., Mass., *verdict,* 21 April 1995.

18. Capron AM. At law: abandoning a waning life. *Hastings Center Rep* 1995;25(4):24–26.

19. Ascension Healthcare Ethics Cases. Available at: http://www.ascensionhealth.org/ethics/public/cases/cases_GL.asp. Accessed December 22, 2007.

20. See Romano L. Staying abreast of tax law. *Washington Post,* April 12, 1994:

> The U.S. Tax Court has agreed that exotic dancer Cynthia S. Hess (aka Chesty Love) can claim her breasts as business assets, which can therefore be depreciated for tax purposes. Hess and her husband claimed a $2,088 deduction in '88 for depreciation on implants that enlarged her—ready?—to a 56 FF. The IRS had rebuffed them, saying that money spent to improve appearance is personal. But Special Trial Judge Joan Seitz Pate found that the breasts are so large and cumbersome that while they did increase her income, Hess didn't get any personal benefit from them. "Petitioner's expenditures were detrimental to her health and contorted her body . . . all for the purpose of making money," Pate wrote in the decision, reports the Associated Press. Before the change, Hess grossed from $416 to $750 per week, but post-enlargement, she made more than $70,000 during 20 weeks in '91. It wasn't all blue skies, however. "In December of 1988, because of the added weight and imbalance created by the implants, petitioner slipped and fell on ice, rupturing one of her implants," the judge wrote. "In addition to medical problems . . . petitioner was ridiculed by people on the street . . . and she was ostracized by most of her family."

21. Imagine a world in which we decided that nonreconstructive cosmetic surgery served a useful societal end but that, because such surgery involved not treatment but enhancement, it should be performed by highly trained technicians rather than by physicians.

22. Brody H, Miller FG. The internal morality of medicine: explication and application to managed care. *J Med Philosophy* 1998;23:384–410.

23. Ladd J. The internal morality of medicine: an essential dimension of the physician-patient relationship. In: Shelp E, ed. *The Clinical Encounter.* Dordrecht: Kluwer Academic, 1983:209–231.

24. Pellegrino ED, Thomasma DC. *A Philosophical Basis of Medical Practice: Toward a Philosophy and Ethic of the Healing Professions.* New York: Oxford University Press, 1981.

25. Kass LR. Regarding the end of medicine and the pursuit of health. *Public Interest* 1975(Summer);40:11–42.

26. Kass LR. Ethical dilemmas in the care of the ill: I. What is the physician's service? *JAMA* 1980;244(16):1811–1816.

27. Kass LR. Ethical dilemmas in the care of the ill: II. What is the patient's good? *JAMA* 1980;244(17):1946–1949.

28. Rhodes R. Futility and the goals of medicine. *J Clin Ethics* 1998;9(2):194–205.

29. Nordin I. The limits of medical practice. *Theoretical Med Bioethics* 1999;20:105–123.

30. Brulde B. The goals of medicine: towards a unified theory. *Health Care Anal* 2001;9:1–13.

31. Nordenfelt L. On the goals of medicine, health enhancement and social welfare. *Health Care Anal* 2001;9:15–23.

32. The goals of medicine: setting new priorities. *Hastings Center Rep* 1996;26(6):S9–S14.

33. Parker-Pope T. Cosmetic surgery used to smooth foreheads might cure migraines. *Wall Street Journal,* December 1, 2000, B1.

34. Miller FG, Brody H. Professional integrity and physician-assisted death. *Hastings Center Rep* 1995;25(3):8–17.

35. *Oxford American Dictionary.* Heald College ed. New York: Avon, 1980.

36. Paola FA. How dead is the federal constitutional right to assisted suicide? *Am J Med* 1998;104:565–568.

37. We have suggested elsewhere (see the work cited in endnote 1) that the term *medically ultra vires* be applied to acts that violate the internal morality of medicine, that the term *ultra fines* be applied to acts that violate the internal morality of medicine because of goal illegitimacy, that the term *ultra modos* be applied to acts that violate the internal morality of medicine because of means illegitimacy, and that the term *ultra nexus* be applied to acts that violate the internal morality of medicine because of means–ends disjunction. The authors are grateful to John Noonan (Associate Professor, Division of Languages at the University of South Florida in Tampa) for explaining that the Latin preposition *ultra* is always followed by accusative case forms; *vires* is, for example, an accusative plural form of the so-called third declension. *Fines, modos* and *nexus* are the accusative plural forms of *finis, modus,* and *nexus* (nominative singular forms). Hence the other phrases coined therein—*ultra fines, ultra modos,* and *ultra nexus.*

38. Clouser KD, Culver CM, Gert B. Malady: a new treatment of disease. *Hastings Center Rep* 1981; 11:29–37.

39. *Patton* [movie]. Twentieth Century Fox, 1970.

40. Fox News. Available at: http://www.foxnews.com/story/0,2933,142687,00.html. Accessed March 22, 2005.

41. See, for example, http://pressherald.mainetoday.com/viewpoints/editorials/050103doctorgov. shtml; http://www.kcadp.org/pdf%20files/Bowling%20PDF/KY%20Board%20Filing.pdf; and http://www.freerepublic.com/focus/f-news/1283670/posts. Accessed March 22, 2005.

42. Robeznieks A. Ethics charges related to executions dropped. *AMA News*, January 31, 2005:21.

43. *Black's Law Dictionary.* Abridged 6th ed. St. Paul, MN: West Publishing, 1991:841.

44. Pellegrino ED. Professionalism, profession and the virtues of the good physician. *Mount Sinai J Med* 2002;69(6):378–384.

45. Latham SR. Medical professionalism: a Parsonian view. *Mount Sinai J Med* 2002;69(6):363–369.

46. Arendt H. What is authority? In: Arendt H. *Between Past and Future.* New York: Penguin Books, 1968:93, 106, 122–123.

47. Condemned prisoner treated and executed. Available at: http://www.deathpenaltyinfo.org/article.php?did=946. Accessed December 28, 2007.

48. Indeed, in a similar case (*Perry v Louisiana,* 498 US 1075 [1990]), the American Psychiatric Association's amicus brief "emphasized the ethical quandaries for psychiatrists and urged the Supreme Court to commute [the prisoner's] death penalty to life imprisonment without possibility of parole. This would allow Perry to receive appropriate care without his psychiatrists having to worry that they would be facilitating his execution." States truly concerned with maintaining the ethical integrity of the medical profession would not force medical practitioners to choose between treating a prisoner-patient's psychosis (and in the process facilitating his execution) and withholding effective treatment.

49. Translation from the Greek by Ludwig Edelstein. From Edelstein L. *The Hippocratic Oath: Text, Translation, and Interpretation.* Baltimore: Johns Hopkins Press, 1943.

50. Project of the ABIM Foundation, ACP-ASIM Foundation, and European Federation of Internal Medicine. Medical professionalism in the new millennium: a physician charter. *Ann Intern Med* 2002;136:24.

Section II

The Provider–Patient Relationship

Chapter 6

Confidentiality

To him that you tell your secret you resign your liberty.

—Anonymous proverb

If you reveal your secrets to the wind you should not blame the wind for revealing them to the trees.

—Kahlil Gibran

Chapter Learning Objectives
At the conclusion of this chapter the reader will be able to:

1. Define *confidentiality*

2. Understand and distinguish the various policy rationales underlying the doctrine of confidentiality

3. Be familiar with protections afforded to confidentiality by the common law and statutory law

4. Be familiar with the cases exploring the limits of confidentiality and the reasoning of the courts therein

5. Understand the limits of confidentiality and be able to recognize situations in which a duty to warn or otherwise protect third parties might exist

In a 1995 article in the *American Journal of Medicine,* Ubel and colleagues rode as observers in hospital elevators, listening for any hospital employee comments that might be deemed inappropriate. They reported that in 36 of 259 one-way elevator trips offering the opportunity for conversation (13.9% of the trips), they overheard 39 inappropriate comments. The most frequent inappropriate comments (18 of 39, or 46%) were violations of patient confidentiality.[1]

The doctrine of confidentiality is a foundational principle in medical ethics. Thus, the Hippocratic Oath reads, in part, "What I may see or hear in the course of the treatment or even outside of the treatment in regard to the life of men, which on no account one must spread abroad, I will keep to myself."[2] More modern statements of ethics also emphasize the fundamentality of the doctrine of confidentiality. Thus, the fourth of the principles of medical ethics of the American Medical Association holds that "A physician shall . . . safeguard patient confidences within the constraints of the law."[3] The Charter on Medical Professionalism (a joint project of the American Board of Internal Medicine

Foundation, the American College of Physicians–American Society of Internal Medicine Foundation, and the European Federation of Internal Medicine) lists a commitment to patient confidentiality as one of ten professional responsibilities:

> Earning the trust and confidence of patients requires that appropriate confidentiality safeguards be applied to disclosure of patient information. This commitment extends to discussions with persons acting on a patient's behalf when obtaining the patient's own consent is not feasible. Fulfilling the commitment to confidentiality is more pressing now than ever before, given the widespread use of electronic information systems for compiling patient data and an increasing availability of genetic information. Physicians recognize, however, that their commitment to patient confidentiality must occasionally yield to overriding considerations in the public interest (for example, when patients endanger others).[4]

The *Guidelines for Ethical Conduct for the Physician Assistant Profession* of the American Academy of Physician Assistants includes a statement on confidentiality, which reads in part:

> Physician assistants [PAs] should maintain confidentiality. By maintaining confidentiality, PAs respect patient privacy and help to prevent discrimination based on medical conditions. If patients are confident that their privacy is protected, they are more likely to seek medical care and more likely to discuss their problems candidly. In cases of adolescent patients, family support is important but should be balanced with the patient's need for confidentiality and the PA's obligation to respect their emerging autonomy. . . . Any communication about a patient conducted in a manner that violates confidentiality is unethical. Computerized record keeping and electronic data transmission present unique challenges that can make the maintenance of patient confidentiality difficult.
>
> PAs should advocate for policies and procedures that secure the confidentiality of patient information.[5]

Privacy and Confidentiality

Privacy and confidentiality are, in some ways, two sides of the same coin. The *right of privacy* is actually a bundle of rights, if you will, including a right against appropriation of one's name or likeness; a right against intrusion upon one's solitude or seclusion; a right against being painted in a false light in the public eye; and, most important for our purposes in this chapter, a right against public disclosure of private facts.[6] Gert, Culver, and Clouser have written that "An individual or group has *privacy* in a situation with regard to others if and only if in that situation the individual or group is normatively protected from intrusion, interference and *information access by others* [italics added]."[7]

Something *confidential* is something "intended to be held in confidence or kept secret."[6(p206)] A *confidential communication* is a "statement made under circumstances showing that the speaker intended [the] statement only for [the] ears of [the] person addressed."[6(p206)] Examples of such communications include "those between spouses, physician-patient, attorney-client, confessor-penitent, etc."[6(p206)] The law protects such confidential communications from forced disclosure on the witness stand at the option of the witness spouse, patient, client, or penitent.

Confidentiality is related to the information-access branch of the privacy bundle of rights.

> People hold information in confidence because the rules of a private situation require them not to reveal that situation. Confidentiality thus refers to a duty within a private situation. Some party—a doctor, nurse, or physician assistant—has the . . . responsibility not to divulge information to inappropriate parties. Privacy is *invaded;* but confidentiality is *violated*—that is, the duty of confidentiality is violated . . . .[7(p126)] (Internal footnotes omitted)

Rationales Underlying the Doctrine of Confidentiality

Why does the doctrine of confidentiality exist? What good flows from it? In fact, a number of rationales underlie the doctrine of confidentiality in the medical context. The first is utilitarian (see Chapter 1). Knowledge that their health care provider owes them a moral and legal duty of confidentiality encourages persons "to seek medical care when they might otherwise avoid doing so out of shame."[8] (Thus, for example, a person with a genital rash might be less likely to seek medical attention if the individual knew that his or her physician was free to share information about the state of his or her genitalia with the public at large.) This benefits the sick, the well (who will, after all, someday be sick), and society as a whole in the form of improved public health.[8]

A second rationale underlying the doctrine of confidentiality is that it furthers the principle of respect for autonomy—in this case, the patient's autonomy over his or her personal medical information.[8,9] The patient decides to whom he or she wishes to disclose personal medical information. To paraphrase Kahlil Gibran, in a world devoid of confidentiality, if you revealed your secrets to the wind you could not blame the wind for revealing them to the trees. The doctrine of confidentiality says that the wind shall not reveal my secrets to the trees and allows me to hold the wind blameworthy if it does so.

The same rationales underlying the existence of the doctrine of confidentiality afford physicians and other health care practitioners (HCPs) reasons to keep confidential the personal medical information of patients. Of course, there are other reasons for HCPs not to violate the duty of confidentiality. Thus, an HCP who has taken an oath containing a confidentiality provision would be contravening a number of moral rules by unjustifiably revealing a confidence.[10] Additionally, HCPs who breach their duty of confidentiality may face legal sanctions.

Legal Protection of Confidentiality

Legal protection of confidentiality includes both common law protections and statutory protections. In general, the *common law* "is a body of law that develops and derives through judicial decisions, as distinguished from legislative enactments."[6(p189)] Conversely, *statutory law* is "that body of law created by acts of the legislature."[6(p983)]

> Most states provide a private cause of action against licensed health care providers who impermissibly disclose [to third parties] confidential information obtained in the course of the treatment relationship. . . . Depending on the jurisdiction, the claim may be phrased as a breach of contract, as an act of malpractice, as a breach of fiduciary duty, as an act of fraud/misrepresentation, or as a breach of a specific civil statute permitting the award of damages. . . . In addition, licensed health care providers who breach the confidentiality of their patients run the risk of professional disciplinary action.[11]

Under the laws of many states, the breach of patient confidentiality by physicians and other HCPs is considered unprofessional conduct (see Chapter 5) and warrants disciplinary action, up to and including license revocation.[8(p120)]

It is important for practicing HCPs to be aware that there exist certain disease-specific state statutes creating confidentiality duties. We shall consider, as an example, the special case of HIV later in this chapter. Additionally, federal law imposes confidentiality requirements on records of patients in federally funded drug and alcohol treatment programs.[8(p121),12]

Case 6-A

A video posted on YouTube in April 2008 showed a noisy Philippine operating room full of doctors and nurses laughing and cheering during the course of an operation to remove a canister of perfume from the rectum of a thirty-nine-year-old male patient. "As a doctor gingerly pulls out the 6-inch long canister from the male patient's rectum, someone shouts, 'Baby out!' amid loud cheers. The doctor then removes the canister cap and sprays the contents toward the crowd of nurses and doctors viewing the procedure."[13] Reportedly "more than 10 people were involved—including staff and medical and nursing students from a nearby operating room," and the video was apparently shot by one of the student nurses.[14] Whose conduct was blameworthy? Why? What consequences might follow?

Analysis

Multiple HCPs and HCPs-in-training breached their professional fiduciary duties to the patient in question. Just as an HCP's access to a patient and his or her medical record is on a "need to know" basis,[15] access to the operating room in this case should have been restricted by the surgeon and nurse in charge to those persons who had legitimate patient-care or pedagogical

Case 6-A (continued)

reasons to be there. The presence of superfluous personnel was an invasion of the patient's privacy. The merrymaking by the operating room personnel at the patient's expense, whether recorded or not, was an affront to his dignity. The HCPs responsible for precepting and serving as role models for the medical and nursing students involved failed miserably. The making of the video without obtaining the informed consent of the patient ran afoul of the principle of respect for autonomy (see Chapter 2) and of the right to informed consent/refusal (see Chapters 8 and 9); its posting on YouTube was an egregious breach of the duty of confidentiality. Even an HCP-in-training should have known better. The episode not only embarrassed the patient involved but also undermined faith in the individual and institutional providers involved and in medicine in general.

Although predicting what consequences might follow from the incident would require knowledge of governing Philippine law, it seems reasonable to suggest that they might include the following: discipline of the medical and nursing students involved, up to and including expulsion; professional disciplinary actions against the licensed HCPs involved; an administrative action against the involved hospital; and a private cause of action for monetary damages against any and all of the above. In fact, on May 14, 2008, it was announced that the Department of Health's regional director had imposed a three-month suspension on two doctors and a nurse in the rectal surgery scandal.[14]

Federal Privacy Regulations: HIPAA

The Health Insurance Portability and Accountability Act of 1996 (HIPAA)[16] delegated to the secretary of Health and Human Services the power to regulate certain aspects of medical privacy. The federal privacy regulations were released in December 2000[17] and revised in 2002.[18]

> In general, the federal privacy regulations impose an obligation to maintain the confidentiality of individually identifiable health information on certain "covered entities," which include health plans, health care clearinghouses, and health care providers who transmit health information in electronic form during certain transactions. These entities must (1) adopt internal procedures to protect the privacy of protected health information; (2) train employees regarding privacy procedures; (3) designate a privacy officer; (4) secure patient records that contain protected information; and (5) ensure that agreements with other entities (called "business associates") include terms requiring the protection of privacy. . . . A violation of the regulations may result in a significant civil penalty or criminal liability or both. The regulations do not provide a private cause of action or remedy.[11(p181)] (Internal citations omitted)

The Limits of Confidentiality: The Duty to Warn or Otherwise Protect Third Parties

You will recall from the discussion of the moral rules (Chapter 3) that not all prima facie violations of moral rules are wrongful. Under certain circumstances, violations of moral rules may be said to be justified. Thus, for example, even the prohibition against killing yields to the right to defend oneself against the use of deadly force. As discussed in Chapter 3,

> Everyone is always to obey the rule unless an impartial rational person can advocate that violating it be publicly allowed. Anyone who violates the rule when no impartial rational person can advocate that such a violation be publicly allowed may be punished. . . . If all informed impartial rational persons would estimate that less harm would be suffered if this kind of violation were publicly allowed, then . . . the violation is strongly justified. . . . If *some but not all* informed rational persons would estimate that less harm would be suffered if this kind of violation were publicly allowed, then . . . the violation is weakly justified. . . . If all informed rational persons would estimate that more harm would be suffered if this kind of violation were publicly allowed, then . . . the violation is unjustified.[19]

So, too, the duty of confidentiality is not absolute. Under certain circumstances, an HCP's duty of confidentiality to the patient must yield to the HCP's conflicting duty to warn or to protect third parties. Because these duties conflict with the duty of confidentiality, they may be conceptualized as exceptions to the confidentiality rule. As was the case with the legal duty of confidentiality, the legal duty to warn or to protect third parties sometimes derives from the common law and sometimes derives from statute.

Statutory Limits of Confidentiality

One of the oldest exceptions to the duty of confidentiality is the required duty of HCPs to report certain communicable diseases—such as HIV/AIDS—to state public health authorities. The policy rationale underlying this exception is the protection of identifiable third parties at risk (e.g., sexual contacts of the infected patient). The same policy rationale underlies statutory duties to report child and elder abuse and the uncontrolled epilepsy of licensed drivers.[8(p122)]

In contrast, the policy rationale underlying another class of exceptions—for example, statutes mandating that HCPs report knife and gunshot wounds—is different. "Here the policy is generally to catch and punish wrongdoers, rather than to protect third parties against continuing or future harms."[8(p123)] Furthermore, the "instrumental *purpose* of protecting confidentiality—encouraging treatment—may be damaged to a lesser degree in the case of such violent injuries, since the victims (like those in any emergency) may be highly likely to obtain treatment out of necessity."[8(p123)]

Common Law Limits of Confidentiality

There are many cases establishing a legal duty on the part of an HCP to protect third parties where the HCP's patient poses a significant danger to others. Traditionally, case law supports the finding of such a duty in patients suffering from contagious disease, in violent psychiatric patients, and in patients with medically related driving impairments. Under the common law, physicians and other HCPs may be liable for harm to third parties when three conditions are met: (1) there exists a "known or reasonably foreseeable hazard that arises in some way from the physician's patient,"[8(p124)] (2) there are foreseeable (not necessarily individually identifiable) third parties placed at risk by the hazard, and (3) the HCP behaves unreasonably under the circumstances.[8(p124)]

The following cases illustrate how some courts have gone about weighing a patient's privacy interests against the health or safety interests of third parties. As you will see, the meaning of "hazard arising in some way from the physician's patient" has been interpreted liberally by some courts as of late, enlarging the scope of the physician's duty to third parties.

Tarasoff v. Regents of University of California (1976)

In 1969, Prosenjit Poddar told his University of California psychologist, Dr. Lawrence Moore, that he intended to kill Tatiana Tarasoff.[20] Dr. Moore attempted to commit Poddar for treatment, but the campus police released him because he appeared rational. Dr. Moore's superior, Dr. Powelson, then directed that no further efforts be made to detain Poddar. Tatiana Tarasoff was not warned of the threats against her. Shortly thereafter, Poddar killed Tatiana Tarasoff.

A criminal prosecution resulted,[21] but Tatiana's family also brought a liability action against the psychologists involved for failure to warn. The legal issue was whether they owed Tatiana Tarasoff a duty to warn. As you will learn in Chapter 15, the law distinguishes between *feasance* (action) and *nonfeasance* (inaction or passivity). When an HCP (or any other person) acts, he must act reasonably or he may be liable for negligence. When someone remains inactive, however, there is no requirement that the inactivity be reasonable under the circumstances.

> Suppose A, standing close by a railroad, sees a two-year-old babe on the track and a car approaching. He can easily rescue the child with entire safety to himself, and the instincts of humanity require him to do so. If he does not, he may, perhaps, justly be styled a ruthless savage and a moral monster; but he is not liable in damages for the child's injury, or indictable under the statute for its death.... The duty to do no wrong is a legal duty. The duty to protect against wrong is, generally speaking and excepting certain *intimate relations* ... a moral obligation only, not recognized or enforced by law.[22] (Italics added)

As you may suspect, the physician–patient (or provider–patient, as the case may be) relationship is indeed one of those intimate relations that impose affirmative duties (i.e., duties to act) on HCPs. In the *Tarasoff* case, however, there was no provider–patient relationship between any of the psychologists and Tatiana Tarasoff. Nevertheless, the court held that the absence of such a relationship was not a bar to liability:

> Although under the common law, as a general rule, one person owed no duty to control the conduct of another, nor to warn those endangered by such conduct, the courts have noted exceptions to this rule. In two classes of cases the courts have imposed a duty of care: (1) cases in which *the defendant stands in some special relationship to* either *the person whose conduct needs to be controlled* or in a relationship to the foreseeable victim of that conduct; and (2) cases in which the defendant has engaged, or undertaken to engage, in affirmative action to control the anticipated dangerous conduct or protect the prospective victim. Both exceptions apply to the facts of this case.[23] (Internal footnotes omitted; italics added)

In other words, the court found that the intimate relation between Poddar and his psychologists was enough to create an affirmative duty to warn his foreseeable victim. *Tarasoff* stands for the principle that once a therapist determines, or in the exercise of reasonable professional judgment should determine, that a patient poses a serious danger of violence to others, he or she bears a duty to exercise reasonable care to protect the foreseeable victim of that danger.

Bradshaw v. Daniel (1993)

As mentioned earlier, an HCP may have a common law legal duty to protect third parties when the patient's condition poses a significant danger to others because of a contagious disease. In *Bradshaw,* patient Elmer Johns was admitted to the hospital in July 1986 with symptoms of Rocky Mountain Spotted Fever (RMSF).[24] Dr. Daniel, the defendant, began him on treatment for the same; notwithstanding, his condition deteriorated and he died. "Although Dr. Daniel communicated with Elmer Johns' wife, Genevieve, during Johns' treatment, he never advised her of the risks of exposure to Rocky Mountain Spotted Fever, or that the disease could have been the cause of Johns' death."[24(p867)]

A week after Elmer's death, Genevieve was admitted with similar symptoms and treated for RMSF. She, too, died, within three days. Dr. Daniel was not Genevieve's physician (it was undisputed that there was no physician–patient relationship between the two). Her family filed suit, alleging that Dr. Daniel had been negligent in failing to warn her of the risk of exposure.

Dr. Daniel defended himself by arguing that he owed his patient's wife no legal duty because, first of all, she was not his patient. Second, although (as we saw earlier) there was precedent for holding physicians liable for injuries to nonpatients caused by contagious diseases, Dr. Daniel pointed out that RMSF is not a contagious disease, because it is not transmitted from one person to another. Consequently, unlike the situation that existed in the *Tarasoff* case, here Dr. Daniel's patient (Elmer Johns) was not the source of the danger to the plaintiff.

Nevertheless, the court held in favor of the plaintiff:

> Returning to the facts of this case, first, it is undisputed that there was a physician-patient relationship between Dr. Daniel and Elmer Johns. Second, here, as in the contagious disease context, it is also undisputed that Elmer Johns' wife, who was residing with him, was at risk of contracting the disease. This is so even though the disease is not contagious in the narrow sense that it can be transmitted from one person to another.... [F]amily members of patients suffering from Rocky Mountain Spotted Fever are at risk of contracting the disease due to a phenomenon called clustering, which is related to the activity of infected ticks who transmit the disease to humans.... Thus, this case is analogous to the *Tarasoff* line of cases adopting a duty to warn of danger and the contagious disease cases adopting a comparable duty to warn. Here, as in those cases, there was a foreseeable risk of harm to an identifiable third party, and the reasons supporting the recognition of a duty to warn are equally compelling here.
>
> *We, therefore, conclude that the existence of the physician-patient relationship is sufficient to impose upon a physician an affirmative duty to warn identifiable third persons in the patient's immediate family against foreseeable risks emanating from a patient's illness. Accordingly, we hold that . . . the defendant physician had a duty to warn his patient's wife of the risk to her of contracting Rocky Mountain Spotted Fever when he knew, or in the exercise of reasonable care, should have known, that his patient was suffering from the disease.*[24(p872)] (Italics added)

Pate v. Threlkel (1994)

In 1987, Marianne New was treated for medullary carcinoma of the thyroid.[25] This cancer "may occur as a sporadic form (usually unilateral) or as a familial form (frequently bilateral), transmitted as an autosomal dominant trait."[26] In 1990, Heidi Pate, New's adult daughter, was diagnosed with medullary thyroid carcinoma. Subsequently, Pate filed suit against the physicians who initially treated Ms. New for the disease, alleging that they knew or should have known of the likelihood that Ms. New's children would inherit the condition genetically. Ms. Pate argued that the physicians had a duty to warn their patient (her mother) that her children should be tested for the disease. Pate further argued that had Ms. New been warned in 1987, Ms. Pate would have been monitored for the condition, and it would have been diagnosed earlier, when it was still curable.

The trial court dismissed Pate's complaint, reasoning that Ms. Pate was not a patient of the defendant physicians and that she "did not fit within any exception to the requirement that there be a physician-patient relationship between the parties as a condition precedent to bringing a medical malpractice action."[25(p280)] The district court affirmed the trial court's dismissal.

The case went to the Florida Supreme Court, which was charged with answering the question, Does a physician owe a duty of care to the children of a patient to warn the patient of the genetically transferable nature of the condition for which the physician is treating the patient?

The court reasoned, first, that the physicians certainly owed a duty of care to their patient Ms. New, and that whether that duty included a duty to warn her of the genetically transferable nature of her disease depended on whether "a reasonably prudent health care provider [would have] warn[ed] [the] patient of the genetically transferable nature of the condition for which the physician was treating the patient."[25(p280)] The court continued:

> The second question we must address in answering the certified question is to whom does the alleged duty to warn New of the nature of her disease run? The duty obviously runs to the patient. . . . In the past, courts have held that in order to maintain a cause of action against a physician, [a special relationship] must exist between the plaintiff and the physician. In other professional relationships, however, we have recognized the rights of identified third party beneficiaries to recover from a professional because that party was the intended beneficiary of the prevailing standard of care. . . . Here, the alleged prevailing standard of care was obviously developed for the benefit of the patient's children as well as the patient. *We conclude that when the prevailing standard of care creates a duty that is obviously for the benefit of certain identified third parties and the physician knows of the existence of those third parties, then the physician's duty runs to those third parties.*[25(pp281-282)]
> (Internal citations omitted; italics added)

Thus, the court found that, if the physician's duty to Ms. New included a duty to warn her of the genetic nature and transmissibility of her disease (a question of fact that would need to be answered by the trial court, to which the case would be sent back), then that duty ran to her daughter Ms. Pate as an intended third-party beneficiary.[6(p1029)]

The court went on, in dictum, to say:

> Though not encompassed by the certified question, there is another issue which should be addressed in light of our holding. If there is a duty to warn, to whom must the physician convey the warning? Our holding should not be read to require the physician to warn the patient's children of the disease. In most instances the physician is prohibited from disclosing the patient's medical condition to others except with the patient's permission. Moreover, the patient ordinarily can be expected to pass on the warning. To require the physician to seek

out and warn various members of the patient's family would often be difficult or impractical and would place too heavy a burden upon the physician. *Thus, we emphasize that in any circumstances in which the physician has a duty to warn of a genetically transferable disease, that duty will be satisfied by warning the patient.*[25(p282)] (Internal citations omitted; italics added)

Safer v. Estate of Pack (1996)

The facts of the New Jersey case *Safer v. Estate of Pack* are as follows.[27] Plaintiff Donna Safer's father, Robert Batkin, was a patient of Dr. George T. Pack in the 1950s and 1960s. In 1956, Dr. Pack operated on Mr. Batkin and performed a total colectomy and an ileosigmoidectomy for multiple polyposis of the colon with malignant degeneration in one area. The discharge summary noted that pathologic examination had revealed the existence of adenocarcinoma developing in an intestinal polyp, and diffuse intestinal polyposis from one end of the colon to the other.

Dr. Pack performed an ileoabdominal perineal resection with an ileostomy on Mr. Batkin in 1961, and in December 1963 hospitalized Mr. Batkin for carcinoma of the colon metastatic to the liver with secondary jaundice. Mr. Batkin died in January 1964 at forty-five years of age. His daughter Donna was ten years old at the time.

In February 1990, thirty-six-year-old Donna Safer was diagnosed with metastatic colon cancer and multiple polyposis. She underwent a total abdominal colectomy with ileorectal anastomosis, a left ovariectomy, and chemotherapy treatment. In September 1991, Ms. Safer obtained her father's medical records, from which she learned that he had suffered from polyposis. She brought suit against Dr. Pack in 1992, alleging negligence on his part in failing to warn of the risk to Donna Safer's health.

The trial court "held that a physician had no 'legal duty to warn a child of a patient of a genetic risk,' "[27(p1190)] reasoning that "genetically transmissible diseases . . . differ from contagious . . . diseases or threats of harm . . . because 'the harm is already present within the non-patient child as opposed to being introduced by a patient who was not warned to stay away.' "[27(p1191)]

The appellate court disagreed, writing "The [trial] judge's view of this case as one involving an unavoidable genetic condition gave too little significance to the proferred expert view that early monitoring of those at risk can effectively avert some of the more serious consequences a person with multiple polyposis might otherwise experience."[27(p1192)] As the Florida Supreme Court had done in *Pate v. Threlkel*, the New Jersey appeals court reversed the trial court's dismissal of the plaintiff's complaint and remanded the case for resolution of certain factual questions. Unlike the approach of Florida in *Pate v. Threlkel*, however, the New Jersey court "decline[d] to hold . . . that, in all circumstances, the duty to warn will be satisfied by informing the patient,"[27(p1192)] leaving open the possibility that such a warning might, in some cases, have to be given directly to the children of the patient.

Case 6-B

Richard is a forty-nine-year-old man who has been married for twenty-four years.[28] He and his spouse have three adult children, and one unexpected child who is eight years old. Recently the relationship between Debra and Richard has become strained. You take care of both of them in your general medical clinic in Florida. Richard has hypertension and Debra has a borderline case of type 2 diabetes.

Richard comes into your office six weeks earlier than his next regularly scheduled appointment, requesting a checkup. He has no particular complaints. He tells you that a couple of weeks ago he had some nonspecific flulike symptoms, but that these have resolved. When you ask why he didn't come in then, he shrugs his shoulders and says, "I don't know, but I'm here now and I want a complete checkup to make sure nothing's wrong with me."

Sensing that Richard is worried about something about which he is not telling you, you tell him that to do a complete checkup you need to start by taking a complete history of everything that has gone on since you last saw him. You learn that on a recent business trip to Las Vegas he had several sexual encounters with prostitutes, and that he is now worried that he might have a sexually transmitted disease. He denies penile lesions, urethral discharge, or swollen inguinal nodes. Richard insists that he be checked anyway. When you ask him what specifically he wants to be checked for, he admits that he cannot get the thought of HIV out of his mind. When you take a more detailed sexual history, you learn that Richard used a condom in his Las Vegas encounters, but that he is nonetheless worried about HIV. You also learn that since returning from Vegas he has had unprotected sex with Debra.

You try to reassure Richard that because he used a condom he has reduced his risk of contracting HIV in Las Vegas. You conduct a physical examination and tell Richard that the exam is completely normal. You suggest ordering some basic lab tests to screen for problems. You also suggest that to put his mind at ease he should consider getting an HIV test. After signing a consent form, Richard is tested.

One week later you see Richard to give him the results of his HIV test. The result is positive. Richard's worst fears are confirmed. During the visit, you mention to Richard that he needs to tell Debra so that she too can seek testing and counseling. Richard seems alarmed at this and says he is not going to tell her. He asks you not to tell her either. How should you handle this situation? Should you breach confidentiality?

Analysis

Because of your physician–patient relationship with Richard, you owe him a duty of confidentiality. On the other hand, the fact that HIV is a contagious disease and that Richard poses a threat to Debra raises the issue of whether you have a duty to warn her. As discussed earlier, breaching confidentiality would arguably violate a number of moral rules, including the moral rule against breaking one's promise, the rule against neglecting one's duty (to the extent that one's professional duty includes a duty of confidentiality), and possibly the rule against breaking the law (depending on the statutory and common law of Florida). In deciding how to proceed, we need to explore two questions: (1) Does Florida case law or Florida statutory law have

Case 6-B (*continued*)

anything to say specifically about the duty of confidentiality or the duty to warn in cases involving HIV? and (2) Would a violation of the moral rules underlying the duty of confidentiality in this case be justified?

With regard to the first question, the answer is yes. Under the Florida Omnibus AIDS Act,[29] when an HIV-infected patient refuses to inform past or present sexual or needle-sharing partners, the HCP has no *legal* duty to warn these third parties,[30] but does have a privilege to warn them. The privilege exists only when the patient discloses the identity of the partner at risk. Also, in order to enjoy the privilege, the HCP must adhere to the protocol prescribed by the Department of Health, which specifies the following:

- Identification of the third party must come from the patient.

- The practitioner must recommend the patient notify the partner, or use the department's notification program, and refrain from activity in a manner likely to transmit the virus.

- Upon the patient's refusal, the practitioner must advise the patient of the practitioner's intent to notify the partner.

- The preceding must be documented, but documentation in the patient's record may not include the name of the third party.

- The practitioner takes full responsibility for notifying the third party in accordance with the protocol. These procedures include protecting to the extent possible the patient's name and privately counseling the third party about HIV infection and the availability of voluntary HIV testing.[31]

Under the act, a provider's unauthorized release of HIV test results is grounds for disciplinary action by his or her licensing body, grounds for a private cause of action for negligence and invasion of privacy, and a first-degree misdemeanor (punishable by up to one year's imprisonment). When the unauthorized release is done maliciously or for monetary gain, the act may instead constitute a third-degree felony (punishable by up to five years' imprisonment).

There is, however, a particularity about this case that changes the legal and moral relationships among the various parties. In this case, unlike in the legal cases discussed earlier, and unlike the situation envisioned in the Florida AIDS Omnibus Act, the third party—Richard's wife Debra—is not simply a third party. She is your patient as well. As a result, you owe her a fiduciary duty—a duty to act in her best medical interests, and the "highest standard of duty implied by law."[6(p432)] One could argue that, even though the Florida AIDS Omnibus Act reportedly "eliminates any legal obligation that may have existed for providers to tell third parties,"[31(p43)] the legislature did not intend for the act to abrogate whatever legal obligations exist for a provider to warn his patients.

Debra should be notified in accordance with the protocol specified in the act. The fact that she is your patient makes the decision to breach confidentiality relatively easier. Even were she not your patient, most persons would probably support the decision to breach confidentiality

(continues)

> ## Case 6-B (continued)
>
> under these circumstances, and the breach would be at least weakly justified (see Chapter 3). Notification will allow her to be tested, to take measures to avoid infection (if she tests negative), and to obtain treatment (if she tests positive).
>
> How might the dilemma in which you find yourself have been avoided? Gert, Culver, and Clouser have written that "physicians should warn patients in advance whenever any . . . diagnostic test suggested to the patient carries with it some risk of loss of privacy. . . . If the HIV+ man knows his wife will be told if [his test result] is positive, then the doctor has not breached any duty of confidentiality toward the patient if he is later forced to tell her."[7(pp188,191)] Indeed, under the Florida AIDS Omnibus Act, HCPs must tell the patient, as part of the process of informed consent (see Chapters 8 and 9) that must precede HIV testing, at least the following information: (1) that HCPs are required by law to report the test subject's name to the local county health department if the HIV test results are positive; (2) that anonymous testing sites are available; and (3) the extent of the confidentiality rights that pertain to the test results. In essence, one can avoid the dilemma of the duty of confidentiality versus duty to warn by recourse to the doctrine of informed consent/refusal (see Chapters 8 and 9).[32]

Conclusion

In Robert Bolt's play *A Man For All Seasons,* Thomas More's wife Alice is angered by his refusal to tell even her his position on the divorce of King Henry VIII. "Make a statement now," she implores him:

> *More.* No—[Alice exhibits indignation.] Alice, it's a point of law! Accept it from me, Alice, that in silence is my safety under the law, but my silence must be absolute, it must extend to you.
>
> *Alice.* In short you don't trust us!
>
> *More.* A man would need to be half-witted not to trust you—but—[impatiently] Look—[He advances on her.] I'm the Lord Chief Justice, I'm Cromwell, I'm the King's Head Jailer—and I take your hand [He does so.] and I clamp it on the Bible, on the Blessed Cross [clamps her hand on his closed fist] and I say: "Woman, has your husband made a statement on these matters?" Now—on peril of your soul remember—what's your answer?
>
> *Alice.* No.
>
> *More.* And so it must remain.[33(p410)]

Looking at this exchange now, having read this chapter, you should be struck by the fact that More's character had no expectation of privacy in a situation (the relationship between husband and wife) that we Americans regard as almost quintessentially private. There was no expectation that the law would protect such communications from forced disclosure on the witness stand. One also appreciates the price paid by those who inhabit a world devoid of privacy and confidentiality—a price measured in the currency of lost intimacy.

Chapter Summary

Confidentiality refers to one's duty in a private situation (e.g., the physician–patient relationship) not to divulge information to inappropriate parties. Interests in utility and autonomy underlie the doctrine of confidentiality. Violations or breaches of confidentiality implicate the moral rules prohibiting the breaking of promises, the breaking of the law, and the neglect of duty. The legal protection of confidentiality includes both common law and statutory protections (including HIPAA). The duty of confidentiality is not absolute; not all breaches of confidentiality are wrongful. Both common law and statutory exceptions to the duty of confidentiality exist. When one of these exceptions is applicable, confidentiality may—and in some cases must—be breached.

Review Questions

1. What is confidentiality? What is privacy? How are they related?
2. Why do we have a doctrine of confidentiality? How does it benefit us?
3. Why is it wrong to breach confidentiality? Explain your answer in terms of ethical theory, the principles of biomedical ethics, or the moral rules.
4. What is common law? What is statutory law? How do they differ?
5. What is HIPAA? Why is it discussed in this chapter?
6. List three exceptions to the legal duty of confidentiality. List two different policy rationales underlying exceptions to the duty.
7. When should a physician or other HCP consider breaching confidentiality? What factors weigh in favor of such a breach?

Endnotes

1. Ubel PA, Zell MM, Miller DJ, Fischer GS, Peters-Stefani D, Arnold RM. Elevator talk: observational study of inappropriate comments in a public space. *Am J Med* 1995;99(2):190–194.
2. The Hippocratic Oath. Available at: http://en.wikipedia.org/wiki/Hippocratic_Oath. Accessed May 25, 2008.
3. American Medical Association. Principles of medical ethics. Available at: http://www.ama-assn.org/ama/pub/category/2512.html. Accessed May 22, 2008.

4. Project of the ABIM Foundation, ACP-ASIM Foundation, and European Federation of Internal Medicine. Medical professionalism in the new millennium: a physician charter. Available at: http://www.annals.org/cgi/reprint/136/3/243.pdf. Accessed May 22, 2008.

5. American Academy of Physician Assistants. The guidelines for ethical conduct for the physician assistant profession. Available at: http://www.aapa.org/manual/23-EthicalConduct.pdf. Accessed May 22, 2008.

6. *Black's Law Dictionary.* Abridged 6th ed. St. Paul, MN: West Publishing, 1991:830.

7. Gert B, Culver CM, Clouser KD. *Bioethics: A Return to Fundamentals.* New York: Oxford University Press, 1997:181–193, p. 183.

8. Hall MA, Ellman IM, Strouse DS. *Health Care Law and Ethics in a Nutshell.* 2nd ed. St. Paul, MN: West Group, 1999:117–131, p. 118.

9. Bok S. *Secrets: On the Ethics of Concealment and Revelation.* New York: Pantheon Books, 1982:119–124.

10. The moral rules that would arguably be contravened under such circumstances include the rule against breaking one's promise, the rule against neglecting one's duty (to the extent that one's professional duty includes a duty of confidentiality), and the rule against breaking the law (see text).

11. Hall MA, Bobinski MA, Orentlicher D. *Health Care Law and Ethics.* 7th ed. Austin: Aspen Publishers, 2007:175–197, p. 179.

12. 42 U.S.C. sec 290dd-2.

13. CBS News. Philippine surgeons goof off on YouTube. Available at: http://www.cbsnews.com/stories/2008/04/16/health/main4020327.shtml?source=RSSattr=Health_4020327. Accessed May 22, 2008.

14. Inquirer.net. DoH suspends 2 docs, nurse in rectal surgery scandal. Available at: http://newsinfo.inquirer.net/breakingnews/regions/view/20080514-136496/DoH-suspends-2-docs-nurse-in-rectal-surgery-scandal. Accessed May 22, 2008.

15. Thus, it was reported in March 2008 that Britney Spears's medical confidentiality had been breached and

> more than 25 employees of UCLA Medical Center face disciplinary action, according to The Associated Press. More than 13 employees are expected to be fired and 12 others, including several doctors, will be disciplined for looking at Spears' UCLA hospital records. There is no evidence that any employee leaked or sold information about Spears. . . . However, merely looking at the confidential records is a violation of state and federal medical privacy laws.

See liveDaily. Hospital says Britney's medical confidentiality violated. Available at: http://www.livedaily.com/blog/1734.html. Accessed May 22, 2008.

16. Pub. L. 104–191.

17. 65 Fed. Reg. 82, 462–82, 829 (Dec 28, 2000).

18. 67 Fed. Reg. 53, 182 (Aug 14, 2002).

19. Gert B, Berger EM, Cahill GF, et al. *Morality and the New Genetics.* Sudbury, MA: Jones and Bartlett, 1996:29–55, pp. 48–49.

20. *Tarasoff v. Regents of U. of Cal.,* 17 Cal. 3d (1976).

21. *People v. Poddar,* 518 P.2d 342 (1974).

22. *Buch v. Amory Mfg. Co.,* 69 N.H. 257 (1897).

23. *Tarasoff v. Regents of U. of Cal.,* 529 P.2d 553, 557.

24. *Bradshaw v. Daniel,* 854 S.W.2d 865 (Tenn. 1993).

25. *Pate v. Threlkel,* 661 So.2d 278 (Fla. 1995).

26. Berkow R, Fletcher AJ, eds. *The Merck Manual of Diagnosis and Therapy.* 16th ed. Rahway, NJ: Merck Research Laboratories, 1992:1086.

27. *Safer v. Estate of Pack,* 677 A.2d 1188 (N.J. 1996).

28. Thanks to Dr. Robert M. Walker for creating this hypothetical. See also pages 189–193 in the work cited in endnote 7.

29. Florida Omnibus AIDS Act. Available at: http://www.doh.state.fl.us/Disease_ctrl/aids/legal/ctforchd.htm. Accessed May 25, 2008.

30. The statute, naturally, concerns itself with legal duties, not moral duties.

31. Hartog JP. *Florida Omnibus AIDS Act: A Brief Legal Guide for Health Care Practitioners.* Florida Department of Health, Division of Disease Control, Bureau of HIV/AIDS, 1999:45.

32. We do not address here the interesting question of what should be done if Richard were to refuse testing upon being told that a positive test result would be disclosed to Debra.

33. Bolt R. *A Man for All Seasons.* In: *Laurel British Drama: The Twentieth Century.* New York: Dell, 1965:353–446.

Chapter 7

Competence

Every human being of adult years and sound mind has a right to determine what shall be done with his own body; and a surgeon who performs an operation without his patient's consent commits an assault, for which he is liable in damages.

—Schloendorff v. Society of New York Hospital

Chapter Learning Objectives

At the conclusion of this chapter the reader will be able to:

1. Explain what competence is and why it matters

2. Understand how competence relates to the principle of respect for autonomy

3. Explain the relationship among understanding, appreciation, rationality, and competence

4. Analyze a situation to determine whether a patient is competent or incompetent

Competence to consent to or refuse treatment is a central concept in U.S. health law and bioethics. It is widely believed that a patient must be fully competent before his consent or refusal is valid. However, despite the wide acceptance of the central role that competence plays in the consent process, there is disagreement not only about how the term should be defined but also about its application to particular cases.

If a patient is judged to be competent to make health care decisions, then, at least in general, her consent to or refusal of a suggested medical intervention is acceded to. If she has been given adequate information about the proposed intervention and no coercion has been employed during the consent process, her consent or refusal is judged to be valid and therefore determinative. It is regarded as legally sanctioned and ethically justified for the physician or other health care professional to proceed with a medical intervention in the presence of a valid consent. However, it is not generally regarded as legally sanctioned or ethically justified to carry out an intervention on a patient who has made a valid refusal. By contrast, if a patient is judged to be incompetent to consent, then, except in emergency situations, a physician or other health care professional should not carry out an intervention even if the patient has agreed to it; rather, some form of surrogate consent should be obtained. Similarly, if a patient who refuses an intervention is judged to be incompetent to refuse, then under some circumstances it is thought to be justified to carry out the intervention nonetheless.

Many definitions of competence have been proposed. Although there is a high degree of agreement among them in how they would classify a random sample of competent and incompetent patients, there are some significant disagreements. Furthermore, these concordant classifications correlate strongly with most persons' intuitions about whether a particular patient's consent or refusal should be acceded to or not. The difficult philosophical problem is to provide an account of competence that will accord with most people's considered judgments about when patients' consents or refusals should be accepted or overruled. In addition to providing a definition of competence, it is also important to provide the criteria by which, in particular cases, its relative presence or absence should be determined.[1]

The Logic of Competence

Before examining various definitions of competence, it is helpful to review some universally agreed upon features of how the term should be used. Persons are often referred to as *competent* or *incompetent*, but this is a somewhat misleading shorthand locution. Competence is task specific: a person is competent or incompetent to make a will, to perform a neurologic examination, or to refuse a suggested medical intervention. It does not follow from the fact that if a person is competent to do X that he is competent to do Y. For example, a somewhat confused man may be competent to eat his breakfast by himself or to tie his shoelaces, but not competent to make a decision about having a radical prostatectomy. A person may even be competent to consent to a rather simple medical intervention (applying a bandage to a cut finger), but not competent to consent to an intervention with a complex spectrum of risks and benefits spread out over time (having a carotid endarterectomy for transient ischemic attacks). No one is competent to do everything, although some persons (the totally unconscious) are not competent to do anything. Saying that a person is *competent* is always shorthand for *competent to do X*.

In discussing the competence that is a necessary requirement for valid consent or refusal, it is crucial to have a clear and precise account of the task that a patient must be competent to perform. The standard way of describing this task is to say that the patient must be competent to consent to or refuse a medical intervention. However, this way of describing the task is ambiguous in important ways. This ambiguity is responsible for the different definitions of competence that have been proposed. As we shall see later, specifying the task in an unambiguous way leads to a more adequate account of competence and also makes clear what criteria should be used to determine whether the patient is competent to perform that task.

Defining Competence to Consent or Refuse

The "Understand and Appreciate" Definition

Various definitions of competence have much in common, but they differ in significant ways. Thus, it is possible, although it seldom happens, for a patient to be competent on one definition but incompetent on another. One thing all definitions have in common is the stipulation that one necessary element of competence be that the patient must understand the factual information she has been given that is relevant to the decision that she is being asked to make. If a patient has been given adequate information in a language that she speaks and in terms that most speakers of that language would understand, but cannot understand what she has been told (because, for example, she is significantly retarded, or because she is suffering from cognitive confusion secondary to a moderate degree of delirium), then even if she does consent or refuse, she is not regarded as competent to make that decision. Valid consents or refusals require understanding, and if a patient does not adequately understand, then one necessary condition of competence has not been satisfied.

Understanding refers to whether a patient has adequately carried out a certain kind of mental process but says nothing about the content of the decision (that is, the consent or the refusal) that the patient actually goes on to make. What is at issue is limited to whether the patient has understood whatever (adequate) information he has been given.

Appreciation refers to whether a patient has adequately carried out another kind of mental process. It concerns more than the patient understanding the information given to her; it requires that she appreciate that the information she has understood is indeed applicable to her at this given point in time. But, like understanding, appreciation says nothing about the content of the decision. One reason a criterion of appreciation has been specified in addition to a criterion of understanding is that on rare occasions patients have delusions that impinge on the consent process and that affect a patient's appreciation but not her understanding. A patient, for example, can fully understand the risks that a suggested intervention carries but also believe that he is Superman and that no harm can befall him. If he consents to a risky procedure with the false belief that he cannot be harmed by it because he is Superman, then it is plausible to say he is not competent to consent because, although he knows the risks, he falsely believes they do not apply to him. *Appreciation* could in fact be regarded as a particular kind of understanding—one could say that *understand* means to understand both the nature of an intervention's risks and benefits and also to understand that they do indeed apply to oneself in the current situation—but usually it is listed as a separate criterion.

Understanding and appreciating are frequently combined into a single "understand and appreciate" (U+A) criterion. It is possible to define competence to consent or refuse using these two formal criteria alone. We call this a *pure U+A* definition. An important feature of defining competence in this way, which is seen by many as its particular strength, is that the patient's actual decision does not enter into the determination of competence. Competence, as defined by U+A criteria, can in theory, and frequently in practice, be determined before knowing whether the patient will consent to or refuse treatment. If the patient understands the (adequate) information she has been given, and appreciates that indeed it applies to her in the current situation, then she is competent, and, absent coercion, whatever decision she makes is determinative and should be respected.[2]

There are advantages to the pure U+A definition of competence that may in part explain its popularity. First, it fits well with the goal that many have of allowing competent patients to make any decision they want. Second, the determination of whether a patient understands and appreciates information is usually relatively easy to make (there are inevitable borderline cases) and can be investigated by briefly quizzing the patient about the content and the pertinence of what he has just been told. If the patient does understand and appreciate, then the physician can simply let the patient decide and behave accordingly. It may seem far more difficult and less objective to determine whether a patient's decision is autonomous or irrational or authentic or to apply some other concept of that ilk (see later in this chapter).

The Inadequacy of the Pure U+A Definition

The problem with the pure U+A definition is that it sometimes gives a result that is so counterintuitive that no responsible physician would act on it. Case 7-A is an example.

Case 7-A

An elderly depressed woman is refractory to antidepressant drug treatment and has lost a significant amount of weight. She is very frightened about the prospect of having electroconvulsive treatment (ECT) and cannot bring herself to consent to the procedure, either verbally or in writing. She does not disagree with her doctor's opinion that she may die without ECT, and she acknowledges that ECT would likely prevent her death, but she still cannot bring herself to consent. She did consent to have ECT when she was similarly depressed several years ago, and she remembers that ECT rather quickly alleviated her depression. She was similarly frightened of ECT on this earlier occasion, but her husband somehow convinced her to consent to the procedure. Her husband is no longer living, and her two grown sons, although they very much want their mother to have ECT, have been thoroughly unsuccessful in influencing her to consent. She understands and appreciates everything her doctor has told her and disagrees with none of it, but she has an irrational fear that prevents her from consenting to ECT.[3]

This patient clearly satisfies the U+A definition of competence.[4] Her refusal to consent was not based on any lack of ability to understand or appreciate information; it was based on the strong irrational fear that she had of the ECT procedure. And yet essentially everyone familiar with this case believed the patient should be given ECT.

Case 7-B provides another example.

Case 7-B

A severely depressed man, weakened by a cardiac disorder, refuses lifesaving treatment for his eminently treatable and potentially reversible cardiac condition. Unlike some depressed patients, he manifests no cognitive delusions or distortions: he understands the relevant information about the likely sequelae of treatment versus nontreatment and appreciates that they apply to him. He refuses all treatments and also nutrition and hydration because he wants to die. He gives, and apparently has, no reason to refuse other than his wish to die, and there is no reason to think his life would not be satisfactory and enjoyable to him if he were to recover from his current condition. The only explanation for his refusal is that he is severely depressed.[3]

This patient also satisfies the U+A definition of competence: he understands and appreciates all of the facts about his situation. His overwhelming desire is to die, and all of his actions (refusing cardiac treatment and refusing nutrition and hydration) are logically consistent with his goal of satisfying his desire to die.

The Irrationality of a Patient's Decision

The woman in Case 7-A suffers from a seriously irrational fear of ECT treatment, and the man in Case 7-B has a seriously irrational desire to die.[5] Most health care professionals (HCPs) believe that these patients' refusals should be overruled. However, if only incompetent patients' refusals can be overruled and if the formal U+A criteria are used strictly and exclusively to define competence, then these patients are both competent to refuse, and the irrationality of their actual choices can play no role in determining their competence.

The U+A definition usually yields a result that coincides with HCPs' judgments about which patients' refusals should be overruled, because people who make seriously irrational treatment refusals usually do so because they do not adequately understand and appreciate the facts about their situation. However, sometimes refusals are made because of irrational fears or irrational desires. Patients like the two just described can irrationally refuse treatment even though they do understand and appreciate all of the relevant information. Irrational fears (phobias) and irrational desires do not always cause the kinds of cognitive distortions that the U+A definition stipulates as the only features that make a person incompetent. If only the refusal of incompetent patients can be overruled, the U+A definition does not allow overruling the patients in Cases 7-A and 7-B. Because the primary point of determining competence is to prevent overruling patients whose decisions should not be overruled but to allow overruling patients whose decisions should be overruled, it is not sufficient for the criteria defining competence to work just part of the time; they must work in every case.

Thus, a dilemma exists. If competent patients can make any treatment decision they want, no matter how irrational, without interference, then competence cannot be defined solely by the use of the formal criteria of understanding and appreciation. As long as whatever formal criteria invoked to define competence do not specify anything about the content of the patient's actual decision, they will allow for cases in which the definition is satisfied even though the patient makes such a seriously irrational decision that nearly everyone would favor overruling the patient.[6,7] It appears that both U+A criteria and the rationality or irrationality of the patient's decision play some role in judgments about competence, and that these two criteria operate to some extent independently.

However, there is a justifiable concern about allowing the rationality or irrationality of the patient's decision to play any role in judgments about competence. Irrationality is often defined in such a way that any decision that deviates from the preferred decision of the HCP is labeled as irrational. When *irrational* is used in this way, the freedom of otherwise competent patients to make their own decisions about whether to accept or reject a proposed treatment is lost. However, if *rational* is used to mean *not irrational*, and no decision is regarded as irrational unless (1) it would result in the patient suffering significant harm for a reason that almost no one with similar knowledge and intelligence would regard as adequate for suffering that harm, and (2) persisting in that decision would result in the person satisfying the definition for having a mental disorder, then the freedom that would be lost is not a freedom that any rational person would want to have.[8]

Modifying the Understand-and-Appreciate Definition of Competence

There are at least three ways in which the criteria discussed previously can be combined to create a definition of competence. The first approach (A) has been discussed: competence can be defined exclusively by U+A (or other formal) criteria. However, within this first approach there are two opposing views about the role of U+A competence in determining whether to overrule a patient's decision. The first view (A1) is to claim that competence defined in this way is determinative: if the patient consents, proceed with the intervention; if the patient refuses, do not proceed with the intervention. Thus, according to this view, the patients described in Cases 7-A and 7-B would both be regarded as competent and therefore would not be treated. Someone who held this view might acknowledge that most persons' intuitions would favor overruling the refusals in cases like these. However, the argument could be made by exponents of this view that it is better in the long run to give everyone unbridled freedom of choice, even if, as a result, some persons make seriously irrational decisions that cause them great harm.

The second position (A2) that can be taken is that although competence should be defined exclusively by understanding and appreciation, and that a finding of competence generally justifies acceding to a patient's decision, the irrationality of the patient's decision should sometimes play an important role in determining whether to override that decision. The claim is that it is ethically justified to overrule the seriously irrational decision of a competent patient.[9] This approach has the advantage of being more congruent with people's widespread intuitions about whether to overrule in actual cases. For example, the patients in Cases 7-A and 7-B would be labeled as competent, but their refusals would be regarded as seriously irrational, and on the basis of that serious irrationality it would be ethically justified to overrule them.[10] The disadvantage of this approach is that the notion of sometimes overruling a competent patient is at variance with the U.S. legal tradition that competent patients' decisions should never be overruled.[11]

A different position (B) that can be taken is to change the definition of competence so that it is no longer defined exclusively in U+A terms. Several theorists have suggested that the definition of competence be plastic and shifting so that it varies with the kind of clinical situation the patient is in.[12] Thus, if a suggested intervention holds the promise of only limited benefit and limited risk (i.e., nothing of great moment is at stake), a patient might be deemed competent to consent or refuse simply on the basis of expressing a choice (a formal criterion). The rationality of a refusal in this situation would not be a factor in determining competence. Even if a patient's refusal was thought to be mildly irrational (i.e., only minor harm would be suffered), he would be deemed competent to refuse. On the other hand, in a clinical situation in which a patient was refusing life-sustaining treatment, it would be necessary for the patient's refusal to be rational for the patient to be deemed competent.

This shifting-definition approach has problems. It is odd to have a key theoretical term change its very meaning from situation to situation. More important, it leads to strange results. For example, two doctors can disagree about the seriousness of a patient's condition because they have a reasonable disagreement about the patient's underlying diagnosis. The patient firmly refuses further diagnostic tests but refuses to discuss his reasons for doing so. One doctor believes the malady from which the patient is suffering is minor and that there is no urgency to conduct additional diagnostic tests unless the clinical situation changes. The other doctor believes it is more probable than not that the patient is suffering from a serious occult disorder and that further tests might be clarifying and even lifesaving. Under the shifting-definition approach, the first doctor could claim that the patient was competent to refuse and the second doctor could claim that the patient was not competent to refuse. The two doctors' disagreement about competence would stem from the differing diagnostic inferences they have made based on the signs and symptoms they observe. However, if *competence* is a mental attribute of persons, which most theorists believe, then changes in competence should vary only with changes in the mental characteristics of the person, not with changes in the person's physical condition. The diagnostic disagreements between the two physicians should be irrelevant in determining the competence of the patient.[13]

Any account of irrationality to be incorporated into the concept of competence must be such that no decision is regarded as irrational if any significant number of persons would regard that decision as rational. All irrational decisions must be such that they would result in the patient suffering significant harm for a reason that almost no one with similar knowledge and intelligence would regard as adequate for suffering that harm. This means that no decision based on religious beliefs that are held by any significant number of people will be irrational. The only irrational decisions are those that would be persisted in by people because of a mental disorder.

Symmetry and Asymmetry of Consents and Refusals

Suppose a patient at a given time consents to a suggested intervention. Using a particular definition of competence, she is judged to be competent to consent. Now suppose nothing about her situation is altered, but after further reflection she changes her mind and refuses the intervention. Is she, automatically, to be judged competent to refuse? Different definitions of competence yield different answers to that question. Under the strict U+A definition, there is a symmetry between consent and refusal. Because competence is judged on the basis of understanding and appreciation and not on the basis of the content of the patient's decision, if the patient is competent to decide in one way, then unless her understanding and appreciation is somehow altered in the interim, she is competent to decide in the other. For example, on the strict U+A definition, the patients in Cases 7-A and 7-B would be judged competent no matter whether they consented to or refused treatment. However, with definition B, if these patients changed their minds and consented to treatment they would be considered competent, but if they refused they would be considered incompetent. Thus there is an asymmetry between consent and refusal.

If a definition of competence makes it possible to always determine whether a patient is competent before the patient's actual decision to consent or refuse is known, then there is symmetry and the definition is one in which understanding and appreciation are determinative. If a definition of competence allows the patient's actual decision to consent or refuse to sometimes determine whether a patient is competent, then there is asymmetry, and irrationality (or some similar normative term) is, in one way or another, being included in the definition of competence. An important question to ask of any definition of competence is whether a patient's competence can be determined before knowing whether the patient has consented or refused.

Competence as the Ability to Make a Rational Decision

If the task that a patient must be competent to perform is described as consenting to or refusing a medical intervention—that is, deciding whether to consent or refuse—then it seems as if there should be symmetry. However, as pointed out earlier, this way of describing the task is ambiguous in important ways. It is not clear what counts as being competent to consent or refuse. Although it is irrational, people often decide to do something without having any information about the consequences of their decision, so it is not clear why everyone agrees that understanding and appreciating the relevant information is necessary for being competent to decide whether to consent to or refuse a medical intervention.

Reflecting on the fact that people do make irrational decisions makes it clear that the task that a patient must be competent to perform is that of making a rational decision about a proposed medical intervention. Thus, we define the competence required for valid consent or refusal as follows: *competence is the ability to make a rational decision.* We noted earlier that competence was task specific. This definition makes clear what the task is: to make a rational decision about the medical intervention being proposed. Thus, competence and rationality should not be defined independently of one another as has been done in the past, but rather should be linked in the way the preceding definition indicates.

Several conditions can take away a person's ability to make a rational decision. Among them are the following:

a. A cognitive disability that prevents the person from understanding the information relevant to making a decision of a certain kind. In the case of medical treatment decisions, this would be the lack of ability to understand the *adequate information* given during the consent process.

b. A cognitive disability that prevents appreciating that the relevant information in (a) does indeed apply to one in one's current situation. The case of Superman, described earlier, is an example of this situation. Superman might well consent to a risky treatment that he would refuse if he did not have the false belief that the risks involved could not happen to him.

c. A cognitive disability that prevents coordinating the information in (a) with the patient's personal rational ranking of the various goods and harms associated with the various available options, insofar as these rankings are relevant.

d. The presence of a mental disorder, such as a mood disorder or a volitional disability, that causes one to make irrational decisions.[14]

If either (a), (b), (c), or (d) is present, then the person lacks the ability to make a rational decision of the particular kind involved, which is to say that she is not competent to make a rational decision of that kind. Thus, the ability to make a rational decision has intellectual, affective, and volitional components.

Each of these four factors may by itself take away a patient's ability to make a particular kind of rational decision. We think this list is exhaustive and thus the absence of all four factors is sufficient to ensure that the patient is competent to make a rational decision of the kind involved. However, more than one of the factors may be present in the incompetent patient. For example, a person may suffer from a delirium that renders him unable to understand the relevant information and also be sufficiently depressed that he would be unable to make a rational decision even if he understood the relevant information.

The vast majority of patients who make irrational treatment decisions are not competent to make rational decisions of the kind involved. Consider a middle-aged man who refuses to have an appendectomy for his acute appendicitis, even though his appendix is in danger of rupturing and causing a possibly fatal peritonitis. It almost always is the case that patients of this kind (1) do not have the cognitive ability to understand the situation, or (2) do not have the volitional ability to consent because of, say, a fear of general anesthesia, or (3) are so depressed because of their situation that, despite their accurate cognitive understanding, they do not have the ability to make this kind of rational decision. Thus, this man will almost certainly be found, correctly, to be incompetent to refuse surgery. Seriously irrational decisions are seldom made by persons who have the ability to make rational decisions of the kind involved, and they are never persisted in unless the person is not competent to make that kind of decision.

However, less seriously irrational decisions are sometimes made by patients who have the ability to make rational decisions. Consider a man who has a wart on the sole of his foot. He is suffering from mild to moderate chronic pain and disability; that is, he limps. The condition can almost always be totally reversed by one or another podiatric procedure, such as blunt excision, that causes only mild brief pain and is nearly risk free. Nonetheless this man suffers from the condition for weeks or months, despite his accurate knowledge of these facts, despite having no adequate reason for delaying treatment, and despite having no mental disorder that interferes with his ability to choose rationally. Thus we could say of him that he is competent, that he has the ability to choose rationally, but that he has made an irrational choice.

Different definitions of competence vary in the way in which they articulate the concepts of competence and rationality. The pure U+A definition of competence sharply distinguishes between competence to make a decision to consent to or refuse a proposed intervention and the rationality or irrationality of the decision made. By contrast, definition B includes rationality or irrationality as a sometimes-important constituent of the definition of competence. Definition B specifies that treatment refusals in high-risk clinical situations must be rational before the person can be regarded as competent to make them, but the definition does not require rational decisions in less risky settings in order to classify patients as competent. Definition C specifies that a person is competent to make a particular medical decision if and only if she has the ability to make a rational decision of the particular kind involved. Being able to make a rational decision of a particular kind has constituent cognitive, volitional, and affective components.

Incorporating the rationality or irrationality of the patient's decision into the account of competence helps bridge the gap that has developed between the specified justifications for two morally similar procedures: overruling patient refusals of medical interventions, and involuntarily committing persons who are deemed dangerous to themselves or others. In most states a person can be involuntarily committed if he is suffering from a mental illness that makes him dangerous to himself or to others. There is no mention of competence, defined as understanding and appreciation or in any other way, in most states' statutory criteria for commitment. The concern is solely with the probability of the person's acting dangerously because of a mental disorder. Acting in that way is exactly what we regard as acting in a seriously irrational way. A sufficient condition for incompetence should be the irrational refusal of a medical intervention because of a mental disorder.

Advantages of Definition C

Definition C has several advantages. First, everyone agrees that competence is task specific, but definition C provides the first explicit statement of the kind of task that competent patients must be able to perform. Defining competence as the ability to make a rational decision explains the common intuition that a high degree of irrationality is a major factor in determining incompetence. By continuing to distinguish between the competence of the patient and the rationality of a particular decision, this definition makes clear that determining incompetence and justifying paternalistic interventions are separate and distinct. Incompetence is not determined by the seriousness of a patient's situation, but the justification for overruling a refusal is. Approaches that simply sort patients into two groups, the competent and the incompetent, seem to consider that no further justification is needed to overrule the refusals of incompetent patients.

Second, unlike the view that irrational decisions of competent patients can be overruled, this definition is consistent with the legal tradition. On definition C, all persons who persist in making seriously irrational decisions are correctly regarded as incompetent.

Third, although we define competence as the ability to make a rational decision, the incompetence of a person to make a kind of rational decision is never determined simply by the irrationality of her decision in the present case. A person is competent to make a rational decision only if both of the following are true: (1) she does not have a cognitive disability preventing her from understanding and appreciating the relevant information or coordinating that information with her own stable values, and (2) she does not have a mental disorder that takes away her ability to make a rational decision. If none of these disabilities, including having a relevant mental disorder, is present, she is competent to make a rational decision, even if she is presently making an irrational decision. Of course, persisting in a seriously irrational decision would show that the person has a mental disorder that takes away her ability to make a rational decision and hence that she is incompetent to make that kind of decision. However, if, for example, a person overcomes a volitional disability that prevents her from consenting to ECT, and consents, then she is competent to make that kind of decision.

The ability to make a rational decision of a certain kind is what people should have had in mind when they accorded competence the primacy it has in the consent process. They did not realize that bare-boned understanding and appreciation of the information presented could exist in the presence of mental disorders that take away from people the ability to make a rational decision of a certain kind. Definition C simply makes explicit what most people already hold. It is understandable that understanding and appreciation were initially selected as criteria for competency: they are fairly easily assessed and they usually do agree with our intuitions about particular cases. This is because the overwhelming majority of patients who lack the ability to make a kind of rational decision lack it because they do not understand and appreciate the relevant information. However, Cases such as 7-A and 7-B force us to realize that understanding and appreciation do not capture the full meaning of the concept of competence as the ability to make a rational decision.

Definition C provides the correct account of the relationship between understanding and appreciation, the rationality or irrationality of the patient's treatment choice, and the concept of competence as an essential feature of valid consent. Neither understanding and appreciation, by itself, nor the rationality or irrationality of the patient's decision, by itself, provides an adequate explanation of the meaning of competence. Combining the two provides a definition of competence that (1) accords with most persons' intuitions about what should be done in particular cases, (2) is linked with a coherent theory about the paternalistic justification for overruling some patients' treatment decisions, and (3) is consistent with the prevailing legal account of the role of competence in valid consent.

Chapter Summary

Competence to consent to or refuse treatment is a central concept in U.S. health law and bioethics, because it is widely believed that a patient must be fully competent before his consent or refusal is valid and because of the principle that the refusal of a competent patient should not be overruled. Competence is task specific: it does not follow from the fact that if a person is competent to do X that the person is competent to do Y. Traditionally, competence has been defined as the ability to understand and appreciate the information given during the consent process (the U+A definition). Unfortunately, there are cases in which a patient who is competent according to the U+A definition irrationally refuses a treatment that almost everyone believes should be administered over his objection. In such cases, the U+A definition forces us to choose between treating the apparently competent patient against his wishes or counterintuitively honoring his irrational wishes.

Defining competence instead as the ability to make a *rational* decision explains both the importance of understanding and appreciation as well as the common intuition that a high degree of irrationality is a major factor in determining incompetence. The ability to make rational decisions has cognitive, volitional, and affective components. A person is competent to make a rational decision only if (1) she does not have a cognitive disability preventing her from understanding and appreciating the relevant information or coordinating that information with her own stable values, and (2) she does not have a mental disorder that takes away her ability to make a rational decision. If none of these disabilities is present, she is competent to make a rational decision, even if she is presently making an irrational decision.

Review Questions

1. Why is competence of ethical importance?

2. How do the terms *understanding* and *appreciation* relate to competence? What is the U+A definition of competence? What are some of its strengths? Its weaknesses?

3. Define *rationality* and *irrationality*. What is the relationship between rationality and competence? Between irrationality and incompetence?

4. When, if ever, is it permissible to disregard a patient's consent to treatment or refusal of treatment?

Endnotes

1. Byron Chell frames the definitional issue similarly: "The trick is to define [competency] so that it helps us do the job that needs to be done. The job in this context is to make decisions involving decision making. We must decide whether or not we will allow the patient to decide. Thus, what are the proper considerations we must keep in mind in making decisions? What criteria should be reflected in a proper definition?" See Chell B. Competency: what it is, what it isn't, and why it matters. In: Monagle JF, Thomasma DC, eds. *Health Care Ethics: Critical Issues for the 21st Century*. Gaithersburg, MD: Aspen, 1998:117–127.

2. Dame Elizabeth Butler-Sloss apparently holds such a position. In a highly publicized case in England, this presiding judge wrote, quoting her own words in an earlier case, "A mentally competent patient has an absolute right to refuse to consent to medical treatment for any reason, rational or irrational, or for no reason at all." See Butler-Sloss E. *Ms B and an NHS Hospital Trust*. 2002 EWHC 429 (Fam) in the High Court of Justice, Family Division.

3. Gert B, Culver CM, Clouser KD. *Bioethics: A Systematic Approach*. 2nd ed. New York: Oxford, 2006:222.

4. In fact, the state in which she was hospitalized (New Hampshire) had a statutory definition of competence that explicitly defined competence in terms of understanding and appreciating, just as these criteria have been defined here. Lawyers who were familiar with the case were of the opinion that the patient should probably be classified as competent to refuse by New Hampshire standards.

5. See Gert B. *Morality: Its Nature and Justification*. Rev. ed. New York: Oxford, 2005, or Gert, Culver, and Clouser, *Bioethics*, for a discussion of irrational fears and irrational desires.

6. Normative terms other than *irrational* could be used, such as *pointless, needlessly harmful, dangerous,* and so forth. We prefer the term *irrational* because its definition has been carefully elaborated. (See Gert, Culver, and Clouser, *Bioethics*.)

7. Other formal criteria could be suggested. "Expressing a choice" is sometimes mentioned (see, e.g., Grisso T, Appelbaum PS. *Assessing Competence to Consent to Treatment*. New York: Oxford, 1998). A patient, for example, might be able to understand and appreciate the relevant information but for some neurologic or psychological reason be unable to express his choice in any way, and therefore understandably be deemed "incompetent to consent or refuse." Another formal criterion sometimes mentioned is the patient's ability to reason logically in justifying

her consent or refusal in terms of her general goals. However, all formal criteria have the same problem: it is possible for a patient to satisfy them and yet make a seriously irrational decision that most observers would feel should be overridden. For example, a seriously depressed patient's most important general and overriding goal may be to die, and thus his refusal of treatment would be a logical extension of his goal.

8. For a full discussion of the definition of mental disorder, see Gert, Culver, and Clouser, "Mental Disorders," in *Bioethics*, pp. 165–190.

9. This is a position that was put forward by Culver and Gert in Culver CM, Gert B. *Philosophy in Medicine.* New York: Oxford, 1982.

10. See Culver and Gert, *Philosophy in Medicine*, for a full explanation of the conditions under which irrational decisions can be paternalistically overruled.

11. That legal tradition itself seems vague and confused, however. See Culver CM, Gert B. The inadequacy of incompetence. *Milbank Q* 1990;68:619–643, pp. 641–642.

12. This position has been advocated by a number of authors. See, for example, Roth LH, Meisel A, Lidz CW. Tests of competency to consent to treatment. *Am J Psychiatry* 1977;134:279-284; Drane J. The many faces of competency. *Hastings Center Rep* 1985;1517–21; and Buchanan AB, Brock DW. *Deciding for Others: The Ethics of Surrogate Decision-Making.* New York: Cambridge University Press, 1989.

13. For a lengthier analysis of shifting-definition approaches, see Culver and Gert, "The inadequacy of incompetence," pp. 632–639.

14. Volitional disabilities are conditions such as addictions and phobias that can interfere with a person's ability to make a rational decision. For example, a patient with a phobia about needles might not be able to consent to have her blood drawn even if she herself acknowledges that it is irrational not to consent to such a low-risk diagnostic intervention. The woman in Case 7-A who dreaded ECT so strongly that she was not able to consent to the one treatment that would probably save her life was suffering from a similar malady and would be judged incompetent on this definition of competence.

Chapter 8

Informed Consent I

At the heart of that Western freedom and democracy is the belief that the individual man, the child of God, is the touchstone of value, and all society, groups, the state, exist for his benefit. Therefore the enlargement of liberty for individual human beings must be the supreme goal and the abiding practice of any Western society.

—Robert F. Kennedy

Chapter Learning Objectives
At the conclusion of this chapter the reader will be able to:

1. Define *informed consent*

2. Apply the principles of medical ethics to the process of informed consent

3. Distinguish between *consent* and *informed consent*

4. Discuss landmark cases that contributed to the development of the contemporary process of informed consent in medical care as well as in research

5. Discuss the historical impact of unethical research that was conducted in Nazi Germany, as well as in the United States, on the development of national and international codes of research ethics

6. List the exceptions to obtaining informed consent

Whereas the parameters of the patient–health care professional relationship are regulated by the principles of medical ethics, informed consent is the practical application of the principle of autonomy, or the person's right to self-determination over his or her own body.[1] There are philosophical as well as legal bases for the development of what is referred to as the *doctrine of informed consent*. The philosophical bases are rooted in ancient Greek philosophy, and the practical bases originated in cases that were litigated during the twentieth century in the United States. This chapter addresses the process of informed consent as it is applied in Western cultures, but more specifically in American medical and research practice. Western norms differ from country to country and from one culture to another; therefore, medical practitioners and researchers must familiarize themselves with the local norms and laws that govern their practice. This chapter outlines the philosophical and legal bases for requiring informed consent that make up the morally valid medical decision-making paradigm.[2,3]

Competent adults have the right to make their own health care decisions under the United States' constitutionally protected right of privacy. This right is grounded in the philosophical principle of autonomy. The practical application of this principle takes the form of informed consent. In addition to the protection afforded by the Constitution, the court system has upheld the right of individuals to make their own health care decisions.[4]

The cases cited in this chapter trace the development of the doctrine of informed consent and give a historical perspective on how case law was pivotal in the way in which this decision-making approach evolved. The process of obtaining informed consent before embarking on the provision of medical care or the conduct of research is rooted in ancient philosophy as well as case law.

The Principles of Medical Ethics

The principles of medical ethics have been central to the code of ethics in medical care, and have been recognized for centuries as major components of trust in the health care professional–patient relationship. As medical research on human subjects has become the basis for developing new treatments and interventions for the prevention and treatment of disease, the health care professional–patient relationship has been a focal area of ethical concern. Conducting research on human subjects has created an inherent conflict of interest for health care professionals who conduct research, and threatened their relationship with their patients. The conflict of interest results from the discrepancy between the goal of health care professionals, namely, to do what is in the best interests of their patients, and the goal of research, which is to develop and test hypotheses and to collect data points to generate generalizable knowledge. Stated otherwise, medical care is for the purpose of benefiting the individual patient, whereas research is conducted for the purpose of benefiting populations.[5] However, the ethical principles that regulate the relationship between health care professional and patient, regardless of context, remain unchanged.

Conflict of physician interest was pronounced in many research projects, such as the Nazi medical experiments conducted by German physicians during World War II and the Tuskegee study for the treatment of syphilis in Tuskegee, Alabama, in the United States (under the auspices of the Public Health Service, the predecessor of the contemporary Centers for Disease Control and Prevention).[6] Although these projects are merely two examples of abuses committed by health care professionals while conducting research, many other research abuses have been thoroughly documented in the published literature.

Beauchamp and Childress identified the four principles of medical ethics as autonomy, beneficence, nonmaleficence, and justice.[7] Whereas Beauchamp and Childress list veracity as a "rule" of ethics,[7(p39)] Perlin[8] prominently lists veracity as a fifth core principle of medical ethics, without which the original four principles would be without much merit. *Veracity* is defined as "truth-telling: the basis of promise-keeping and other fiduciary relationships; the premise of an open health care professional-patient relationship."[8(p10)] Without having access to the (known) truth, people cannot make informed decisions, thereby nullifying the principle of autonomy, a cornerstone of the informed consent process of decision making.

Autonomy

The term *autonomy* is rooted in Greek culture and philosophy and was first developed to describe the rights of cities and states to self-govern. The term was later extended to the right of individuals to privacy and individual choice over what happens to their bodies based on their own values. The basis of this principle is that individuals have the freedom to act in ways that are consistent with their own beliefs, provided that such freedom does not interfere with others' free will.[7] This principle is therefore not absolute; it is limited if exercising one's autonomy interferes with the rights of others to exercise theirs. Autonomous decision making is particularly valued in Western culture and is routinely referred to in the United States as the basis of informed consent to consent to or to refuse medical care as well as to participate or not in research.

Research has documented some cultural groups' preferences for what is referred to as a "family-centered model" of decision making. This model advocates giving people a choice of whether to exercise their right to make their own health care decisions or to defer to members of their social milieu to make decisions for them.[9] Beauchamp and Childress still view this model of decision making as autonomous because members of these cultural groups are freely choosing to defer their right to decide to others.[7] They view the exercise of autonomy as the "right" to choose, rather than the "duty" to choose. Individual state informed consent laws and institutional legal counsel may prohibit deferral (by adult competent individuals) to others for consenting to medical or research procedures, or both; therefore, medical practitioners and researchers must consult their own state laws to resolve the conflict between the American standard of an individual-based decision making model and this cultural-diversity-based extended model of autonomous decision making.

Autonomous decision making can be exercised only by individuals who have reached the age of majority (18 and older) and those whose decisional capacity is intact. Parents and legal guardians exercise the right to autonomy on behalf of minor children, and decisions for incapacitated individuals are made by proxy decision makers, usually the legal next of kin as identified by state law, or by individuals who are appointed through legal procedures. Although complete autonomy in decision making is not practical because people consult others and are subject to being influenced by them, choices are considered autonomous when the choice is intentionally exercised, when there is understanding of the choice, and when the choice is not coerced by others.[7]

Beneficence

Generally acting in ways that benefit others is a moral obligation, although specific acts of beneficence are not necessarily obligatory. People are not obligated to help others in any one particular situation, particularly if helping places them in danger, but acting in helpful ways toward others exemplifies the principle of *beneficence*. This principle is frequently the motivating factor influencing health care providers in their work with individuals with whom they come in contact in the context of their professional activities. Beneficent acts are acts of kindness, mercy, charity, altruism, love, and humanity. These acts also include protecting and defending the rights of others, preventing harm from occurring to others, helping the disabled, and rescuing individuals who are in danger.[7]

One undesirable outcome of pure beneficence is *paternalism*. There is an inherent conflict between the health care professional's sense of moral obligation to help others, and the principle of respecting others' right to make their own health care decisions. As the informed consent laws delineate health care professionals' obligation to respect their patients' rights to autonomous decision making, acts of beneficence (by health care professionals) must yield to respecting autonomous decision making. Deference to autonomy reflects the American legal and clinical practice of obtaining informed consent before medical procedures and interventions are initiated, although this approach is not without its critics.

Nonmaleficence

Whereas beneficence is exemplified by actions, *nonmaleficence* is more passive. This ethical principle dictates the obligation "not to inflict harm on others."[7(p113)] This principle is often associated with the Hippocratic edict, but it is in fact inferred from other passages rather than a reflection of a literal translation of any part of the traditional oath recited by physicians. Some philosophers rank nonmaleficence as a higher principle than beneficence, because it is more important to avoid inflicting harm on others than it is to do good deeds. However, there is a need to balance the risk, burden, or harm imposed by the deed versus the benefit that could be gained from it. An example is in a comparison of the harm of swelling that is caused by injecting medication via a needle in a person's arm versus the benefit that will result from the patient receiving the injected medication or vaccine. In this case, the beneficent act (receiving benefit from the medication) ranks higher than the maleficent act (swelling)—thereby ranking beneficence higher than nonmaleficence in this case.[7]

The balance between beneficence and nonmaleficence in the context of research is addressed by the Belmont Report, which argues that the goal of doing no harm can only be reached by learning what is harmful. Research on human subjects is justified by the assertion that knowledge of whether the benefits outweigh the harms can only be achieved through experimentation that involves human subjects.[10]

Justice

The fourth and last ethical principle is *justice*. In the context of medical care, this principle is labeled *distributive justice* because it addresses the fair and just distribution, by some system, of beneficial scarce resources, such as organs that are available for transplantation "to each person an equal share; to each person according to need; to each person according to effort; to each person according to contribution; to each person according to merit; to each person according to free-market exchanges."[7(p228)] However, justice in research refers at least in part to the just distribution of the *burden* of research in an effort to avoid exploiting some individuals (research participants) to benefit the general population. In an effort to ensure that justice is served in research, the burden (and ultimate benefit) of participating should be distributed among all potential beneficiaries, including women, children, and older adults. Those who benefit from the results of research should also share the burden of participating in the development of the science leading to the desired results.[10] Historical examples of exploitation of some classes to benefit others include experimentation on the poor in public institutions to benefit those who have private funding (the rich); prisoners without their consent (in Germany as well as in the United States), including the Nazi experiments in concentration camps;[11] the Tuskegee study of untreated syphilis in the United States; and many others.[12]

The awareness of the need to obtain informed consent from patients receiving medical interventions as well as from subjects participating in research, developed simultaneously, although for different reasons. In medical intervention, informed consent was developed to ensure that patients participated in the decisions affecting their own fate, whereas informed consent to participate in research was developed to protect human subjects from the actions of unscrupulous researchers.

Historical Medical Cases Leading to Informed Consent

Among the many informed consent cases resulting in court decisions that helped to shape current methods of medical decision making, Devettere[12] cites the following four landmark cases: *Schloendorff* (1914),[13] *Salgo* (1957),[14] *Canterbury* (1972),[15] and *Candura* (1978).[16] Faden and Beauchamp[2] cite a fifth case, that of *Natanson* (1960).[17] Each of the five cases is described in this section to illustrate its unique incremental contributions to the contemporary doctrine of informed consent.

Schloendorff (1914)

This landmark case is widely cited because for the first time in documented medical history, a judge (Justice Cardozo) established a patient's right to give voluntary consent to medical intervention. Mrs. Mary E. Schloendorff agreed to have her physician examine her under anesthesia to determine whether a diagnosed fibroid tumor was malignant. She specified that she was not consenting to the removal of the tumor. While she was anesthetized (for the expressed purpose of being examined), the surgeon removed the tumor without her expressed consent. Mrs. Schloendorff sued the hospital because the surgeon operated on her against her repeatedly expressed wishes. This case generated the following quote by Justice Benjamin Cardozo, an eloquent and well-respected justice: "Every human being of adult years and sound mind has the right to determine what shall be done with his own body; and a surgeon who performs an operation without his patient's consent commits an assault, for which he is liable in damages, except in cases of emergency where the patient is unconscious, and where it is necessary to operate before consent can be obtained."

Salgo (1957)

The *Salgo* decision marks the birth of the doctrine of informed consent as it is now known. The term *informed consent* was first used in this case. Mr. Salgo consented to undergo a diagnostic procedure to locate the source of chronic leg pain. A dye that had the potential to cause paralysis was injected in his leg. Upon experiencing paralysis, he sued his doctor, claiming that he was not informed about paralysis being a risk or possible complication of the dye injection. In the doctor's defense, it was argued that if patients were informed of all the possible complications they would become frightened and would not consent to treatment. The court did not accept this defense and ruled that simple consent is not sufficient for medical procedures. Sufficient disclosure of possible risks and complications (i.e., informed consent) was necessary for patients to be making autonomous decisions.

Natanson (1960)

Mrs. Natanson suffered severe burns resulting from radiation subsequent to a mastectomy. Although Mrs. Natanson had consented to the radiation, she sued her physician because he did not disclose to her its possible harm or the alternatives to the treatment. This case confirms the need for full disclosure and emphasizes the need for offering patients alternatives to the treatments proposed by their health care providers.

Canterbury (1972)

Mr. Canterbury developed paralysis after he fell off his hospital bed while urinating, subsequent to having surgery on his back. The court held that Mr. Canterbury should have been told of the risk of paralysis even though it was not clear whether the paralysis was caused by the surgery or was a result of the fall. Faden and Beauchamp hail this case as the most influential of all the informed consent cases.[2] The physicians knew about the potential paralytic effect that could result from the procedure that Mr. Canterbury received, but this information was not disclosed to him. He consented to the surgery without being sufficiently informed of all the possible consequences of that surgery. Although his consent was an expression of his right to self-determination, he made his decisions without the benefit of full disclosure.

This case makes the distinction between the different standards, or levels, of disclosure. The court decided that the "professional standard"[2(p135)] was not sufficient for Mr. Canterbury to make an informed decision. In this case, the court advocated the use of the "reasonable person standard."[2(p135)] These standards are outlined in more detail later in this chapter.

Candura (1978)

After initially consenting to the amputation of her gangrenous leg, Mrs. Candura changed her mind. Her daughter filed a petition with the court to become her legal guardian so she could sign the informed consent form for her mother and have the surgery performed against her mother's wishes. The court decided that Mrs. Candura was not incompetent and that she had the capacity to make her own health care decisions, even though her decision might have seemed irrational to others. Mrs. Candura's decision prevailed. The significance of this case is in its illustration that the court system will uphold the right of adult competent patients to make health care decisions even when such decisions are viewed by others as not being in the patient's own best interest.

The landmark cases just discussed paved the way for the development of a legal mechanism to ensure that health care professionals obtain informed consent from their patients before they provide medical treatments. To protect patients' right to privacy, the doctrine of informed consent, with its five elements, was developed and is used as the standard in the United States.

Notorious Research Giving Rise to the Attention Paid to Informed Consent

The following cases exemplify the horrors that result from conducting unethical research, as defined by the lack of subjects' informed consent to participate in research or by the obtaining of inadequate and flawed consent.

The Nazi Experiments

In an attempt to help the war effort in World War II, German physicians conducted research on the prisoners confined to concentration camps. Their justification was that the prisoners were to die anyway, so why not conduct the experiments to further science that would help soldiers in the field? Pence briefly lists a few experiments, including the following: the deliberate infection of wounds to test the efficacy of newly developed antibiotics, the injection of prisoners with blood tainted with typhus to test the efficacy of vaccines, the shooting of inmates to study gunshot wounds, the deprivation of inmates of food and water to study the effects of malnutrition and dehydration, and the immersion of Jewish and Russian prisoners in icy water to develop revival techniques for the benefit of pilots who were shot down during the war.[18] In the 1947 Nuremberg trials, twenty-four physicians were charged with conspiracy to commit war crimes against humanity, war crimes, crimes against humanity, and membership in a criminal organization for their role in participating in the human experimentation in concentration camps without the knowledge or consent of the research subjects. Although some of the defendants were executed, others were sentenced to varying numbers of years in prison, and others were acquitted.[19] The most renowned researcher in the Nazi experiments, Josef Mengele, fled to Brazil and was never captured or tried in the Nuremberg tribunals. He was most infamous for his experimentation on twins to study genetics to develop a superior race. Mengele died in 1985 without ever facing justice for the war crimes that he committed.[18]

The Tuskegee Study

The most infamous unethical medical research in U.S. history carried the official title of the "Tuskegee Study of Untreated Syphilis in the Negro Male."[6] The Tuskegee syphilis study has been used over the last half century to exemplify egregious violations of human rights and ethical practice in research, particularly because the process of research ignored the subjects' right to consent to their participation in research, and serves as an example of past exploitation of poor black subjects for the benefit of the affluent white population.

In an attempt to study the effects of untreated syphilis, the United States Public Health Service (the predecessor to the contemporary Centers for Disease Control and Prevention [CDC]) launched a study in 1932 on 600 African American residents of Tuskegee, Alabama, 399 of whom were diagnosed with syphilis, and 201 control subjects who were not infected. The study was led by the surgeon general, Raymond Vonderlehr, and touted as an excellent opportunity to observe untreated latent syphilis from the time of diagnosis to the time of death. The study was to last approximately six months, but was extended past the initial study period and lasted forty years. All the study participants were black and largely illiterate; hence, their chances of staying within Macon County, Alabama, were good, allowing them to be observed with no interruption or opportunity to be lost in the general population. The subject population did not include a treatment group for scientific comparison, and was therefore later considered scientifically flawed. The subjects in the control group were often included in the study group when they converted from being syphilis free to being syphilitic—another scientific flaw in the design of the study. The subjects were not closely observed by anyone other than by a nurse, Eunice Rivers, who was the only constant member of the study research team. Because observation was sporadic, some of the study subjects were able to get treatment for their syphilis outside of the study protocol, therefore nullifying the purpose of the study (i.e., the study of untreated syphilis).

The study yielded no new insights regarding the development of syphilis and its effects because the effects of having untreated syphilis were already well known in the medical community, since effective treatment of syphilis had not been possible until penicillin became widely available in 1948. What added to the atrocity of this study was the deception that continued throughout the study. The subjects did not consent to be part of experimental research; in fact, they were told that they were receiving treatment for syphilis—a diagnosis the subjects knew they had. They were told that they had "bad blood" and that they were getting treatment to cure their bad blood. Such "treatments" included undergoing painful and risky spinal taps, a diagnostic procedure, not a treatment for syphilis or for any other medical condition. The view that contracting syphilis was a symptom of immoral behavior contributed to the inertia that was rampant throughout the Tuskegee study.

The study continued until 1972, when Peter Buxtun, a venereal disease investigator employed by the CDC, contacted Jean Heller, a reporter for the Associated Press. Members of Congress were enraged to discover that exclusively black and illiterate men were being used as research subjects without their consent, and this media exposé resulted in an abrupt halt of the study by Congress. One year later, attorney Fred Gray filed a class-action lawsuit on behalf of the Tuskegee study subjects citing racism as a motive for the study and outlining the unethical behaviors that had been supported by a governmental agency that was charged with protecting the health of the public. In 1974, the case was settled out of court, and the surviving study participants and their families were financially compensated for the deception by the government and for enduring the devastating effects of untreated syphilis. It was concluded by critics of the Tuskegee study of untreated syphilis that more was learned about racism than about syphilis, and that there is a great need for understanding how individual and societal values affect professional behavior.[20]

In 1997, President William Jefferson Clinton offered an apology to participants in the Tuskegee study and their families, stating, "What the United States did was shameful, and I am sorry."[18(p226)] One major benefit resulting from the Tuskegee study was the research community's new zeal to ensure that research participants give their consent to participate in research.

Hepatitis at the Willowbrook State School

Although consent was obtained from parents, *inadequate consent* was cited as a major concern in the hepatitis studies conducted in the Willowbrook State School in New York. This institution housed retarded children who were difficult to care for in their parents' homes. The parents' consent was obtained to engage their children in research that subjected them to being deliberately infected with the hepatitis virus to aid in the development of a vaccine—as a condition of admission to the school. Although the parents did, in fact, consent to having their children participate in the studies, the ethics of obtaining consent under the duress of needing to institutionalize their children has been questioned. The researchers felt that infecting the children was justified because most of the admitted children became infected with hepatitis within one year of admission anyway, and the deliberate infection simply allowed for more controlled observation and follow-up. The conditions of overcrowding and the fact that many of the children were not toilet trained were factors that contributed to the rapid, and perhaps inevitable, transmission of the hepatitis virus. The ethics of the research was also questioned because it is difficult to conclude that infecting children with a virus that can eventually destroy one of the vital organs (the liver) can ever be justified. The studies were conducted between 1956 and 1970.[12]

Cancer Research at the Jewish Chronic Disease Hospital

In a study conducted at the Sloan-Kettering Cancer Center in New York and funded by the center, the U.S. Public Health Service, and the American Cancer Society, twenty-two patients were infected with cancer cells to determine the cause of the weakened immune system in patients suffering from cancer. The aim of the study, conducted by Dr. Chester Southam, was to determine why cancer patients are less able than healthy people to fight cancer. The consent process to participate in this study was questioned because some of the patients did not have decisional capacity to consent, and others were not given full disclosure about being injected with cancer cells. The consent process was not documented, and the physician-researcher did not get permission from the hospital research committee to conduct the study.[12]

Violation of the informed consent process has not been limited to medical research. Ethical concerns have been raised by researchers and ethicists alike because of the deception practiced by some social and behavioral researchers. Examples of these studies include Stanley Milgram's[21] psychological study of subjects yielding to authority,[22] and the notorious observational study of men's sexual behaviors in public restrooms by Laud Humphreys.

Laud Humphreys' Tearoom Study

For his doctoral dissertation in sociology from Washington University, Laud Humphreys set out to study men's impersonal sexual behaviors in public restrooms in St. Louis, Missouri, and he published his findings in a book entitled *Tearoom Trade: Impersonal Sex in Public Places.*[23] This study has been cited as the type of research that exemplifies unethical behavior in social and behavioral research, and it enraged Washington University officials to the point that they threatened to withdraw Humphreys' doctorate degree.

Humphreys visited public restrooms and acted as a "watchqueen" to observe men seeking sexual gratification from other men without engaging in the social pleasantries customary in sexual relationships.[24] He was interested in studying the lives of these men and did not reveal the real purpose of observing them, a fundamentally unethical research behavior because of the deceptive nature of his involvement with them.[25] He was later able to track the men one year after his observations ended through their car license plates, and he visited them in their homes to interview them. He disguised his appearance, and visited them under the false pretenses that he was conducting a "social health survey," collecting intimate information about their families, employment, socioeconomic status, and other private matters.[22] Adler and Adler summarized critics' ethical objections to Humphreys' study as follows: he deceived his subjects by claiming to be a lookout or a watchqueen, rather than a researcher; his concerns were only for himself as a researcher rather than for the privacy of his "subjects"; he did not consider the social costs of being exposed as a consumer of homosexual activities; and he underestimated the government's power to force him to identify his research subjects because they were engaging in socially unacceptable, as well as illegal, activities.[26]

Although Humphreys' study clearly had its outspoken critics on ethical grounds, others have been supportive of it because he tackled a sensitive social subject that other researchers had ignored or avoided studying, and they applauded his efforts to conduct very difficult social research in a meticulous manner to conceal and protect the identities of his study participants. Humphreys was later awarded the C. Wright Mills Award from the Society for the Study of Social Problems for his "contribution to the study of critical social issues."[26(p389)]

In response to the abuses that have occurred over the years in conducting research, the standards of ethical conduct of research were developed. The most frequently cited standards and codes are the Nuremberg Code, the Declaration of Helsinki, and the Belmont Report. Historical accounts of medical research led to the regulation of research conduct that "was born in scandal and reared in protectionism."[27(p106)]

International Research Regulations

The Nuremberg Code (1947)

Consequent to the Nuremberg tribunals, the Nuremberg Code of ethical behavior in research was developed, which lists ten basic requirements of research on human subjects.[19] The first requirement, and perhaps the most crucial, is that "the voluntary consent of the human subject is absolutely essential" (the principle of autonomy).[28] Other requirements are as follows: the research must yield fruitful results to continue (the principle of beneficence); animal experimentation must precede experimentation on humans; there must be assurance that unnecessary physical and mental suffering and injury are avoided (the principle of nonmaleficence); there must be assurance that there is no knowledge that the experiment will inevitably result in disabling injury or the death of the participant; risk must be minimized (the principle of justice); the subject must be protected from injury, disability, or death; researchers must be well trained and have the necessary skills to conduct the research; human subjects must be assured that they are at liberty to bring the experiment to an end; and the researcher must end the experiment if continuation would inevitably bring injury, disability, or death to the human subject.[28] The Nuremberg Code laid the foundation for universal research ethics standards, but lacked enforcement powers.

The Declaration of Helsinki (1964)

Although the Nuremberg Code was a good start, giving researchers basic guidelines to conduct ethical research, it did not tackle some fundamental aspects of research. To address these deficiencies, the Declaration of Helsinki was developed in 1964 by the World Medical Association (WMA).[29] It was revised by the WMA General Assembly in 1975, 1983, 1989, 1996, 2000, and 2002; another iteration was published in 2004, with an anticipated additional revision and ratification scheduled for October 2008.

The Declaration of Helsinki is considerably more detailed than the Nuremberg Code's ten requirements, because it has thirty-two paragraphs and requirements. It specifically addresses international research. It includes and expounds on all the edicts of the Nuremberg Code, but also adds the need to obtain assent from incompetent human subjects in addition to obtaining consent from their legal representatives. Incompetent human subjects are defined as subjects who are younger than eighteen, and subjects whose decisional capacity is not intact as a result of physical and/or mental medical conditions. The Declaration emphasizes the health care professional's obligation to consider the subject's best medical interest first in the words "the health of my patient will be my first consideration," thus establishing at the outset of the Declaration that it is not permissible to harm individual human subjects for the benefit of the general population. Positive as well as negative results must be either published or made available to the public, and sources of funding and conflicts of interest must be declared. A significant contribution of the Declaration of Helsinki is the establishment of the standard of submitting research protocols to "a specially appointed ethical review board" to provide comment, guidance to the researchers, and approval for the research prior to the initiation of research and to approve the continuation of research. This standard has evolved into the formation of the contemporary institutional review board (IRB), with the inclusion of members representing scientists, medical specialists, ethicists, and the community.[30]

An American Research Regulation: The Belmont Report (1979)

The Belmont Report was developed in 1979 by the National Commission for the Protection of Human Subjects of Biomedical and Behavioral Research.[10] It was built on the ethical principles of autonomy, beneficence, and justice, codifying the Nuremberg Code and the Declaration of Helsinki into one decree that is published in the *Federal Register*, thus particularly applying to U.S. researchers.

In addressing the principle of autonomy, the Belmont Report incorporates the right of competent individuals to exercise autonomous decision making, in addition to protecting the rights of subjects whose autonomy is diminished. These two components are combined in one principle labeled "respect for persons." Beneficence is the second ethical principle in the Belmont Report, which acknowledges two components of beneficent acts:

avoiding harm and maximizing the potential benefits. Balancing the value of the benefits to be gained from the research and the harms to which the research exposes human subjects may be necessary to assess whether the research is beneficent or maleficent. Thus, "difficult choices" may have to be made by researchers and IRBs when assessing whether research should go forward or be halted. The final principle listed in the Belmont Report is justice. There is agreement between the three codes (the Nuremberg Code, the Declaration of Helsinki, and the Belmont Report) that the burden of research ought to be shared by the classes of people who would benefit from the results of the research, thus stopping the practice of burdening poor subjects in public medical facilities with participating in research while diverting the benefits to private patients who are treated in private facilities.

Consequences of Violating the Ethical Principles of Research

The purpose of conducting research in an ethical manner is to ensure that human subjects are protected from harm. Absent this protection, institutions that sponsor the research may be subject to litigation and to disruption of their research activities. Violating the ethical principles of research may result in harmful consequences to the subject, such as loss of employment or interference with relationships. Vulnerable subjects, such as the institutionalized elderly, may also be harmed by giving consent to participate in research when they do not possess the competence to make informed decisions.[31] The institutions sponsoring research may also suffer grave consequences as a result of violating informed consent protocols. For example, in January 2000, the Food and Drug Administration placed the human gene therapy research being conducted at the University of Pennsylvania on an indefinite clinical hold when a subject, Mr. Jesse Gelsinger, died and the process of his informed consent was not well documented.[32] Researchers who engage in unethical research may also suffer negative personal consequences, such as dismissal from employment, loss of tenure, inability to publish research results, and loss of grant sponsorship. Conducting research in an ethical manner protects research institutions, human subjects, and the researchers who study them.

The Doctrine of Informed Consent

The lack of informed consent has been viewed as a major violation of research subjects' rights in many studies cited for unethical behavior, and the need to obtain informed consent from research participants was central to the Nuremberg Code, the Declaration of Helsinki, and the Belmont Report. In 1966, Henry K. Beecher published a landmark article in the *New England Journal of Medicine* listing twenty-two experimental research studies that were conducted in American "medical schools, university hospitals, private hospitals, governmental military departments (the army, the Navy, and the air Force), governmental institutes (the NIH), Veterans Administration hospitals, and industry" for which informed consent was not appropriately obtained.[28(p1354)] It is important to note that all cited studies were conducted after the Nazi experiments era and the development of the Nuremberg Code, and that in spite of the availability of documents giving researchers guidelines for ethical research conduct, violations of subjects' right to make autonomous decisions (as exemplified by their giving informed consent) remained widespread.

Informed consent has become the cornerstone of ethical behavior when conducting research because it is the practical application of the ethical principle of autonomy, or respect for persons. Whereas obtaining informed consent from patients receiving medical care from their health care providers originated in case law,[4] informed consent to participate in research is grounded in the Nuremberg Code and subsequent laws and regulations.[5]

Informed consent to participate in research encompasses the same elements of consent as for medical procedures: disclosure, understanding, voluntariness, competence, and finally signing the informed consent document. Each element is described in detail here.

Disclosure

Disclosure of information to patients and research subjects is a necessary component of consent. According to Beauchamp and Childress, there are three standards of disclosure: the professional practice standard, the reasonable person standard, and the subjective standard.[7] The *professional practice standard* is determined by the medical community and emphasizes the patient's best medical interest. Expert witnesses are in the best position to determine whether this standard has been upheld or violated. This standard is frequently criticized because it assumes that the health care professional is capable of determining what is in the patient's best interest. This standard was cited by the physicians in their defense in the *Canterbury* case discussed earlier. The court expressed preference for the use of the *reasonable person standard,* which supposes a "hypothetical reasonable person."[7(p148)] It takes into consideration the patient's need for information, rather than the health care professional's opinion of the patient's needs. Respecting the patient's autonomy and his or her right to self-determination is central to this standard. The difficulty with this standard is that it is difficult to determine what (or who) is a reasonable person. The preferred standard of disclosure is referred to as the *subjective standard*. This standard indicates that for the principle of autonomy to be maximized, the level of disclosure of relevant information should be tailored to the patient based on his or her individual needs. Information should be presented at a level that the person understands, based on intellectual ability, and taking into consideration cultural differences, functional limitations, and language barriers.

The disclosure of relevant information to help the research participant in making an informed decision is also necessary. Disclosure must first state that the subject is consenting to participate in "research," and must describe the research and its goals, what the subject is expected to do, how long the subject is expected to be in the study, how many other subjects are expected to participate, what the risks of participating are, what potential benefit the subject may gain, what alternatives are available to the subject, how the subject will be compensated (if at all), the costs that the subject may incur, how the subject's confidentiality will be protected, how the research results will be disseminated, and finally why the subject was selected to be asked to participate.[5] Although the duty of disclosure is met by giving information, if the subject does not understand what is being disclosed, then disclosure is of limited value.

Understanding

Related to the concept of disclosure, but even more important, is the concept of understanding. Health care professionals and researchers need to ensure the existence of an atmosphere that encourages patients or subjects to ask questions and clarify ambiguous information. Understanding clearly implies that if the patient has difficulty understanding the English language, an interpreter needs to be provided. If the patient has difficulty hearing or seeing, assistive devices need to be made available to ensure that thorough understanding is occurring and that the communication between the health care professional and the patient is optimized.

Because much research is technical and may be difficult for the average person with no formal medical training to comprehend, researchers are obligated to ensure that potential subjects understand what they are being asked to consent to do. One requirement of informed consent forms is that they be written at a readability level that is commensurate with the potential subject pool. Studies have consistently shown that informed consent forms are written at a college level of comprehension, whereas the general population has been reported to read at a fifth grade level.[5] The informed consent form is only one aspect of the informed consent process, however, and must be viewed in the context of the entire process. Potential subjects must be given an opportunity to discuss the research protocol with their regular health care professionals, families, and friends, and they must be given contact information of researchers and their team members for the purpose of answering questions before consenting to participate in the research, and subsequently during the conduct of research.

Voluntariness

Voluntary participation in treatment and research is essential to the concept of autonomy and self-determination. Patients can make reasoned choices when they are not manipulated or coerced to undergo procedures they are resisting.[3] In attempting to persuade a patient to undergo medical treatment, the health care professional may permissibly exercise some influence over the patient's final decision, but he/she may not be coercive.

"[V]oluntary consent of the human subject is absolutely essential" is the first point in the Nuremberg Code, which shows the importance of ensuring that subjects are not consenting to being research participants under duress.[33] In addition to the voluntary requirement of participation, the Nuremberg Code requires that subjects be informed of their right to terminate their participation in the research at any time they feel that they have "reached the physical or mental state, where continuation of the experiment seemed . . . to be impossible."[33] Groups that have been viewed as being particularly vulnerable to involuntary participation in research through coercive measures are prisoners, women, the elderly, racial and ethnic minorities, the socially and socioeconomically disadvantaged, the mentally ill, and the institutionalized. Special protections must be put in place to ensure that these groups are in fact volunteering to participate in research rather than being coerced by others because of their vulnerabilities.

Competence

The concept of competence is elusive because individuals may have the competence to perform some functions and at the same time may not be competent to perform others. In 1978, the case of Mr. Robert Quackenbush was decided in his favor based on the judge's decision that Mr. Quackenbush was competent, albeit lacking decisional capacity at times.[34] Mr. Quackenbush was a seventy-two-year-old patient who needed amputation of his gangrenous leg. His capacity to make health care decisions fluctuated, and there was no consensus of medical opinion among the psychiatrists who evaluated his ability to make health care decisions. The court decided that although Mr. Quackenbush did not maintain decisional capacity at all times, his competence was not in question. It concluded that the decisions Mr. Quackenbush made during times of lucidity were valid, and needed to be followed by his physicians.[35]

The President's Commission for the Study of Ethical Problems in Medicine and Biomedical and Behavioral Research also makes the distinction between *decisional incapacity*, a medical determination that can fluctuate, and *incompetence*, which is a more durable legal determination. Decisional capacity means that the individual has values and goals, has the ability to communicate and to understand information, and has the ability to reason.[36]

Research subjects whose decisional capacity appears to be impaired as a result of the use of drugs or alcohol should be temporarily excluded from participating in the research and from giving informed consent. Consent obtained under conditions of impairment is not legally "informed" because the subject lacks the capacity to understand relevant information.[37] Understanding basic information relevant to participating in research, such as the consequences of participation, and the ability to assess the burdens and benefits of participation may not be possible while one is impaired by the use of drugs and alcohol.

In the provision of medical care, when there is a question about an individual's ability to comprehend the given information, an assessment of that individual's ability to make decisions is necessary before consent forms are signed. Making health care decisions for those who lack competence is done by following legal standards. According to Jonsen, Veatch, and Walters, the President's Commission recognizes best interest, substituted judgment, and reasonable judgment as the acceptable standards for decision making by proxies.[36] Substituted judgment is based on the proxy's knowledge of what the patient's wishes would have been, best interest is simply based on promoting what is good for the patient, and both standards are guided by what is considered reasonable by medical standards.

When individuals' competence is intact, they have the right to autonomous decision making. However, individuals who have lost their competence retain the right to autonomous decision making, albeit exercised through different mechanisms—that is, autonomous decisions made on their behalf by others, such as proxy decision makers as allowed by state law. For example, autonomous decision making for minors is exercised on their behalf by their parents or legal guardians. Similarly, the autonomy of once competent but now incompetent adults may be exercised by proxy decision makers as permitted by state law or through their previously expressed wishes in advance directives (living wills and formal designations of surrogate decision makers), in concordance with their values (see Chapter 14, "End-of-Life Decision Making"). Incompetence, as defined in law, means that the person is not capable of autonomous decision making because of intoxication, mental or physical disability, or inability to think rationally and exercise the right to self-determination.

Determining a subject's ability to consent to participating in research depends entirely on the type of decision that is required. For example, the same individual might be deemed to possess the decisional capacity to consent to social and behavioral research that entails completing a survey, while at the same time being deemed to lack the decisional capacity to consent to medical research that requires a brain biopsy. The justification for assigning different levels of competence relates to the level of risk that is incurred by participating in research by completing a survey versus the risk incurred by consenting to a brain biopsy. Competence to participate in research must be assessed based on the level of understanding that is required to make an informed decision.[5] All adults are presumed competent to make autonomous decisions unless challenged by acquaintances such as family members, friends, health care professionals, or researchers (see Chapter 7, "Competence").

Informed Consent Forms

The final step in the process of informed consent is the signing of the consent form, documenting that the individual agrees to participate in a procedure or therapeutic intervention. Although the patient's signature is the standard indication that the patient has consented, it is not an essential component of the consent process. The law requires that the informed consent process take place, but some patients are, for example, incapable of signing. Additionally, consent forms are for the most part drafted to apply to medical procedures, but the duty to obtain informed consent is not limited to situations involving procedures. In such cases, the health care professional may document in the patient's medical record that the informed consent process has taken place. Devettere emphasizes the need for proper documentation of the informed consent process as a reminder of its importance and as a symbolic portrayal of patient participation in decision making.[12]

Obtaining informed consent from research subjects must be viewed as a process rather than as a one-time event. Rather than viewing informed consent to have been obtained because a form was signed, the signed consent form should instead be viewed only as evidence that the process of informed consent has occurred. Berg asserts that signing the consent form "must become less an empty ritual and more a meaningful social practice."[5(p189)] The consent of research subjects throughout the study must be ongoing to ensure that subjects remember that they are participating in research, that their continuous participation is entirely voluntary, and finally that consent can be withdrawn at any time.

Exceptions to the Doctrine of Informed Consent

Informed Consent and Cultural Differences

Some elements of the informed consent doctrine may conflict with the beliefs and habits of subcultures in the United States. For example, full disclosure of medical information and seeking consent from the individual patient are two ways in which members of certain subcultures are not in agreement with the majority culture. Cultures that emphasize hope, such as the Navajo tribe, opt to receive limited information. Disclosure of the risks of medical treatment and discussion related to delivering bad news are not acceptable to members of the Navajo tribe. It is their belief that thought and language have the power to shape reality and to control events, and that discussing potential complications may in fact precipitate their occurrence.[38] Discussing negative information with members of the Navajo tribe may be viewed as potentially harmful, and therefore needs to be reexamined within the context of informed consent. Members of other cultures may find the strict application of individual autonomy unsuitable and may prefer a family-centered approach to medical decision making. However, in 1982, the President's Commission "found a universal desire for information, choice, and respectful communication about decisions"[36(p464)] The form in which communication occurs should be tailored to the individual patient based on his or her cultural preferences.

Competing Claims

Competing claims may override the doctrine of informed consent when the best interests of society or of the individual are at stake. Faden and Beauchamp outline five recognized exceptions to the informed consent requirement: public health emergencies, medical emergencies, the incompetent patient, therapeutic privilege, and the patient waiver.[2] Each of these exceptions is detailed here.

Public Health Emergencies

To protect the interests of the public and of society, such as in the case of epidemic disease, the government may breach the rights of individuals. The case of tuberculosis is an example. To this day, patients who are diagnosed with tuberculosis may properly be coerced into receiving treatment. The disease is airborne and is easily transmitted by casual contact. Quarantine and forced treatment are two strategies that have been successfully used, and can be enforced through the court system. Mass, compulsory immunizations at times of epidemics are another example of this public health exception to informed consent. There are limits to the state's right to so intervene when contagion is not likely, such as in the case of the spread of AIDS. AIDS cannot be transmitted by casual contact; thus, the public is not at immediate risk of infection. Thus, confinement and involuntary treatment of AIDS patients are, in general, not justifiable.

Medical Emergencies

In matters of life and death, when the patient is not able to consent due to incapacity that resulted from the medical emergency, the health care professional is relieved from the responsibility of obtaining informed consent. In cases where preservation of life is not at stake, the health care professional is obligated to seek consent from an appropriate proxy.

Incompetence

As a rule, incompetence is a legal determination. Adult individuals are presumed competent unless determined otherwise by a judge in a court of law. Minors are not capable of giving informed consent except when they have engaged in activities that presume their competence, such as marriage, or engaging in sexual activity and requesting medical treatment for venereal disease. When decision making is required and incompetence is established, state law dictates the procedures for obtaining informed consent from appropriate proxies.

Therapeutic Privilege

The concept of therapeutic privilege is controversial because it borders on the practice of paternalism and should, therefore, be used sparingly. Health care professionals may use this privilege of limited disclosure when complete disclosure can be proved to be harmful to the patient. The courts have struggled with this concept, and its interpretation varies between jurisdictions. The courts caution that this privilege should not be widely used because it interferes with the patient's right to self-determination.

Waiver
Waiving the right to make decisions is an informed choice made by the individual in question. When a patient exercises this decision, the health care professional may not be required to obtain informed consent from the patient. The patient has the right to defer his or her decision making to anyone he or she wishes. This is the patient's constitutionally protected right to privacy. Although this right is guaranteed by the U.S. Constitution, it can potentially be abused by health care professionals. The potential for paternalism abounds.

Chapter Summary

Maximizing patients' right to autonomous health care decision making is ensured through the process of informed consent. The doctrine of informed consent also applies to human subjects who participate in research. There are few exceptions to the doctrine, and these must be used with caution to minimize the possibility of manipulation and paternalism by researchers and physicians.

Obtaining written informed consent from patients and from research subjects protects them from paternalism and from manipulation and unscrupulous practices. It can also protect health care professionals and the institutions where they practice and conduct research from litigation, although written consent may not always be necessary. The informed consent process can be used as a tool to enhance patients' and research subjects' understanding of the proposed treatments and research and their consequences.

The doctrine of informed consent is based on ancient philosophical principles, and its practical application occurred incrementally as a result of successful litigation against health care professionals and researchers who did not ensure the active participation of their patients and research subjects in decision making involving them. Informed consent is codified in state law as well as in the regulations that developed to ensure the active participation of patients and research subjects in the decisions that affect them.

Review Questions

1. What are the principles of medical ethics?

2. How are the principles of medical ethics related to the development of the doctrine of informed consent?

3. List the landmark cases that were instrumental in the incremental development of the contemporary process of obtaining informed consent.

4. Name the most notorious research studies that were cited for violating the standard of obtaining informed consent.

5. What are the elements of informed consent?

6. What are the differences between the best interest standard and the substituted judgment standard in proxy decision making?

7. What are the exceptions to obtaining informed consent?

Endnotes

1. Portions of this chapter have been reprinted with permission. Reprinted portions have been integrated throughout the chapter from the following: Osman H. History and development of the doctrine of informed consent. *Int Electr J Health Educ* 2001;4:41–47. Available at: http://www.iejhe.org.

2. Faden R, Beauchamp R. *A History and Theory of Informed Consent*. New York: Oxford University Press, 1986.

3. Pellegrino ED, Thomasma DC. *The Virtues in Medical Practice*. New York: Oxford University Press, 1993.

4. Osman H. History and development of the doctrine of informed consent. *Int Electr J Health Educ* 2001;4:41–47.

5. Berg JW, et al. *Informed Consent: Legal Theory and Clinical Practice*. 2nd ed. New York: Oxford University Press, 2001.

6. U.S. Department of Health and Human Services, Centers for Disease Control and Prevention. U.S. Public Health Service syphilis study at Tuskegee. 2007. Available at: http://www.cdc.gov/tuskegee/. Accessed May 2008.

7. Beauchamp TL, Childress JF. *Principles of Biomedical Ethics*. 5th ed. New York: Oxford University Press, 2001.

8. Perlin TM. *Clinical Medical Ethics: Cases in Practice*. Boston: Little, Brown and Company, 1992.

9. Blackhall LJ, Murphy ST, Frank G. Ethnicity and attitudes toward patient autonomy. *JAMA* 1995;274:820–825.

10. National Institutes of Health. *The Belmont Report: Ethical Principles and Guidelines for the Protection of Human Subjects of Research*. 1979. Available at: http://ohsr.od.nih.gov/guidelines/belmont.html.

11. Lifton RJ. *Medical Killing and the Psychology of Genocide: The Nazi Doctors*. New York: Basic Books, 1986.

12. Devettere RJ. *Practical Decision Making in Health Care Ethics*. 2nd ed. Washington, DC: Georgetown University Press, 2000.

13. *Mary E. Schloendorff, Appellant, v. The Society of the New York Hospital*. Court of Appeals of New York, 211 N.Y. 125; 105 N.E. 92. Decided April 14, 1914.

14. *Salgo v. Leland Stanford Jr. Univ. Bd. of Trustees,* 317 P.2d 170 (Cal. Ct. App. 1957).

15. *Canterbury v. Spence,* 464 F.2d 772 (D.C. Cir. 1972).

16. *Lane v. Candura,* 376 N.E.2d, 1232, 6 Mass. App. Ct. 377 (1978).

17. *Natanson v. Kline,* 350 P.2d 1093 (Kan. 1960).

18. Pence GE. *Medical Ethics: Accounts of the Cases That Shaped and Define Medical Ethics*. Boston: McGraw Hill, 2008.

19. The President and Fellows of Harvard College. *Nuremberg Trials Project: A Digital Document Collection*. 2003. Available at: http://nuremberg.law.harvard.edu/php/docs_swi.php?DI=1&text=medical.

20. Brandt AM. Racism and research: the case of the Tuskegee syphilis study. *Hastings Center Rep* 1978;8(6):21–29.
21. Milgram S. Behavioral study of obedience. *J Abnorm Soc Psychol* 1963;67:371–378.
22. Punch M. Politics and ethics in qualitative research. In: Denzin NK, Lincoln YS, eds. *Handbook of Qualitative Research*. Thousand Oaks, CA: Sage, 1994:83–97.
23. Humphreys L. *Tearoom Trade: Impersonal Sex in Public Places*. New York: Aldine, 1975.
24. Sieber J. Laud Humphreys and the tearoom sex study. 1977. Available at: http://web.missouri.edu/~bondesonw/Laud.html. Accessed October 20, 2007.
25. Fontana A, Frey JH. Interviewing: the art of science. In: Denzin NK, Lincoln YS, eds. *Handbook of Qualitative Research*. Thousand Oaks, CA: Sage, 1994.
26. Adler PA, Adler P. Observational techniques. In: Denzin NK, Lincoln YS, eds. *Handbook of Qualitative Research*. Thousand Oaks, CA: Sage, 1994.
27. Levine C. Changing views of justice after Belmont: AIDS and the inclusion of "vulnerable" subjects. In: Vanderpool HY, ed. *The Ethics of Research Involving Human Subjects: Facing the 21st Century*. Frederick, MD: University Publishing Group, 1996:106.
28. Beecher HK. Ethics and clinical research. *New Engl J Med* 1966;274:1354–1360.
29. The World Medical Association Ethics Unit. Declaration of Helsinki. 2007. Available at: http://www.wma.net/e/ethicsunit/helsinki.htm.
30. The World Medical Association. World Medical Association Declaration of Helsinki: ethical principles for medical research involving human subjects. 2004. Available at: http://www.wma.net/e/policy/b3.htm.
31. Kayser-Jones J, Koenig BA. Ethical issues. In: Faber F, Gubrium A, Sankar A, eds. *Qualitative Methods in Aging Research*. Thousand Oaks, CA: Sage Publications, 1994.
32. Ciment J. Gene therapy experiments put on "clinical hold." *BMJ* 2000;320:336.
33. U.S. Government Printing Office. *Trials of War Criminals Before the Nuremberg Military Tribunals Under Control Council Law No. 10*. 1949. Available at: http://www.hhs.gov/ohrp/references/nurcode.htm.
34. *In re Quackenbush,* 156 N.J.Super.282,383 A.2d 785, 788.
35. Furrow BR, et al. *Health Law: Cases, Materials and Problems*. 3d ed. St. Paul, MN: West Publishing, 1997.
36. Jonsen AR, Veatch RM, Walters L. *Source Book in Bioethics: A Documentary History*. Washington, DC: Georgetown University Press, 1998.
37. President's Commission for the Study of Ethical Problems in Medicine and Biomedical and Behavioral Research. *Making Health Care Decisions*. Washington, DC: U.S. Government Printing Office, 1982.
38. Carrese JA, Rhodes LA. Western bioethics on the Navajo reservation: benefit or harm. *JAMA* 1995;274:826–829.

Chapter 9

Informed Consent II

Freedom is the Right to Choose, the Right to create for oneself the alternatives of Choice. Without the possibility of Choice, and the exercise of Choice, a man is not a man but a member, an instrument, a thing.

—Thomas Jefferson

Chapter Learning Objectives

At the conclusion of this chapter the reader will be able to:

1. Define *battery* and explain how it relates to consent and informed consent

2. Recognize and explain the emergency exception to the rule that requires that consent be obtained prior to a medical touching

3. Recognize and explain the extension doctrine and how it relates to the rule that requires that consent be obtained prior to a medical touching

4. Recognize and define *ghost surgery* and explain how it relates to battery and consent

5. Explain the diverse consequences of a health care provider mistakenly believing a patient has consented to a medical touching

6. Explain the doctrine of informed refusal and recognize situations in which its dictate applies

7. Recognize and explain the ways in which consent may and may not be used to modify the terms of the health care provider–patient relationship

8. List, recognize, and discuss novel disclosure obligations, including health care provider experience, nontechnical characteristics of health care providers (e.g., substance abuse and HIV infection), and financial conflicts of interest

The preceding chapter dealt with the basics of the doctrine of informed consent. This chapter rounds out our understanding of the doctrine by exploring its legal roots. Additionally, it builds upon the material introduced in the last chapter by examining more recent advances in the doctrine, including, for example, some novel disclosure obligations.

Battery and Consent

"In 1957 the California Supreme Court held that an action arising from a physician's failure to give a patient sufficient information to make an informed decision should sound in negligence [and] not battery."[1] Consistent with that decision, modern informed consent law is negligence based. However, "early cases . . . involving patient consent spoke almost exclusively of battery."[1] The historical roots of the informed consent doctrine, therefore, lie in the law of battery.[2]

Battery

Battery is an intentional tort and is defined as "intentional and wrongful physical contact with a person without his or her consent that entails some injury or offensive touching."[3] Stated otherwise, battery is the intentional infliction of harmful or offensive contact with the person of another without the other's consent. A *tort*, in turn, is "a legal wrong committed upon the person or property [of another] independent of contract."[3] An *intentional tort* is a "tort or wrong perpetrated by one who intends to do that which the law has declared wrong."[3] The tort of negligence, in contrast, is one in which the wrongdoer or tortfeasor "fails to exercise . . . care in doing what is otherwise permissible."[3] We shall deal extensively with negligence in Chapter 15, which discusses health law.

Whether a suit is brought as a negligence suit or as a battery may matter a great deal to the health care provider who is the object of the suit. First of all, the statute of limitations often differs. Second, punitive damages are almost never available to plaintiffs in negligence suits, but may be had in suits involving intentional torts. Also, under the terms of some medical malpractice insurance policies, intentional torts are excluded from coverage.

Battery and Intent

We should take a moment here to explore more precisely the nature of the *intent* element of battery. Under the definition of battery, what must a defendant have intended?

One possibility is that the defendant must have intended "injury or offense." This will not do, however. Imagine that while riding a subway, I turn to a woman I do not know who is sitting next to me and I kiss her. In defending myself against a claim of battery, it will do me no good to say that I meant no harm or offense. It is a battery all the same. The law, therefore, does not require that one guilty of a battery have intended injury or offense.

Another possibility is that the defendant must have intended the physical contact or touching. If we return to our subway hypothetical, such intent is clearly sufficient, but is it necessary? Consider another scenario. I am playing soccer in the park with some friends when I see an old nemesis walking past. His head down, he does not see me. I kick the ball forcefully in his direction, intending that it will pass near his face and startle him. Alas, my aim is not what it used to be, and the ball strikes him in the face. Battery? Yes! The fact that it is a battery means that the law does not require that I intended the physical contact or touching. It is enough that I intended to produce some physical or mental effect on the plaintiff.

Problems with Consent: Battery or Negligence?

The modern approach to consent and informed consent is to distinguish between situations in which consent to a procedure is not obtained—battery—and those in which consent to the procedure has been obtained but is substandard or flawed—negligence. Thus,

> [i]n the typical informed consent claim, the patient has given technical consent to being "touched" by the defendant but argues that consent would not have been given if appropriate disclosures had been made. Courts generally reject battery claims because the patient has "consented" to the touching. In most jurisdictions, battery claims are reserved for those situations in which (1) the patient has not consented to any procedure at all, (2) the health care provider performs a completely different procedure than that for which consent was given, (3) the health care provider performs a procedure on the wrong area of the body, or (4) a different, unconsented-to provider performs the procedure.[4]

With this in mind, consider the following cases in light of what you have learned so far about consent and informed consent.

Case 9-A

Mrs. Mohr consulted Dr. Williams about a right ear disorder.[5] Dr. Williams examined the ear. At the same time, he attempted to examine the left ear, but was unable to do so completely because of cerumen. Mrs. Mohr submitted to general anesthesia on the understanding that Dr. Williams would operate on the diseased right ear. After examining both ears under general anesthesia, Dr. Williams decided that the left ear was in worse condition than the right, and so operated on the left ear only. When she awakened and learned what had happened, Mrs. Mohr sued Dr. Williams. What are Mrs. Mohr's possible arguments? What are Dr. Williams's possible defenses?

Analysis

Mrs. Mohr could bring a negligence action (i.e., her consent to surgery was not informed), alleging that Dr. Williams's disclosures regarding the surgery were substandard. Alternatively, she could bring a battery claim by arguing that she did not consent to any surgery on her left ear. Because we shall have more to say about negligence and informed consent in Chapter 15, let's focus on the battery claim here.

What might Dr. Williams say in his own defense? Looking again at the definition of battery (the intentional infliction of harmful or offensive contact with the person of another without the other's consent), he might try arguing that his contact with the person of Mrs. Mohr was neither harmful nor offensive because he actually ameliorated her left ear disorder. That argument will not succeed, because courts have decided that, as a matter of law, unconsented-to medical touchings are offensive. He might try arguing that he did not intend

(continues)

Case 9-A (*continued*)

any harm or offense, but as we saw previously, the definition of battery does not require intent of that kind. The only plausible argument he can make in his own defense is that Mrs. Mohr did in fact give consent.

What might that argument look like? He could argue that Mrs. Mohr's consent was *express*, and that she in effect consented to surgery on her diseased ear, and it just so happened that her left ear was more diseased than her right. The court, while rejecting the argument, wrote that the "contention [was] not without merit."[5]

Alternatively, Dr. Williams could argue that Mrs. Mohr's consent was *implied* by law. He could make two arguments in this regard. First, the law will imply consent when a patient unable to give consent (because of unconsciousness, etc.) presents in an emergency situation and "immediate treatment is required to prevent more serious harm."[4] Here, the court wrote, the evidence did not "justify the court in holding, as a matter of law, that [Mrs. Mohr's ear disorder] was such an affliction as would result immediately in the serious injury of the plaintiff, or such an emergency as to proceed without her consent."[5] In short, consent could not be inferred under the emergency exception because there was no emergency.

Second, the law will also imply consent under the extension doctrine. Under that doctrine, as explained by the Supreme Court of North Carolina in *Kennedy v. Parrott*,

> In major internal operations . . . the consent—in the absence of proof to the contrary—will be construed as general in nature and the surgeon may extend the operation to remedy any abnormal or diseased condition in the area of the original incision whenever he, in the exercise of his sound professional judgment, determines that correct surgical procedure dictates and requires such an extension of the operation originally contemplated. This rule applies when the patient is at the time incapable of giving consent, and no one with authority to consent for him is immediately available.[6]

Unfortunately for Dr. Williams, the extension doctrine is not applicable either, because the "diseased condition of the plaintiff's left ear was not discovered in the course of an operation on the right, which was authorized, but upon an independent examination of that organ, made after the authorized operation was found unnecessary."

Because none of Dr. Williams's defenses were persuasive, Mrs. Mohr prevailed in her battery claim.

Case 9-B

Urologist Dr. Pirozzi advised his patient Mr. Perna to have surgery for removal of kidney stones.[7] Mr. Perna agreed, requesting that Dr. Pirozzi perform the surgery, and signed a consent form naming Pirozzi as the operating surgeon and authorizing him, "with the aid of unnamed 'assistants,' to perform the surgery."[7] Two days later the surgery was performed by Drs. Del Gaizo

Case 9-B (*continued*)

and Ciccone, partners of Dr. Pirozzi, who was not himself present. Mr. Perna sued Drs. Del Gaizo and Ciccone. What is the nature of his claim against them?

Analysis

Regarding the claim against Drs. Del Gaizo and Ciccone, the court considered "the nature of the claim resulting from the performance of the operation by a physician other than the one named in the consent form, so-called 'ghost surgery.'" The court wrote, "If the claim is characterized as a failure to obtain informed consent, the operation may constitute an act of medical malpractice; if, however, it is viewed as a failure to obtain any consent, it is better classified as a battery." Again, since we shall have more to say about negligence and informed consent in Chapter 15, let's focus on the battery claim here.

Del Gaizo and Ciccone might argue that Mr. Perna did consent to the surgery and that consequently there cannot have been a battery. However, Perna's consent to being operated upon by Pirozzi is nontransferable. As the Supreme Court of New Jersey wrote in its review of this case, "Absent an emergency, patients have the right to determine not only whether surgery is to be performed on them, but who shall perform it. A surgeon who operates without the patient's consent engages in the unauthorized touching of another and, thus, commits a battery."[7] This is consistent with the previous discussion, in which it was stated that an action in battery will lie where a different, unconsented-to provider performs the procedure.

Case 9-C

Ms. Tisdale was told by her family physician that she needed a dilation and curettage (D&C) for a missed abortion.[8] A second opinion was required before her insurer would agree to pay for it. The company referred her to Dr. Pruitt. Ms. Tisdale so informed Dr. Pruitt's receptionist, who noted this on the chart. Dr. Pruitt did not read the chart. He placed Ms. Tisdale on the exam table, examined her, and proceeded to do the D&C. The procedure lasted about five minutes, during which Ms. Tisdale was upset and crying. It was not a completely satisfactory D&C, and a second one was needed, and was done by her family physician in the hospital under general anesthesia. At trial, Dr. Pruitt testified that the patient was "just absolutely docile I guess, and I just assumed that she was acquiescing, but I thought that I had her consent and her . . . very informed consent." Ms. Tisdale testified that, if fully informed, she would not have consented to have a D&C done in the office that day because "I had known Dr. Pruitt for about fifteen minutes . . . and I would never consent to have something that painful done in an office." What are Ms. Tisdale's possible arguments against Dr. Pruitt? What are Dr. Pruitt's defenses?

(*continues*)

Case 9-C (*continued*)

Analysis

Similar to the cases discussed previously, the plaintiff can argue that she did not consent to the D&C and that, consequently, Dr. Pruitt committed a battery against her. Alternatively, she can argue that any consent that was found to have been given was uninformed, and that therefore Dr. Pruitt was negligent. As before, we shall focus on the battery claim here.

What are Dr. Pruitt's defenses to the battery claim? Recalling that battery is the intentional infliction of harmful or offensive contact with the person of another without the other's consent, and keeping in mind all we have learned so far, it would seem that Dr. Pruitt must defend by arguing that Ms. Tisdale's consent to his performing the D&C was implied by her silence and passivity. This case affords us an opportunity to explore in greater detail the nature of the consent element in the legal definition of battery.

"If it reasonably seemed to the defendant that the plaintiff consented, consent will be held to exist *regardless of the plaintiff's subjective state of mind*. That is, it is the *objective manifestations* by the plaintiff that are taken into account—a not surprising rule, since defendants are not mind readers."[9] Where the defendant, instead, makes an unreasonable mistake about consent—concluding that a plaintiff has consented when no reasonable person would so conclude under the circumstances—then a battery will be held to have occurred.

So the question becomes, Was Dr. Pruitt's belief that Ms. Tisdale had implied consent—by her silence and passivity—reasonable under the circumstances? The jury did not think so. As noted earlier, Dr. Pruitt's receptionist indicated on Ms. Tisdale's chart that she was there for a second opinion. In order to characterize Dr. Pruitt's mistake regarding consent as reasonable, one would have to argue that it is reasonable for a doctor not to read a patient's chart before doing a procedure on that patient.

Informed Refusal

Consider the 1980 case of *Truman v. Thomas*.[10] Mrs. Truman died at the age of thirty in 1970 of cervical cancer. Dr. Thomas, a family physician engaged in a general practice, had seen Mrs. Truman frequently between 1964 and 1969, but never performed a Pap smear on her. Mrs. Truman's two children sued Dr. Thomas for his failure to perform a Pap smear on their mother. Dr. Thomas testified that he did not specifically inform Mrs. Truman of the risk involved in refusing to undergo such a test, but rather told her, "You should have a Pap smear." He further testified, "I am sure we discussed it with her so often that she couldn't fail to realize that we wanted her to have a complete examination."

This is a fascinating case. At first glance it looks like a run-of-the-mill negligence case, in that the plaintiffs are alleging that Dr. Thomas was negligent in not performing a Pap smear. But the reason he failed to perform the Pap is that Mrs. Truman refused to consent to it, and as you will recall from the preceding chapter, "Every human being of adult years and sound mind has a right to determine what shall be done with his own body."[11] The plaintiffs, however, responded that their mother refused the potentially lifesaving Pap smear because Dr. Thomas's disclosure regarding the Pap smear was inadequate or substandard. The plaintiffs argued, "It is the duty of a physician to disclose to his patient all relevant information to enable the patient to make an informed decision regarding the submission to *or refusal* to take a diagnostic test [italics added]."[10] In other words, their argument is that this case is actually about informed consent and that "Dr. Thomas breached his duty of care to Mrs. Truman when he failed to inform her of the potentially fatal consequences of allowing cervical cancer to develop undetected by a [P]ap smear."[10] Unlike the informed consent cases we have seen so far, the plaintiff here *refused* the procedure in question and was injured as a result of the refusal rather than the procedure; thus, the case is more accurately characterized as being about *informed refusal.*

This was the first well-known case of its kind. One of the issues the court needed to decide was whether consent and refusal were two sides of the same coin that should be treated alike or whether they should be distinguished and treated differently. The plaintiffs, of course, argued in support of the former position. Dr. Thomas argued in favor of the latter:

> Dr. Thomas contends that . . . the duty to disclose applies only where the patient consents to the recommended procedure. He argues that since a physician's advice may be presumed to be founded on an expert appraisal of the patient's medical needs, no reasonable patient would fail to undertake further inquiry before rejecting such advice. Therefore, patients who reject their physician's advice should shoulder the burden of inquiry as to the possible consequences of their decision.

Dr. Thomas's position was not without merit, but in the end the court sided with Mrs. Truman. Accordingly, patient refusals must be handled by physicians as if they were patient consents—that is to say, the patient refusing a test or procedure must be fully informed of the consequences of that decision, including all material risks, benefits, and alternatives.

Using Consent to Modify the Terms of the Health Care Provider–Patient Relationship

Next we take up the issue of when and how consent may be used to modify the terms of the health care provider–patient relationship.

As a matter of public policy, patients cannot consent to negligent treatment. "Generally speaking, releases of liability or waivers of the right to sue for medical negligence, signed at the time of treatment [by patients], are unenforceable as contrary to public policy."[4(p414)] The seminal case in this regard is *Tunkl v. Regents of University of California.*[12]

In *Tunkl*, defendant hospital presented to all incoming patients a document entitled "Conditions of Admission," which provided that the patient release the hospital from liability for negligent or wrongful acts. [The Supreme Court of
California] observed that the "would-be patient is in no position to reject the
proffered agreement, to bargain with the hospital, or in lieu of agreement to find
another hospital." Thus, the patient had no realistic choice but to assent to a
standardized agreement under which he waived his right to recover from negligently inflicted injuries.[13]

If enforced, the "agreement" in *Tunkl* would have had the effect of lowering the legal
standard of care. The Supreme Court of California, however, held that the hospital's
exculpatory agreement, signed on admission, was unenforceable as an adhesion
contract.

On the other hand, courts will enforce releases from liability (and hence allow patient
consent to modify the terms of the health care provider–patient relationship) when
medical care departs from standard practice for a good reason. We discuss four such
reasons here.

First, "releases are . . . commonly obtained and enforced when patients leave the hospital against medical advice ('AMA')."[4(p414)] Second, releases are obtained and enforced
when patients with decisional capacity refuse medical treatment. In the case of *Shorter v.
Drury*, the Washington Supreme Court held that a document signed by a Jehovah's
Witness patient releasing providers from responsibility for the consequences of that
patient's refusal of blood products constituted an enforceable assumption of risk.[14]

Third, under some circumstances the law will recognize the efficacy of covenants not
to sue in cases involving experimental care or alternative medicine. Under New York law,
for example,

> [w]here a patient voluntarily agrees to undergo an experimental and inherently
> dangerous surgical procedure, the parties may covenant to exempt the physician
> from liability for those injuries which are found to be the consequences of the
> non-negligent, proper performance of the procedure. . . . That is to say, that an
> experimental procedure which, because of its inherent dangers, may ordinarily be
> in and of itself a departure from customary and accepted practice (and thus pos-
> sibly actionable as malpractice) even if performed in a non-negligent manner,
> may be rendered unactionable by a covenant not to sue.[15]

In *Schneider v. Revici*, patient Edith Schneider sought treatment for breast cancer with
unconventional therapy from Dr. Emanuel Revici, "who treats cancer patients with 'non-
toxic,' noninvasive methods that have not been adopted by the medical community." After
Mrs. Schneider signed a consent form characterizing Revici's treatment procedures and
medications as "investigatory" and releasing Revici from all liability, Dr. Revici began
treating her with selenium and dietary restrictions. After fourteen months of such treat-

ments, the tumor increased in size and metastasized, and Mrs. Schneider underwent a bilateral mastectomy and sixteen months of conventional chemotherapy. In the subsequent action against Dr. Revici, one of the issues was whether Mrs. Schneider's release of Dr. Revici from liability was void as against public policy. On appeal, the court held that it was not, writing: "We see no reason why a patient should not be allowed to make an informed decision to go outside currently approved medical methods in search of an unconventional treatment."[16]

Finally, "[r]eleases from liability or covenants not to sue for negligent care are also valid if signed *after* the harm occurs and the claim arises. This is how parties settle a dispute."[4(p415)]

Expanding Frontiers: Novel Disclosure Obligations

In all of the informed consent and informed refusal cases we have seen up until now, the emphasis has been on whether the provider adequately disclosed to the patient information intrinsic to the procedure in question. In other words, the focus has been on whether the provider "has disclosed: '(1) the nature of the procedure, (2) the risks and hazards of the procedure, (3) the alternatives to the procedure, and (4) the anticipated benefits of the procedure.'"[17] In the materials that follow, we shall consider whether the provider's disclosure obligations extend beyond the scope of the procedure itself. In other words, should health care providers have a legal duty to disclose to patients material risks that result from the provider rather than from the procedure itself? As the name of this section suggests, these are developing areas in the law of informed consent.

Health Care Provider Experience

Should health care providers have a legal duty to disclose to patients material risks that result from the provider's experience?

Johnson v. Kokemoor was a case concerning plaintiff Donna Johnson, who underwent a computed tomographic scan to determine the cause of her headaches.[18] Based on the results of the scan, she was referred by her family physician to the defendant, Dr. Kokemoor, a neurosurgeon in the Chippewa Falls area. He diagnosed an enlarging aneurysm at the rear of the plaintiff's brain and recommended surgery to clip the aneurysm. The defendant performed the surgery in October of 1990. Ms. Johnson, who had no neurologic impairments preoperatively, was rendered an incomplete quadriplegic as a result of the surgery.

In the trial that followed, Ms. Johnson introduced evidence that Dr. Kokemoor had overstated his experience in performing the particular type of aneurysm surgery she required, including evidence that, when asked about that experience,

> he replied that he had performed the surgery . . . "several" times; asked what he meant by several, [he] said "dozens" and "lots of times."

> In fact . . . the defendant . . . had operated on basilar bifurcation aneurysms only twice and had never operated on a . . . basilar bifurcation aneurysm [as large as] . . . the plaintiff's.[18] (Footnotes omitted)

In the trial court (the Circuit Court of Chippewa County), Ms. Johnson prevailed, with the jury finding (1) that Dr. Kokemoor had failed to adequately inform her of the risks and advantages of her surgery, and (2) that a reasonable person in Ms. Johnson's position would have refused surgery by Dr. Kokemoor had she been adequately informed.

Dr. Kokemoor appealed the verdict, and the court of appeals reversed the decision of the trial court. On appeal to the Supreme Court of Wisconsin, that court reversed the decision of the court of appeals and wrote:

> What constitutes informed consent in a given case emanates from what a reasonable person in the patient's position would want to know. This . . . is the prudent patient standard. . . .
>
> In this case, the plaintiff introduced ample evidence that had a reasonable person in her position been aware of the defendant's relative lack of experience in performing basilar bifurcation aneurysm surgery, that person would not have undergone surgery with him. . . . We conclude that the [trial] court did not erroneously exercise its discretion in admitting evidence regarding the defendant's lack of experience and the difficulty of the proposed procedure. A reasonable person in the plaintiff's position would have considered such information material in making an intelligent and informed decision about the surgery.[18]

Johnson v. Kokemoor would seem to stand for the proposition that provider-associated risks may be material and that health care providers may have a legal duty to disclose those risks to patients.

Other jurisdictions that have considered the issue, however, have not adopted this broader view of informed consent. Consider, for example, the case of *Duttry v. Patterson*.[19] In that case, the plaintiff (Ms. Duttry) consulted with the defendant (Dr. Patterson) regarding whether she needed surgery for her esophageal cancer. Ms. Duttry claimed that, in the course of that consultation, she asked Dr. Patterson about his experience performing the surgical procedure in question. Patterson allegedly answered that "he had performed this particular procedure approximately once every month,"[19] and Ms. Duttry consented to surgery.

Three days after the surgery, which involved the resection of portions of Ms. Duttry's esophagus and stomach, a leak and subsequently a rupture developed at the site of the surgery. Ms. Duttry ultimately underwent emergency surgery.

In the trial that followed, Ms. Duttry tried to introduce evidence that Dr. Patterson had performed the surgical procedure in question only nine times in the preceding sixty months, but the trial court ruled such evidence inadmissible because it was irrelevant to the issue of informed consent. The trial court "reasoned that the only information that a physician must impart to a patient to obtain informed consent is information relative to the risks of the procedure itself."[19]

The jury returned a verdict in favor of Dr. Patterson. On appeal, the Superior Court disagreed with the trial court and concluded that evidence regarding Dr. Patterson's surgical experience and his alleged misrepresentations to Ms. Duttry was relevant to the issue of informed consent.

On further appeal to the Pennsylvania high court, the Supreme Court of Pennsylvania agreed with the trial court and reversed the Superior Court. They wrote:

> [T]he Superior Court found it critical that Patterson's alleged misinformation was given in response to a specific question posed by Duttry. The majority held that where a patient requests information regarding the physician's experience, then the physician must answer that question accurately in order to obtain the patient's informed consent. . . .
>
> We are unpersuaded by the Superior Court's reasoning. The expansive approach taken by the Superior Court below is in opposition to this commonwealth's traditional view that the doctrine of informed consent is a limited one. We have historically demanded that a physician acquaint the patient only with "the nature of the operation to be performed, the seriousness of it, the organs of the body involved, the disease or incapacity sought to be cured, and the possible results.". . . Thus, we hold that evidence of a physician's personal characteristics and experience is irrelevant to an informed consent claim.[19] (Internal footnotes omitted)

The Court, aware of the questions raised by its position on this issue, went on, writing:

> Our holding should not, however, be read to stand for the proposition that a physician who misleads a patient is immune from suit. Rather, we are merely stating that the doctrine of informed consent is not the legal panacea for all damages arising out of any type of [wrongdoing] by a physician. . . . [O]ther causes of action provide avenues for redress to the injured patient. For example, . . . in situations . . . in which the physician allegedly provides inaccurate information regarding his experience in performing a procedure, the plaintiff may have a cause of action for misrepresentation.[19]

Why did *Johnson* and *Duttry* answer differently the question of whether the legal doctrine of informed consent should be broadened to include information regarding health care provider experience? Part of the explanation may reside in the fact that Wisconsin and Pennsylvania have distinct legal traditions; perhaps public policy differences underlie the divergent results. Alternatively, the explanation for the discrepant holdings may be grounded in the factual differences between the two cases. It should be kept in mind that, as pointed out in *Johnson v. Kokemoor,*

[Johnson's] neurosurgical experts testified that even the physician considered to be one of the world's best aneurysm surgeons, who had performed hundreds of posterior circulation aneurysm surgeries, had a reported morbidity and mortality rate of ten-and-seven-tenths percent when operating upon basilar bifurcation aneurysms comparable in size to [Johnson's] aneurysm. Furthermore, information in treatises and articles which [Kokemoor] reviewed in preparation for the plaintiff's surgery set the morbidity and mortality rate at approximately fifteen percent for a basilar bifurcation aneurysm. The plaintiff also introduced expert testimony that the morbidity and mortality rate for basilar bifurcation aneurysm operations performed by one with [Kokemoor's] relatively limited experience would be between twenty and thirty percent.[18]

Thus, in *Johnson* a strong evidentiary basis was provided for the conclusion that the provider-specific information at issue was information that "add[ed] to the risks inherent in [the] procedure and [would have] suggest[ed] to the patient that a viable and possibly preferable alternative to the procedure may [have been] having the procedure performed by another provider."[17] In *Duttry* it is not as clear—at least from a reading of the Pennsylvania Supreme Court's opinion—that Patterson's relative lack of surgical experience was shown to have added to the risks inherent in the surgical procedure.

Nontechnical Characteristics of the Provider

Should health care providers have a legal duty to disclose to patients material risks that result from the nontechnical characteristics of the provider? Herein we consider two such characteristics: substance abuse and HIV infection.

Substance Abuse

In *Hidding v. Williams*, the plaintiff, Paul Hidding, underwent a decompressive laminectomy (L3 to sacrum).[20] As a result of the surgery, he was rendered incontinent of stool and urine. Hidding filed suit against Dr. Williams alleging, among other things, that the doctor had been negligent in advising him of the risks of surgery. At trial, the district court judge found in favor of Hidding and awarded him $307,006.50 in damages. On appeal, the Court of Appeal of Louisiana, Fifth Circuit, wrote:

> The district court judge found as a matter of fact that Dr. Williams abused alcohol at the time of Paul Hidding's surgery. Based on both fact and expert testimony the court concluded that this condition [re]presented a material risk to the patient, the increased potential for injury during surgery, that was not disclosed. Had the risk been disclosed, [the plaintiff] would have selected another course of treatment. Thus by failing to disclose his chronic alcohol abuse Dr. Williams violated the informed consent doctrine.[20]

Contrast the outcome of this case with that obtained in *Albany Urology Clinic v. Cleveland*.[21] In the latter case, the plaintiff (Mr. Cleveland) consulted the defendant (Dr.

Trulock) about a mass on the ventrum of his penis. After Cleveland signed an informed consent form, Trulock surgically removed the mass, which turned out not to be cancerous. Postoperatively, Cleveland developed a painful deformity of the penis that rendered him unable to engage in sexual intercourse.

Cleveland sued Trulock and threw the legal equivalent of the kitchen sink at him. Cleveland's complaint included "an assertion that Trulock had fraudulently concealed . . . his 'illegal use and abuse of cocaine . . .' at the time of Cleveland's treatment."[21] At trial, the evidence indicated that during the general period of Cleveland's treatment, Trulock used drugs "outside of work and when he was not on call."[21] The jury found for Cleveland on the claim for fraudulent concealment of cocaine abuse, but the trial court granted Trulock's motion for a judgment notwithstanding the verdict,[22] holding that the claim must fail because, as a matter of law, Trulock had no duty to disclose his cocaine abuse. The court of appeals reversed the trial court, and the Supreme Court of Georgia granted certiorari.[23]

The Supreme Court of Georgia held that, "absent inquiry by a patient or client, there is neither a common law nor a statutory duty on the part of either physicians or other professionals to disclose to their patients or clients unspecified life factors which might be subjectively considered to adversely affect the professional's performance."[21] Consequently, the failure to make such a disclosure did not provide the basis for a fraud action, nor did it "vitiate a patient's consent so as to authorize an action for battery."[21] In this 2000 opinion, the court pointed out that under Georgia common law, "Prior to 1988, Georgia physicians were not required to disclose to their patients any of the risks associated with a particular medical treatment or procedure."[21] In 1988 the Georgia General Assembly had enacted an informed consent statute changing the common law rule and requiring that medical care providers disclose to their patients, prior to surgical or diagnostic procedures, the indications for the procedure, the nature of the procedure, the material risks associated with the procedure, alternatives to the procedure, and the consequences of refusal.[24] The court decided that the statute was to be strictly construed and that, since its "plain and explicit terms" did not cover the situation in question, the common law rule (no disclosure required) would control.[21]

HIV Infection

In *Estate of Behringer v. Medical Center at Princeton*, the plaintiff, Behringer, was an otolaryngologist (ENT) on the medical staff of the Medical Center when he was diagnosed with acquired immunodeficiency syndrome (AIDS).[25] In response, the Medical Center temporarily suspended his surgical privileges. As a condition of lifting the suspension, the Medical Center required that Behringer disclose to his patients that he was seropositive for the human immunodeficiency virus (HIV) in the process of obtaining informed consent to surgery from them. Subsequently, relying on an opinion by the Council on Ethical and Judicial Affairs of the American Medical Association (AMA) suggesting that physicians with infectious diseases should not engage in activities creating a risk of disease transmission to others, the Medical Center adopted a new policy for HIV-seropositive health care workers. Under that policy, physicians or health care providers with known HIV seropositivity would be permitted to treat patients at the Medical Center, but would not be permitted to perform procedures posing any risk of HIV transmission to patients. Behringer never again operated at the Medical Center.

Behringer's estate brought an action against the Medical Center alleging, among other things, that the restrictions it had placed upon his surgical privileges were discriminatory. The court held that the Medical Center had "properly required the plaintiff, as a physician with a positive diagnosis of AIDS, to secure informed consent from any surgical patients . . . as a condition of vacating the temporary suspension of plaintiff's surgical privileges."[25] In reaching its decision, the court considered the risk (probability) of HIV transmission from the health care provider to the patients, as well as the severity of the consequences to the patient should transmission occur. Additionally, the court wrote:

> It is the court's view that the risk of [HIV] transmission is not the sole risk involved. The risk of a surgical accident, i.e., a needlestick or scalpel cut, during surgery performed by an HIV-positive surgeon, may subject a previously uninfected patient to months or even years of continual HIV testing. Both of these risks are sufficient to . . . requir[e] disclosure. . . .
>
> . . . If there is to be an ultimate arbiter of whether the patient is to be treated invasively by an AIDS-positive surgeon, the arbiter will be the fully informed patient.[25]

Payment Incentives and Financial Conflicts of Interest

Should health care providers have a legal duty to disclose to patients material risks that result from existing financial conflicts of interest (COIs)?

In *Shea v. Esensten*, plaintiff Patrick Shea consulted his primary care physician regarding chest pains he had experienced that had necessitated his hospitalization while on an overseas business trip.[26] Notwithstanding Shea's complaints of chest pain and dyspnea and his extensive family history of heart disease, his physician told him that referral to a cardiologist was unnecessary because of his age (forty); the physician's recommendation remained unchanged even after Shea offered to pay for the cardiologist himself. Mr. Shea died within a few months of heart failure.

> Mr. Shea had been an employee of Seagate Technologies, Inc. . . . Seagate provided health care benefits to its employees by contracting with a health maintenance organization (HMO) known as Medica. . . . Medica required Seagate's employees to select one of Medica's authorized primary care doctors[, of whom Mr. Shea's family doctor was one]. [Under the terms of the plan, b]efore Mr. Shea could see a specialist, . . . Medica required . . . a written referral from his primary care doctor. Unknown to Mr. Shea, Medica's contracts with its preferred doctors

created financial incentives that were designed to minimize referrals. Specifically, the primary care doctors were rewarded for not making covered referrals to specialists, and were docked a portion of their fees if they made too many. According to Mr. Shea's widow . . . , if her husband would have known his doctor could earn a bonus for treating less, he would have disregarded his doctor's advice, sought a cardiologist's opinion at his own expense, and would still be alive today.[26]

Shea's widow commenced an action asserting, among other things, that Medica's nondisclosure of its financial incentives violated its fiduciary duties. The district court dismissed the complaint, and Mrs. Shea appealed.

On appeal, the U.S. Court of Appeals for the Eighth Circuit wrote:

> Although the district court acknowledged Medica's duty of loyalty, the court felt the compensation arrangements between Medica and its doctors were not material facts requiring disclosure. We disagree. From the patient's point of view, a financial incentive scheme put in place to influence a treating doctor's referral practices . . . is certainly a material piece of information. . . . Thus, we conclude Mr. Shea had the right to know Medica was offering financial incentives that could have colored his doctor's medical judgment about the urgency for a cardiac referral.[26]

Other courts faced with the financial COI issue have decided differently. *Neade v. Portes* was a case involving Anthony Neade, a hypertensive, hyperlipidemic obese smoker with a family history of heart disease.[27] In August 1990, at age thirty-seven, he complained to his primary care physician, Dr. Steven Portes, of chest pain radiating to his arm associated with dyspnea. Portes hospitalized him for three days, during which time he underwent testing that included a thallium stress test and an electrocardiogram. Dr. Thomas Engel (presumably a cardiologist) found the test results to be normal and attributed the chest pain to a hiatal hernia and/or esophagitis.

In the six weeks following his hospitalization, Neade saw Dr. Portes on three occasions, "complaining of continued chest pain radiating to his neck and arm. Relying on the results of the thallium stress test and EKG . . . Dr. Portes informed Neade that his chest pain was not cardiac related."[27]

In October 1990 Neade returned, complaining of stabbing chest pain. Dr. Portes asked his associate, Dr. Huang, to examine Neade. Based on that examination, Dr. Huang recommended that Neade undergo cardiac catheterization and coronary angiography. Dr. Huang, however, did not have hospital privileges; in any event, Portes, as Neade's primary care physician, "was responsible for ordering any necessary . . . additional tests." He did not do so.

In June 1991 Neade returned, again complaining of chest pain. This time Portes asked another associate, Dr. Schlager, to see him. Dr. Schlager, too, recommended an angiogram, but again Portes did not authorize the angiogram. In September 1991, Neade suffered a massive myocardial infarction and died nine days later.

Neade's wife brought suit, alleging (1) that Portes was negligent in relying on the thallium stress test and failing to order an angiogram, and (2) that Portes breached his fiduciary duty to Neade by failing to disclose (to Neade) that he (Portes) had financial incentives not to order the angiogram. Regarding the latter allegation, Neade's wife contended that, under an agreement between Chicago HMO (Neade's health insurer) and Dr. Portes's primary care group, the former would pay the latter $75,000 per year (the so-called Medical Incentive Fund). This money was to be used to pay the costs of patient referrals and medical tests.

> Pursuant to the contract between Dr. Portes, Primary Care and Chicago HMO, any portion of the Medical Incentive Fund that was not used for referrals or outside tests would be divided at the end of each year between Primary Care's full time physicians and Chicago HMO, with the physicians receiving 60% of the remaining money and Chicago HMO receiving 40%. If the Medical Incentive Fund was exhausted prior to the end of the year, Dr. Portes and his group would be required to fund any additional consultant fees and outside tests.[27]

The trial court held that the evidence regarding Dr. Portes's financial incentives was not relevant to the negligence claim against him (claim 1),[28] and dismissed the second claim because it found that "there existed no cause of action against a physician for breach of fiduciary duty."[27]

Mrs. Neade appealed, and the appellate court sided with her on both issues—that is, on the relevance of the evidence regarding financial incentives to the malpractice claim (the first claim) and on the existence of a cause of action for breach of fiduciary duty by a physician (the second claim).

Dr. Portes appealed to the Supreme Court of Illinois. The court dealt with the two claims in reverse order. Regarding claim 2, the Supreme Court of Illinois declined "to recognize a new cause of action for breach of fiduciary duty against a physician for the physician's failure to disclose HMO incentives in a suit brought against the physician for medical negligence."[27] In so deciding, the court relied partly on the argument that claim 2 (the breach of fiduciary duty claim) was duplicative of claim 1 (the medical malpractice claim), an argument that the U.S. Supreme Court had earlier found persuasive in *Herdrich v. Pegram*.[29] Regarding claim 1, the Supreme Court of Illinois held that evidence of the Medical Incentive Fund might be relevant if Dr. Portes testified at trial, because such evidence would bear on his credibility as a witness.

Chapter Summary

Battery is the intentional, harmful, or offensive touching of another without his or her consent. Whereas early consent cases were grounded in the law of battery, modern informed consent law is negligence based. Nevertheless, modern medical providers can still be sued for battery if (1) the patient has not consented at all, (2) the medical provider performs a procedure other than the one to which the patient consented (including, for example, the right procedure on the wrong part of the body), or (3) an unconsented-to medical provider performs the procedure.

Patient consent to medical procedures may be express or implied, as, for example, under the emergency or the extension doctrines. When a medical provider makes a mistake about consent, the outcome of the case will depend on the reasonableness of the mistake. In cases in which the defendant's mistake is reasonable, consent will be held to exist and there is no battery. In cases in which the defendant's mistake is unreasonable, then a battery will be held to have occurred. Modern cases treat informed refusal and informed consent as two sides of the same coin. Consequently, patients refusing a recommended test or procedure must be fully informed of the consequences of that decision, including all material risks and benefits of the refusal and alternatives thereto.

A patient's consent—given at the time of treatment—to release a medical provider from liability for medical negligence is void as against public policy. Courts will enforce releases from liability where medical care departs from standard practice for good reasons, including patients leaving the hospital against medical advice, patients exercising their right to refuse medical treatment, and patients seeking experimental care or alternative medicine. Also, releases from liability for negligent care are valid if signed *after* the harm occurs and the claim arises.

More recently, the frontiers of informed consent law have been tested and courts have considered whether medical providers have a legal duty to disclose to patients material risks that result not from the procedure being consented to but from some characteristic of the medical provider himself or herself (e.g., medical provider experience, provider substance abuse, provider HIV positivity, or the existence of financial incentives). Courts have largely split on these novel disclosure obligations.

Review Questions

1. What is battery? When health care providers are sued because of problems involving consent, what kinds of cases does the law deal with as negligence cases? As battery cases?

2. What is the emergency exception? What is the extension doctrine? How do they relate to consent and informed consent?

3. What does the term *ghost surgery* mean? Is consent for a health care provider to perform a medical procedure transferable to another provider?

4. How does the law handle those situations in which the health care provider, believing he or she had obtained consent from a patient who did not mean to consent, performs a medical procedure on that patient? Is it a battery? Negligence? Neither?

5. How does informed refusal differ from informed consent? How are they alike?

6. In *Truman v. Thomas,* Dr. Thomas argued that "since a physician's advice may be presumed to be founded on an expert appraisal of the patient's medical needs, no reasonable patient would fail to undertake further inquiry before rejecting such advice," and that consequently, "patients who reject their physician's advice should shoulder the burden of inquiry as to the possible consequences of their decision." Why do you think this argument was unpersuasive? Do you believe that patients presume that their physicians' advice is always based solely on their medical needs?

7. Is a patient's consent to a provision releasing his or her health care provider from liability for future negligence effective? Why or why not?

8. List four ways in which consent can be used to modify the terms of the health care provider–patient relationship.

9. As part of the informed consent process, must a health care provider disclose to the patient the extent of his or her experience with the procedure under consideration? Does it matter whether the patient makes specific inquiry?

10. As part of the informed consent process, must a health care provider who is an active substance abuser disclose this to the patient? Should such persons be practicing medicine, or any of the allied health professions, to begin with?

11. As part of the informed consent process, must a health care provider who is HIV positive disclose this to the patient? Does the nature of his or her practice make a difference? Suppose he or she is a psychiatrist? An internist? An acupuncturist? A surgeon?

12. As part of the informed consent process, must a health care provider disclose any financial conflicts of interest that incentivize undertreatment (e.g., HMO arrangements) to his or her patient? What if it is overtreatment of the patient that is being incentivized (e.g., fee for service)? When, if ever, should such disclosure be made? How? By whom?

Endnotes

1. Consent to and refusal of medical treatment. In: Sanbar SS, Gibofsky A, Firestone MH, et al., eds. *Legal Medicine.* 5th ed. St. Louis: Mosby, 2001:245–267, p. 256. *The chapter was written by a committee of the editors (see above), who gratefully acknowledged the past contributions of Emidio A. Bianco, MD, JD, and Harold L. Hirsch, MD, JD.*
2. For a discussion of battery, see Franklin MA, Rabin RL. *Tort Law and Alternatives: Cases and Materials.* 4th ed. Mineola, NY: Foundation Press, 1987:759–815. See also Emanuel S. *Torts.* 3rd ed. Larchmont, NY: Emanuel Law Outlines, 1988:9–14.
3. *Black's Law Dictionary.* Abridged 6th ed. St. Paul, MN: West Publishing, 1991:104.

4. Hall MA, Bobinski MA, Orentlicher D. *Health Care Law and Ethics.* 7th ed. Austin, TX: Aspen Publishers, 2007:215.
5. *Mohr v. Williams,* 95 Minn. 261, 104 N.W. 12 (Sup. Ct. Minn. 1905).
6. *Kennedy v. Parrott,* 243 N.C. 355, 90 S.E.2d 754 (Sup. Ct. N.C. 1956).
7. *Perna v. Pirozzi,* 92 N.J. 446, 457 A.2d 431 (Sup. Ct. N.J. 1983).
8. *Tisdale v. Pruitt,* 394 S.E.2d 857 (Ct. App. S.C. 1990).
9. Emanuel S. *Torts.* 3rd ed. Larchmont, NY: Emanuel Law Outlines, 1988:9–14.
10. *Truman v. Thomas,* 611 P.2d 902 (Sup. Ct. Cal. 1980).
11. *Schloendorff v. Society of New York Hospital,* 105 N.E. 92 (NY 1914).
12. *Tunkl v. Regents of U. of Cal.,* 383 P.2d 441 (Cal. 1963).
13. *Madden v. Kaiser Foundation Hospital,* 552 P.2d 1178 (Cal. 1976).
14. *Shorter v. Drury,* 695 P.2d 116 (Wash. 1985).
15. *Colton v. New York Hospital,* 414 N.Y.S.2d 866, 876 (Sup. Ct. N.Y. 1979).
16. *Schneider v. Revici,* 817 F.2d 987 (2d Cir. 1987).
17. *DeGennaro v. Tandon,* 873 A.2d 191, 196 (Conn. App. 2005).
18. *Johnson v. Kokemoor,* 545 N.W.2d 495 (Wis. 1996).
19. *Duttry v. Patterson,* 771 A.2d 1255 (Pa. 2001).
20. *Hidding v. Williams,* 578 So. 2d 1192 (La. Ct. App. 1991).
21. *Albany Urology Clinic v. Cleveland,* 272 Ga. 296, 528 S.E.2d 777 (Ga. 2000).
22. A "judgment notwithstanding the verdict" is also known as a j.n.o.v., or a judgment *non obstante veredicto.* It refers to a "judgment entered by order of the court for the plaintiff (or defendant) although there has been a [jury] verdict for the [other party]." See *Black's Law Dictionary,* p. 730.
23. A party wishing a higher court to hear its case, where appeal to that higher court is not a matter of right but of discretion, files a petition for a writ of certiorari. "If the writ is denied, the [higher] court refuses to hear the appeal and, in effect, the judgment below stands unchanged. If the writ is granted [by the higher court], then it has the effect of ordering the lower court to certify the record [of a particular case] and send it up to the higher court. . . ." See *Black's Law Dictionary,* p. 1109.
24. O.C.G.A, section 31-9-6.1 (a) (1)-(6).
25. *Estate of Behringer v. Medical Center at Princeton,* 592 A.2d 1251, 1255 (N.J. Super. Ct. Div. 1991).
26. *Shea v. Esensten,* 107 F.3d 625 (8th Cir. 1997).
27. *Neade v. Portes,* 739 NE2d 496 (Ill. 2000).
28. In other words, the court was saying that the standard of care under such circumstances is what it is (i.e., either an angiogram was indicated or it was not), and the existence or nonexistence of financial incentives has nothing to do with the standard of care. But see our discussion of the standard of care in Chapter 15, particularly our discussion of the best judgment rule. Under that rule, could an argument be made that evidence of financial incentives is relevant?
29. *Herdrich v. Pegram,* 530 U.S. 211 (2000). Two points should be made here. First, in *Herdrich*—a discussion of which is beyond the scope of this chapter—the U.S. Supreme Court was not faced with the question of whether a failure to disclose financial incentives is a violation of fiduciary duty. In a footnote therein, however, the Court did suggest that failing to disclose financial incentives might violate the Employee Retirement Income Security Act (ERISA). See footnote 8, and see Hall, note 9 on p. 1134. Second, as was pointed out by Chief Justice Harrison in his dissent in *Neade v. Portes,* "In this case . . . the negligence and breach of fiduciary duty counts . . . are not identical. As the appellate court correctly recognized, 'It is conceivable that a trier

of fact could find both that Dr. Portes was within the standard of care and therefore not negligent in relying on the thallium stress test and the EKG in deciding that an angiogram was not necessary and also that Dr. Portes did breach his fiduciary duty in not disclosing his financial incentive arrangement and, as a proximate result thereof, Neade did not obtain a second opinion, suffered a massive coronary infarction, and died.' " (See *Neade,* 303 Ill. App. 3d, p. 814.)

Section III

Ethics Across the Lifespan

Chapter 10

Ethics and Genetics

I'll never understand what possessed my mother to put her faith in God's hands, rather than her local geneticist.

—Vincent, in *Gattaca*

Chapter Learning Objectives
At the conclusion of this chapter the reader will be able to:

1. Identify the ethical issues raised by genetic medicine

2. Discuss the implications of genetic testing for individuals, families, and research

3. Defend an ethical position concerning genetic testing

4. Apply ethical reasoning to future issues in genetic medicine

---

Case 10-A

Your patient, AB, has had amniocentesis because she is older than thirty-five years. The results reveal a male fetus with an apparently balanced translocation karyotype. Parental blood chromosome studies are indicated, and AB is found to be a translocation carrier. One month later, AB's sister, CD, comes to you for an evaluation of her poor pregnancy history, which includes a stillbirth with multiple congenital anomalies and three first-trimester miscarriages. If AB has inherited the translocation from a parent, CD may also be a translocation carrier. Because of her experience, she refuses any invasive prenatal diagnostic testing. She is unaware of the results of her sister's testing.

This chapter is devoted to an examination of the ethical issues that have arisen as a result of the recent scientific developments in the field of human genetics. The concept of a concerted effort to map and sequence the human genome was introduced in 1985. The fifteen-year Human Genome Project, begun in 1990 and completed ahead of schedule, in 2003, exemplifies the rapid developments in human genetics. Studies of the long-range ethical, legal, and social implications of the project were supported by three percent of the funds allocated to the project.[1]

Much of the following discussion is based on the assumption that the information generated by genetic testing has a significance that is greater than that of other medical information, a point of view called *genetic exceptionalism*.

Does Genetic Information Warrant Special Treatment?

Genetic Exceptionalism

Genetic exceptionalism is the concept that genetic information is qualitatively different from other medical information and therefore requires a higher level of protection. This difference is based on its "uniquely personal and uniquely powerful" characteristics.[2] Some individuals view genetic information as more central to the core being of humans than other types of information about us. It is believed that genetics can reveal who we really are. The arguments in support of the position of exceptionalism are presented by Thomas Murray,[3] and can be summarized as follows:

- The impact genetic information can have on others
- The risks for stigmatization and discrimination
- A resulting attitude of genetic determinism

Information that has a genetic basis can affect not only the individual whose information it is, but others as well. Although it may be an individual who is subject to genetic testing, the results of those tests reveal information that may be shared by other people. Of course, our genes are inherited from our parents, so we share fifty percent of them with each parent. A positive test result for the BRCA1 gene (a known gene for breast cancer) or for a translocation chromosome does not tell us from which side of the family it came. We also share half our genes with our siblings and our children. A positive genetic test result, then, has implications for them as well. There is a risk that any one of these family members may carry the BRCA1 gene or the chromosome translocation. The extended family (aunts, uncles, cousins, grandparents, etc.) may also be at increased risk for carrying the same genetic finding, a risk that is lower than fifty percent or twenty-five percent, but still increased above that of the general population. Genetic information about one member of the family can reveal risk information about others who may not have been aware of it, such as CD in Case 10-A, and who may not want that information. The argument regarding shared genes can be extended to include racial and ethnic groups. People have a risk for a number of genes in common with others of the same ethnic background, such as the genes for Tay-Sachs disease[4] in the Ashkenazi Jewish population or thalassemia[5] in the Mediterranean populations, or of the same race, such as sickle hemoglobin[6] in the black population or cystic fibrosis[7] in Caucasians.

The results of genetic testing can have not only health implications but also social implications. Genetic information can be predictive of possible future illness. Genetic tests can identify disease-causing genes in healthy people. Positive BRCA1 test results, for example, imply a risk for breast, ovarian, and other cancers that is increased above that of people who do not carry the mutation. It does not determine whether or when a mutation carrier will become affected. Testing done prior to an individual's having symptoms of a disorder is called *presymptomatic testing*. Genes that have a high rate of penetrance,[8] such as the gene for Huntington disease,[9] and therefore a greater degree of predictability of disease, can also be identified. Predictive tests are not diagnostic tests, whereas presymptomatic tests may be. The knowledge of the results of these tests can make an individual vulnerable on many personal and social levels.

History has taught us that access to genetic information can lead to the misuse of that information in the stigmatization of and discrimination against individuals. The eugenics movement,[10] employers, and insurance companies have all been implicated in discriminating against those who are already affected or who may be affected in the future. Genetic exceptionalism requires that special protections be put in place to ensure the privacy of genetic information and to prevent discrimination against vulnerable individuals.

It can be argued that the reasons that are presented to support genetic exceptionalism are much more social than scientific.[11] A corollary to the worry that without special protection people could be "blamed" for their DNA is the danger that genetic exceptionalism may lead to genetic essentialism or determinism.[12] *Genetic determinism* is the notion that genes determine and explain everything about a person. It strengthens the perception that understanding and controlling genetics will eradicate illness, as well as the perception that because people are shaped by their genes, they have no responsibility for their behavior.

Genetic exceptionalism has its proponents and critics. Whether or not we support the position that genetic information is different from other medical information, there has been a movement in medicine that includes ethical considerations of the implications of genetic testing.[13] Genetics has stimulated much conversation and debate about the ethical challenges in research and medicine. Foster and colleagues worry that as genetics becomes more integrated into medicine, or becomes routinized, there will be a loss of the broader moral reflection on genetic issues that has been encouraged to date, as well as the special ethical protections and clinical practices that developed largely because of genetic exceptionalism in medicine, research, and clinical care.[14] The following discussion includes a closer look at some of the ethical issues that have been identified and the clinical practices that have been developed based on the view that genetic information has special qualities that are personal, sensitive, and familial and could lead to misuse or abuse of the information.

Two ethical issues that are strengthened from a position of genetic exceptionalism are privacy and prevention of discrimination.

Privacy
From a privacy perspective, the autonomous ability to have control over one's own genetic information is central. A desire for genetic privacy suggests that there are fears of discrimination, social stigma, familial problems, and loss of control over one's identity and of freedom from interference in private choices.[12(p277)] Individual privacy rights concerning information would include the right *not* to:

- Have one's genetic information collected without permission
- Have one's genetic information used for an unauthorized purpose
- Have one's genetic information disclosed to a third party
- Know one's own genetic information (if one didn't want to)[15]

A person's medical information can be found recorded in his or her medical records. It is not unusual for society to protect special information that is maintained in written form. Medical records containing information about mental health treatment or HIV test results have long been afforded extra privacy protection.

Your patient, CD, relying on your respect of her privacy, can be confident that you will not do any testing on her without her permission. Her sister, AB, knows that her medical records with her chromosome test results will not be released to anyone she does not want to know about them. Are AB and CD correct in these assumptions? This raises the questions of who should have access to genetic information and why. These issues will be discussed later in this chapter.

Prevention of Discrimination

There is a concern about the use and misuse of genetic information. We cannot control or determine the genes we inherit. Genetic information is immutable. Consequently, it is unfair to allow this information to be used to cause harm to an individual. Past social injustices have shown, though, that unanticipated social harms can be caused by the misuse by third parties of our personal characteristics. Although there is very little modern data to support the fear that genetic information will be used to discriminate against individuals, the possibility of that happening is ever present.

Only some positive genetic tests are actually diagnostic of illness. On the other hand, not all illnesses have a genetic marker. Having a genetic predisposition is not the same as having a diagnosis of disease. A woman with a family history of breast cancer and a positive BRCA1 test has an increased risk for, but may never get, breast cancer. This concept is not always well understood, which makes it especially vulnerable to misuse in the areas of insurance and employment.

Insurance companies claim that they should have access to all of a person's relevant information. They want to prevent an individual with a positive genetic or diagnostic test from hiding, or not disclosing, that information before buying extremely large amounts of insurance. This does not seem to be the case in life insurance, however.[16] The insurance industry considers the classification of individuals neutral because it is for purposes of underwriting. Individuals with equivalent risks should be treated the same. The public, however, considers the adverse treatment of asymptomatic individuals to be unfair.[16(p354)]

Employers also claim to have a legitimate interest in having access to medical information that may affect the health and therefore the performance of employees. Employees with genetic susceptibilities have the potential for lost productivity and increased costs associated with disease. Using the ethical principle of avoiding harm, the employer would try to protect the health and safety of the individual employee and others working with him or her. Employees, on the other hand, are concerned that they would be excluded from jobs because of their medical information. The ethical principle of justice supports equal opportunities in employment.

The harms that can follow from the fear of genetic-based discrimination include the reluctance to take tests that could be important in identifying risks and leading to health interventions. Research can also suffer when people do not participate because of the fear of losing control over personal information. There should be a balance between personal control and unwarranted uses of genetic information without restricting the clinical and research value of genetic technology and information.

Whose Information Is It?

Case 10-B

Ms. EF has been identified as a carrier of a cystic fibrosis mutation. Her husband, GF, refuses testing, claiming he was tested during his first marriage and found not to carry a mutation. You remember testing him during his first marriage and know that he is indeed a carrier of the delta F508 mutation. His first wife was not a mutation carrier, so they were not a couple at risk for having a child with cystic fibrosis. You think that either he never learned about his carrier status, he did not understand the information given to him about it, or he does not want to share it with his new wife.

The Individual

The debate about who owns genetic information is more about privacy than about ownership. Privacy is not the same as sole ownership of information. Most specific genetic information is obtained by examining and testing an individual. Does that individual own his or her information? Many individuals choose to keep the results of their genetic tests private. Ms. AB in Case 10-A decided not to share her test results with her sister. Mr. GF in Case 10-B seems to have made the same decision. When a person has a skeletal dysplasia, such as achondroplasia,[17] his or her genetic status for that gene is obvious to everyone else. If the genetic information is not obvious and may not become apparent until some future time, such as with Huntington disease, most people have an expectation of privacy regarding that information.[18] Many will express their autonomy by choosing not to share it with others.

When an individual is found to have a disease-specific gene, such as cystic fibrosis, his or her family members have an up to fifty percent risk of also being gene carriers.

They do not receive personal carrier status or a diagnosis on the basis of the individual's test. For disorders that are apparent or may affect one or more family members, such as breast cancer, interested family members can pursue their own testing without the need to know the original patient's genetic status.[19] For disorders that are not apparent or for which there is no family history, without specific risk information, testing may not be done or may be delayed. In Case 10-B, GF may in fact be communicating a desire not to know his genetic status by denying knowledge of it. It would benefit his children, who are at risk for having cystic fibrosis, to have his genetic information conveyed to their doctor. For those affected children, not knowing they are at risk for cystic fibrosis could cause them harm by delaying their care and exacerbating their health problems.

We should consider other possible harms done by not sharing genetic information with family members. Ms. CD in Case 10-A may be a translocation carrier like her sister. Without having this knowledge, she is at risk of going through the heartbreak of having another unanticipated miscarriage or stillborn child with multiple congenital anomalies. On the basis of her pregnancy history, chromosome testing would be appropriate, and could be offered without disclosing her sister's test results. If the situation were reversed and CD was a translocation carrier, her pregnancy history would be known to AB, who could then be offered chromosome analysis on that basis. In general, the harms of not sharing genetic information with relatives do not usually lead to immediate or grave damages to others. When genetic information could lead to interventions that reduce morbidity and mortality from disease, individual privacy could result in harm to others. Limiting disclosure would be unjust. Encouraging altruism is one approach to the individual-versus-family (or control-versus-access) conflict.

The Family

Individual autonomy has been challenged by genetic medicine. Individuals are members of families, who have inherited their genetic information from common ancestors. Family members have an interest in the genetic test results of relatives and can claim a right to know the nature of familial genetic information. Some pedigrees or family trees have multiple branches. When considering who owns or has a right to "familial" genetic information, we have to define *family*. This can be problematic. Families may share as much as fifty percent or a little as eight percent of their genes and still be at risk for the same diseases. We see this clearly when cousins marry. The percentage of children born with problems from cousin relationships is higher than in the general population. Defining a relative as anyone who shares a specific number of genes is arbitrary. Lucassen considers family members to be "account holders" using a joint account model.[20] Because genetic information is shared by a family, she claims that confidentiality and privacy should not apply to the individual but to the family. She argues that if anyone should own genetic information, it should be all those who inherit it.

Duty to Warn

The position that families have the right to the genetic test results of relatives raises the specter of a duty to warn. Although this question has been addressed by several U.S. courts, we will focus on the ethical issues of such a duty. When asked, ninety-five percent of patients said they would tell family members who were at risk for the same genetic disorder if the patient perceived the information would be useful to those relatives.[21] If family members have a right to the genetic information that those few individuals do not want to share, whose responsibility is it to notify ("warn") them when the information has implications for their health status? The health care provider is the most obvious choice. We have to weigh the benefits and harms of taking on that responsibility. Sharing patient information without permission is a breach of confidentiality. The harms to the patient of such a breach include the disruption of the patient–provider relationship. There are also social harms to the patient, including the psychological impact and the interference with family relationships. When asked why they would choose not to tell their relatives, patient responses included concern for altering family dynamics, protecting relatives from the knowledge, estranged family relations, refusal to accept a genetic etiology, and guilt.[22]

A duty to warn would also impose burdens on the health care provider. Nonmaleficence would suggest that the health care provider's responsibility is to protect vulnerable individuals, such as those who have just received a genetic diagnosis or have a genetic disease, against the imposition of family or professional views. Being responsible to third parties with whom there is no professional relationship puts the health care provider in an untenable, adversarial relationship with his or her patients. The definition of at-risk relatives again becomes an issue. Identification of current and future relatives who may at some time have an unspecified risk is a potentially unlimited responsibility. Some suggest that a health care provider should notify at-risk relatives when there is an imminence of harm from the genetic disorder and where those relatives can be identified.[23] When the harms to the patient are not outweighed by the harms to the family, patient confidentiality would argue against the family's right of access to the patient's genetic information and the breach of confidentiality it would require. The situations in Cases 10-A and 10-B involve pregnancies, which limit the number of relatives involved and the time frame in which the health care provider can work. The provider's communication to the patient of the familial risk of genetic problems and encouragement to share that information with relatives would satisfy any ethical obligations to the family.

Researchers

Researchers also have an interest in genetic information. Most people are willing to allow personal genetic information to be used in medical research. Historically, tissue samples removed from an individual have been considered to be donations made to the researcher. Property rights have been asserted, however, by individuals whose tissue has been used to generate personal gain for the researcher or the researcher's institution, and who are asking to share in the profits. In a California case, the court concluded that the individual gave up control of his tissue once it was removed through surgery.[24] Policy reasons for not recognizing individual property rights in genetic material include the possible inflation in the cost of research, which could result in a decrease in the development of medicines, for example, and an increase in the cost to the consumer. A decrease in participation in clinical research has also been cited as a harm resulting from creating a personal property right in genetic material.

The Special Case of Monozygotic Twins

A unique situation is that of monozygotic twins, who share all their genes. Testing one twin will reveal information about the other.

> **Case 10-C**
>
> Mr. JL has requested predictive testing for Huntington disease. His mother, her brother, and their father have died from the disease. JL has a 1 in 2 chance of having inherited the gene. The family history reveals that he has a twin brother, KL, who lives in another state. JL's physician wonders whether he needs the participation or permission of KL prior to testing JL.[25]

From a privacy perspective, each twin is an individual with the freedom to know or not know his genetic status. The effects on an individual of this knowledge can change the way he thinks about himself and can influence the decisions he makes about life choices. The twins in Case 10-C may not agree, however, about having the test for Huntington disease. To deny testing to one twin because the other does not want to know his own genetic status gives the second twin unjustified control over the first. The nonconsenting twin should not have veto power over the decision of the other. Both the desire to know and the desire not to know would seem to be of equal importance. If the health care provider does not provide testing, he is violating his patient's freedom to know. If the harm that is to be prevented by not doing the testing (i.e., respecting KL's right not to know) is not unquestionably significantly greater than the harm caused (i.e., not respecting JL's autonomy), then JL's request for testing should be honored.[26] Prior to making a testing decision, all reasonable efforts should be made to have the twins work out an arrangement that allows both to satisfy his wishes as far as possible.

Clinical Applications of Genetic Testing

Deciding what constitutes a genetic test is not easy, and definitions vary widely, as can be seen in the genetic privacy laws of the various states.[27] Genetic testing covers an array of techniques, and is used in health care to confirm a suspected diagnosis or predict the risk for genetic diseases. Testing can be useful at different life stages:

- Heterozygote carrier testing may identify a couple at risk for an autosomal recessive disease.

- Prenatal testing may identify an affected fetus.

- Newborn screening programs identify infants with treatable metabolic disorders.

- Presymptomatic testing identifies those at risk for adult-onset disorders.

Reprogenetics

Of all of the possible uses of genetic tests, prenatal diagnosis has stimulated the most discussion. The combination of genetics and reproductive techniques, when used in a clinical setting, has been called *reprogenetics*.[28] Several techniques are used to detect genetic disorders, most of which are generally effective and accurate. These include preimplantation genetic diagnosis, maternal serum screens, chorionic villus sampling, and amniocentesis.

In general, some claim that prenatal diagnosis is so closely linked to abortion that it is necessary to assume the acceptability of patient choice regarding abortion before even considering performing any procedures.[29] Abortion, however, is not a consideration for everyone. Relief of anxiety, preparation for the birth of an affected child, consideration of adoption, and preparation for medical treatments have also been suggested as reasons for utilizing prenatal diagnosis. Some families have a high risk for having an affected child, such as an at-risk couple for Tay-Sachs disease. Prenatal diagnosis can remove a risk that may be perceived as totally unacceptable. Because most test results are normal, pregnancies that may never have been attempted or that would have been ended early are continued to term. Prenatal diagnosis enhances reproductive choice and increases an individual's autonomy.[30]

Some thinkers maintain that parents have a responsibility not to bring a disabled child into the world.[31] Prenatal diagnosis can be seen as eugenics in disguise by determining, in effect, which lives are valuable and which are not.[30] It can also be seen to express certain attitudes toward disabled people. If the diagnosis of disability is negatively valued on prenatal diagnosis, that attitude can carry over to people living with that disability. There is a negative attitude, or implied disrespect, for those individuals who are disabled.[32] These prenatal diagnostic techniques are thus seen as being used for impairment prevention.

Although negative valuations of the lives of disabled individuals are often based on prejudice, sometimes they are based on evidence. Some impairments not only make life more limited and burdensome for the affected individual but also create burdens for those who care for them. Some disabled people do have a very poor quality of life, as do their caretakers. Undergoing prenatal diagnosis and abortion when the results are positive is not inevitably discriminatory or prejudiced against disabled people.[33]

Case 10-D

Ms. MN has a two-month-old son affected with Wiskott-Aldrich syndrome.[34] Her brother died of the same disease. The patient learns through a parent support group of the success of bone marrow transplantation from an HLA-matched sibling donor as a cure for Wiskott-Aldrich syndrome. She asks you to help her conceive an unaffected HLA-identical fetus that after birth can be the source of bone marrow for use in transplantation into the affected child.

Preimplantation genetic diagnosis (PGD) is done on one or two cells that have been removed from an eight-cell embryo created through in vitro fertilization (IVF). The DNA from these cells is analyzed to ascertain which embryos carry a specific disease mutation or chromosome abnormality. Those embryos without the mutation or chromosome abnormality are then implanted in the uterus. The timing of PGD helps couples avoid having to make a decision about evaluating quality of life or maintaining a pregnancy when the future is unclear. It also avoids the burdens that are associated with disease. For the adult, it eliminates any physical complications from abortion. An important variation on the use of PGD is for nondisclosing diagnosis. For families with Huntington disease who do not want to know the parent's own gene status but also do not want to pass the gene to the next generation, PGD can be helpful. Only embryos with normal huntingtin genes can be implanted without the family learning the genetic status of other embryos or the number of embryos available.[35]

Are there unacceptable uses of PGD? The patient in Case 10-D wants to use PGD to create a child for the purpose of saving another, not necessarily because she wants another child. The DNA studies would be done not solely to identify a disease mutation, but to find a specific non-health-related trait that will not be pertinent to that child. The use of PGD to comply with the patient's request can be considered a first step in the nonmedical application of this procedure. Selection of non-health-related traits can also be called enhancement. The techniques used for PGD and IVF are costly. Access to enhancement techniques will be available to those who can afford them. This access will be unequal and therefore unfair. Parents with resources could increase the chances that their children will succeed in life by making them taller, smarter, or stronger. This could increase the gap between those who have resources and those who do not.[36] Despite widespread intuitive objection to using PGD, it can be justified in terms of parental autonomy and falls within the value of family planning.[37]

Sex Selection

Prenatal diagnosis has been used as a vehicle for the selection of a fetus of a specific sex. Sex selection has its supporters and detractors. The principal medical reason is the known or suspected risk for a sex-linked genetic disorder. MN of Case 10-D could have requested the identification of only female fetuses if an HLA-compatible bone marrow donor for a cure was not available. When PGD is used for independent medical reasons, with no danger found to the child or mother, sex selection should be allowed.[38] More generally, sex selection is supported by those who see it as a mechanism for increasing the happiness of parents who could fulfill their desire for a child of a particular sex. Other arguments in support of sex selection include the following: it may help slow population growth (families would reach their goals of a balanced family more quickly), it enables parents to fulfill religious and cultural expectations (demonstrating multicultural sensitivity), and children would feel more wanted by the family (because they have been chosen).

There are many arguments against prenatal sex selection, the most common being that it reflects and contributes to negative attitudes about and discrimination against women, whether the reasons given are personal, social or cultural.[39]

Screening

Genetic testing is often confused with genetic screening. Evaluating an individual for a specific gene or mutation because of personal or family indications, for example, is genetic testing. Screening entails testing all members of a population when there is no evidence that any given individual has that gene or mutation. Common screening programs include Rh and ABO typing of pregnant women to identify Rh-negative women who may become sensitized to a positive fetus during pregnancy. Newborn screening programs are found in all states, and include metabolic disorders that when identified at birth can be successfully treated. The ethical issues raised by screening programs are similar to those that can be found in any genetic testing situation.[40]

Workplace Screening

Case 10-E

In its manufacturing process, XYZ Company produces high levels of respiratory irritants on site. The company plans to screen all its employees for alpha$_1$-antitrypsin deficiency,[41] regardless of their personal or family histories of lung disease. The rationale for this screening is a public health argument: the company is identifying individuals who are at greater risk than the average employee for suffering adverse effects from exposure, and can prevent injury to that employee by removing the employee from the environment that could cause him or her harm. XYZ Company also employs pilots who deliver the finished products to other countries.

Employers have an interest in genetic testing for reasons that are not related to the interests of patients. Justifications for workplace screening usually involve the greater good, that is, public health or safety. The cost to a company of hiring employees who have increased risk of genetic disease is also a concern for employers. Although XYZ Company may have used the results of its screening to advise employees of potential risks, individuals may have been inappropriately excluded from job opportunities. Genetic tests have poor predictive value in most cases. Screening employees to exclude them from the workforce because they may develop a genetic disorder in the future raises the ethical issues of privacy and prevention of discrimination. XYZ Company may decide to screen its pilots for Alzheimer disease.[42] Involuntary screening raises informed consent and privacy issues. Coerced testing violates the principle of autonomy. A more effective approach to protecting the public's safety would be routine testing of a worker's actual capacity to function in a job that is sensitive to safety. Respect for autonomy would require that employees be apprised of the testing program, asked to give informed consent, and allowed to decide how they will incorporate the test results into their career plans.[43]

Predictive Testing in Childhood

Asymptomatic individuals can be tested for genetic disorders prior to the onset of disease. The issue of doing such testing for children has received much attention, and is the basis of twenty-seven guidelines and position papers.[44] Potential benefits of testing children include medical issues such as early and effective preventive therapies and clarification of diagnosis. Psychosocial issues include reduction of uncertainty and the ability to make realistic plans for the future. Future reproductive issues could be raised by such testing. The harms to children from genetic testing include, among others, lack of preventive or therapeutic interventions, alteration of self-image or family dynamics, and the possibility of coerced decisions.[45] In general, the availability of medical benefit to the child is the most important justification for performing predictive and presymptomatic testing, regardless of the timing of the onset of the disease. Testing a child with a family history, but no personal history, of Huntington disease, therefore, would be discouraged, whereas testing a child with a family history of familial adenomatous polyposis[46] is recommended. The absence of medical benefit is the most important justification for respecting the child's autonomy and deferring testing until the child is able to make his or her own decision regarding whether to undergo testing.

Unexpected Findings

Case 10-F

Your patient, OP, Jr., needs a bone marrow transplant. Tests done on the family in search of a donor indicate that OP, Sr., is not OP, Jr.'s biological father. The family was not aware that the testing they were having performed could reveal this information.

Genetic testing can reveal more information than a patient may expect or want to have revealed. Patients may learn more than the answers to the questions originally asked of the testing. As in Case 10-F, nonpaternity is not an uncommon finding when family studies are done. Also, in the course of testing for one disease, information regarding another disease may be discovered. Once the health care provider has test results, what should he or she do with the information? We have to weigh the benefits and harms of sharing the information with the family members. The provider–patient relationship requires confidentiality. It also requires that we not break promises to or deceive the patient. If the family comes to see you as a group, the family unit is the patient. Withholding information from the family could be considered dishonest, patronizing, and disrespectful of the autonomy of the family members. The information belongs to the individuals involved.

If OP, Jr., in Case 10-F is a minor, then who should have the information: his mother, his father, or both? You would not know whether the family is aware of the situation, or whether the information would be detrimental to the family's continued well-being. We also have to respect the patient's autonomy. An adult OP, Jr., may or may not want to have his family relationships disrupted. He has a right not to know that OP, Sr., is not his biological father. Your responsibility to your patient is to tell the truth. The American Society of Human Genetics has recommended that family members not be informed of nonpaternity findings unless the determination of paternity was the purpose of the testing.[47]

If OP, Sr., in Case 10-F had Huntington disease, and the question was whether OP, Jr., was a gene carrier, the finding of nonpaternity would have major significance for OP, Jr.'s future. Some genetic information may also be used by the family to decide whether or not to have prenatal diagnosis. If OP, Jr., was unaware of the lack of risk for himself, unnecessary prenatal testing would constitute a harm to a pregnancy. In that situation, the rule prohibiting harm or risk of harm would require sharing the nonpaternity finding with OP, Jr. If the information does not influence health or treatment decisions, disclosing it could be counterproductive or harmful. In some situations, this position could lead to erroneous risk assessment.

The health care provider should avoid having to make determinations regarding whether and to whom the results should be given at the time the test results become available. Including the possibility of unexpected results from the genetic tests in the informed consent process would alert family members and allow them to determine how such results should be communicated, and with whom the provider should discuss them.[48]

Behavioral Genetics

Human behavioral genetics seeks to understand the genetic and environmental contributions to variations in behavior. Actions (e.g., novelty seeking) as well as states of mind (e.g., schizophrenia) are types of behaviors. Most human traits are distributed in a continuous fashion, illustrated by the bell-shaped curve. These represent complex traits that are the result of an interaction between genes and the environment. Large genetic influences on complex traits can result from the accumulation of the small effects of many genes interacting with many environmental factors over time.[49]

One goal of behavioral genetics is to reduce suffering. Because some of the traits that are under study are used for social purposes, behavioral geneticists guard against the use of their results to justify a status quo that may be unfair. The differences on IQ tests among children of different races have been used to maintain a racial hierarchy. Behavioral genetics studies of the influence of socioeconomic status (SES) on IQ scores illustrate that genetic differences depend on the SES of the person taking the test. Researchers found that genes help explain the differences in scores among the high-SES children, but not among the low-SES children. Social interventions have been put in place based on these studies.

The classic methods used to study the relationship between genes and the environment use identical and fraternal twins who are raised together or apart. Identical twins have been found to be more alike than fraternal twins for traits such as height, intelligence, and schizophrenia. These studies help researchers understand the extent to which differences among people are genetic. Molecular studies are then used to identify the specific genes associated with particular traits, and new technology allows for the study of how genes affect these traits. Concerns have been expressed about the study of human differences through behavioral genetics research, in that it may undermine the concept of moral equality. Another concern is that the results of studies might be used to justify inequalities in the distribution of social power.[50]

Uses of Genetic Techniques

Pharmacogenomics

People respond to drugs in different ways, and genetic variations among patients can account for differences in the degree of success with particular treatments. Drug metabolism can be influenced by an individual's gene mutations or polymorphisms. Warfarin, for example, is effective in reducing blood clots. It has a narrow therapeutic range, and determining the proper dose is difficult. Adverse drug reactions lead to emergency room visits. The variability in response to warfarin has been attributed to variation in the genes that produce the enzymes that metabolize warfarin. Tests that predict a response to therapy are referred to as *pharmacogenomics*. Improving the monitoring, safety, and efficacy of warfarin use can be achieved through pharmacogenetic testing of patients. Pharmacogenetic tests differ from conventional genetic tests in that they involve a drug as well as the disease that drug is being used to treat.[51] Ethical issues that are raised concern treatment choices, privacy, "orphan" genotypes, and race. Physicians do not treat all patients with the same medications. The choices are usually made based on which medications would best help a particular patient. The scientific basis for the choices rests on observation or research. If people feel they are not receiving what they consider to be the appropriate treatment for their disease, they could become angry and hostile.

Research for pharmacogenetics requires large numbers of participants. Privacy issues then become important. Those individuals who have genotypes that are not found to be responsive or who have adverse reactions to the tested drug—that is, those with orphan genotypes—will not be benefited by the research. There is evidence that members of different ethnic groups react on average differently to some drugs.[52] Public perceptions of pharmacogenetic testing are important because resistance could lead to patients not receiving the best care or the most beneficial medications, or having serious adverse reactions to medications. Pharmacogenetic tests may enable patients to know more about their condition, to feel more in control of their treatment, and to ultimately receive better care.[40] The medical benefits of pharmacogenetics seem to outweigh any special harms.

Therapeutics

Researchers can alter animals genetically and reproduce them reliably. Genes can be added to the genome to create drug-producing animals, or genes can be inactivated to produce animal models of human diseases. Normal functioning genes can also be inserted into human cells to treat or cure single-gene disorders. The vectors used in gene replacement therapy are often viruses. Ethical issues have been raised by this form of therapy that are different from those raised by other treatments. When the host cells are somatic cells, the results are the treatment of the individual. The duty to produce more benefits than harm is the same as for any form of treatment. Some harms that have been reported include inflammatory responses to the vectors that may limit their repeated use. Unforeseen or latent harms have also been reported. In treating children with severe combined immunodeficiency disease (SCID)[53] using retroviral gene therapy, three children developed leukemia, and one died. Use of adenoviral gene therapy for an adult with ornithine transcarbamylase deficiency (OTC)[54] resulted in his death.[55]

When gene therapy involves germ line cells, whether by intention or inadvertently, it affects the individual being treated as well as all his or her offspring. Although successful treatment would cause little alarm, future effects are unpredictable and might not appear for generations. The line between the elimination of deleterious genes and perfecting the human genome in general raises the issue of the slippery slope of enhancement.[56] Some of the harms may include disruption of the normal functions of proto-oncogenes[57] or tumor suppressor genes,[58] resulting in mutagenesis that could be independent of where the insertion occurred. Vectors can cause a broad range of effects that may have public health implications, such as the introduction of dangerous genes into the gene pool. In correcting genes that cause disease in an individual, there may be a loss of hereditary information, genetic variation that is important for the population. It may also eliminate the possibility of the combination of the target disease gene with other genes that could have resulted in population benefits.[59] Using gene transfer to treat genetic disease is endorsed with two restrictions: no changes should be made that would be passed on to the patient's children, and no attempts should be made to exceed the restoration of normal.[60]

The boundary between using genetic therapeutic techniques for the treatment or cure of disease and using them to produce enhancements is controversial. Some claim that gene therapy is an abuse of medicine or a form of social cheating that undermines the social value of achievements. Besides the unapproved, off-label uses of these techniques and the harms that could ensue, moral concerns are raised by changing a single individual and not addressing the social biases that underlie the perceived need for enhancement.[60]

Designer Babies

Prenatal diagnosis is a powerful tool. Prenatal information, preimplantation genetic diagnosis, and selection could be applied in the future to traits such as personality or intelligence. How far do the rights of parents extend when having children? Do parental rights include the designing of their descendents? Some theorists treat enhancements as a matter of individual liberty, because the harm to others is supported only by speculative arguments. If a legitimate purpose of medicine is to improve a patient's psychological and social well-being, prenatal diagnosis in conjunction with techniques developed to treat disorders could be used to enhance a child's characteristics. Taller, smarter, faster, and stronger children could be designed. Genetically superior people would be the goal. The boundary between what is ordinary human variability and what is pathology is being blurred. How tall is tall? Is a man who is five feet ten short? Would six feet six be better? The concern that is raised is about attitudes toward life that stress competition, mastery, and control, and leave little room for alternative ways of living.[61]

As with other uses of this technology, access to the technology would be driven by the market, and therefore access to enhancements would be unequal. Parents with resources would be able to obtain the enhancements for their children, and thus increase their chances for success. Such designer children would be better able to succeed in a competitive society, again further increasing the gap between the haves and have-nots. Using reprogenetics for enhancement suggests that parents are bowing to the unjust norms of society (e.g., that a genetic height of five feet ten is short). Will such enhancement encourage parents to have unrealistic expectations for their children? And, if a height-enhanced child does not use that height to succeed in life—say, he becomes a musician—have the parents failed the child or has the child provoked greater disappointment?[36]

Cloning

Cloning is a technique for duplicating biological material. It can be used to create identical copies of an entire cell (a cell line) or to produce complete genetically identical animals, such as twinning. In 1997, a sheep named Dolly was introduced to the world.

Dolly was produced using the cloning technique of somatic cell nuclear transfer, the cell used coming from an adult animal. This raised the specter of human cloning. Cloned children would be individuals who were genetically identical to the donor. The ethical issues raised by the manipulation of humans were considered morally unacceptable.[62] Ethical issues raised by cloning as a method to produce children include safety, individuality, family integrity, and treating children as objects.[63] Social concerns other than those for children, such as opening another door to eugenics and the manipulation of others, have been countered by arguments regarding the protection of personal choice, the maintenance of privacy, and the freedom of scientific inquiry, as well as the encouragement of the development of new biomedical breakthroughs.[64]

Direct-to-Consumer Marketing

Case 10-G

Ms. RS came across an advertisement on the Internet for genetic testing that would improve the care of her skin and make her look younger. She received her results along with an offer for skin care products that were said to be tailored to her results. She has come to you because she cannot afford the expensive skin products and has become very anxious about the present and future state of her skin.

Advances in genomic medicine offer improved care and prevention of many diseases. Consumers have been shown to have unclear and confused notions about the value of genetic testing, and express many of the same concerns that have already been discussed, such as privacy and discrimination.[65] Superimposed on this background is the marketing of genetic tests directly to consumers (DTC). For a fee, private companies will generate genetic information for any individual about himself or herself. Advertising genetic testing to consumers began almost unnoticed and without regulatory oversight.

In a free market system, individuals should have the autonomy to pursue their own genetic testing and companies should be allowed to provide that service. The companies that offer DTC testing seem to differ in terms of the services provided and their approach to testing. In a survey of DTC websites, it was found that companies are not providing enough information for consumers to make well-informed decisions. Some sites offer tests with little evidence of clinical value, such as the one Ms. RS found.[66] Advertisements make use of themes of choice, hope, fear, and peace of mind to validate patients' worries about genetic risks. They appeal to the individual's desire for control over confusing and complex concepts.

Both the testing process and the results from these tests can be questioned. Use of samples collected at home makes it difficult to verify the source of the sample, the method of collection, and the reliability of the results. Test information, such as sensitivity and specificity, that is available from certified laboratories is not always present on the DTC website. The potential for harm to the consumer includes unnecessary anxiety or fear from misunderstanding the results. Genetic testing often requires the expertise of specialists to explain and interpret the results. Obtaining DTC tests is also limited to those who have computers and access to the Internet, as well as the financial means to order testing. This raises concerns about fairness and access.[67]

DTC tests allow some individuals freedom of access, as well as autonomy to choose testing. The expectation of confidentiality is greater when the testing is done at home. There is also a sense of privacy and control over the information when it is acquired in this manner. A secondary benefit may be that patients such as Ms. RS will go to see their doctors for more information or to discuss genetics and genetic testing.

A free market will regulate itself. If people do not want DTC testing, they will not purchase it. However, if consumers do not have the information needed to make decisions about testing, then the harms of doing DTC testing seem to outweigh the benefits. Educating the public about existing privacy protections and the benefits of genetic testing in a clinical setting will go a long way toward eliminating consumer demand for DTC genetic testing.[68]

Chapter Summary

Rapid advances in clinical applications and research in human genetics have presented challenges to medical professionals, ethicists, and the general public. The technology developed for the Human Genome Project has been applied to both clinical medicine and medical research. This chapter explored the challenges raised with regard to privacy and confidentiality. There has been an increased awareness that the large amount of health information now available to caregivers and researchers can be a great benefit. Understanding the advances in genetics and the implications for health care will be important for the present and future generations.

Genetic information could be used to prevent or delay the onset of disease, alleviate the burden of illness, or assist people in planning their futures. However, genetic information can also have economic and social harms for individuals and for groups. The use of genetic information for purposes that are not related to research or health care, such as for employment and insurance decisions, resource allocations, or biological enhancements, raises issues regarding the harms and benefits to individuals, families, and society. The variety of interests in and the complexity of the problems engendered by genetics were introduced in this chapter. There is no single answer to any of these issues. Consideration of the issues raised by genetic testing, treatment, and research has not resulted in consistent positions or uniform policies. The promise of genetic medicine needs to be accompanied by a continuing discussion of the ethical issues raised.

Review Questions

1. What is the impact of genes in determining our futures?

2. Is there a difference between taking a family medical history and asking for the results of genetic tests? If yes, what is that difference?

3. Should an individual have complete control over his or her genetic information? If no, who should have access to or use of this genetic information?

4. Is a monozygotic twin who requests genetic testing for himself required to get the approval of his twin?

5. What ethical concerns arise from possible eugenic uses of genetic information?

6. Should the conduct of genetic research be influenced by a concern for the social good?

7. To what extent will the developments in genetics increase the gap between the haves and have-nots with respect to access to health care?

8. Are the issues raised by pharmacogenetic tests different from those raised by genetic tests concerned with the diagnosis of disease?

9. Do parents have a duty to bear only children with the best opportunities for success in life?

10. Should genetic tests be performed if no treatment for the tested disorder is available? If yes, under what circumstances? If no, are there any exceptions?

11. What are the boundaries between the treatment of genetic disorders and genetic enhancement?

12. Does the influence of genes on behavior suggest that an individual is not free to choose particular actions?

13. Are there any aspects of genetic testing that should be commercialized? Should the federal government regulate the commercialization of genetic testing?

Endnotes

1. Cahill GF. A brief history of the Human Genome Project. In: Gert B, et al., eds. *Morality and the New Genetics*. Boston: Jones and Bartlett, 1996:1–28.
2. Annas G, Glantz LH, Roche PA. Drafting the Genetic Privacy Act: science, policy and practical considerations. *J Law Med Ethics* 1995;23:360–365.
3. Murray TH. Genetic exceptionalism and "future diaries": is genetic information different from other medical information? In: Rothstein MA, ed. *Genetic Secrets: Protecting Privacy and Confidentiality in the Genetic Era*. New Haven, CT: Yale University Press, 1997:60–73.
4. Tay-Sachs disease is an autosomal recessive disease caused by a deficiency of the enzyme hexosaminidase A. One in thirty Ashkenazi Jews have been found to carry this gene.

5. Thalassemia is an autosomal recessive hemoglobinopathy caused by mutations in either the alpha- or beta-chain genes controlling the synthesis of hemoglobin. The highest incidence of beta-thalassemia is found in Cyprus (14%) and Sardinia (12%).

6. Sickle cell anemia is caused by a mutation in the HBB gene that results in hemoglobin S production, with variable degrees of hemolysis and vascular occlusion. Eight to ten percent of African Americans are gene carriers. In West Africa the carrier frequency is twenty-five to thirty percent.

7. Cystic fibrosis is the most common life-limiting disease in Caucasians (carrier frequency of from one in twenty-two to one in twenty-eight). This autosomal recessive disease is caused by an abnormality in cystic fibrosis transmembrane conductance regulator (CFTR) function, resulting in lower airway inflammation and infection and pancreatic insufficiency.

8. *Penetrance* is the characteristic of a gene to be apparent in an individual who carries that gene.

9. Huntington disease is an autosomal dominant progressive neurologic deterioration caused by the expansion of a CAG repeat in the protein huntingtin gene. Onset is typically in the second or third decade, but can occur earlier or later.

10. *Negative eugenics* is the elimination of deleterious genes. *Positive eugenics* is the systematic improvement of the human race. Eugenics has been attempted as a social engineering solution to combat social problems. Ostensibly based on legitimate scientific studies, most claims made by proponents of eugenics were based on unfounded extrapolation of genetic findings, poor scientific studies, and sometimes only assumptions.

11. Rothstein MA. Genetic exceptionalism and legislative pragmatism. *Hastings Center Rep* 2005;35(4):27–33.

12. Everett M. Can you keep a (genetic) secret? The genetic privacy movement. *J Genet Counsel* 2004;13(4):273–291.

13. See, for example, the opportunities from the Ethical, Legal, and Social Issues (ELSI) part of the Human Genome Project.

14. Foster MW, Royal CDM, Sharp RR. The routinization of genomics and genetics: implications for ethical practices. *J Med Ethics* 2006;32:635–638.

15. Wright T. *Project on Genetic Testing: Submission to the Ontario Law Reform Commission*. Toronto: Information and Privacy Commission/Ontario, 1992:1–5.

16. Rothstein MA, Anderlik MR. What is genetic discrimination, and when and how can it be prevented? *Genet Med* 2001;3(5):354–358.

17. Achondroplasia is an autosomal dominant skeletal dysplasia characterized by short stature with disproportionately short arms and legs, a large head, and characteristic facial features.

18. Lucassen A. Should families own genetic information? Yes. *BJM* 2007;335:22.

19. Clark A. Should families own genetic information? No. *BJM* 2007;335:23.

20. Lucassen A. Genetic information: a joint account? *BMJ* 2004;329:165–167.

21. Weiss JO, et al. Whom would you trust with your genetic information? *J Hum Genet* 1997;61(4):A24.

22. Forrest K, Simpson SA, Wilson BJ, et al. To tell or not to tell: barriers and facilitators in family communication about genetic risk. *Clin Genet* 2003;64:317–326.

23. See, for example, President's Commission for the Study of Ethical Problems in Medicine and Biomedical and Behavioral Research. *Genetic Screening and Counseling: Ethical and Legal Implications*. Washington, DC: Government Printing Office, 1983:41–88.

24. *Moore v. Regents of the University of California*, 51 Cal.3d 120, 271 Cal. Rptr. 146, 793 P.2d 479 (1990).

25. Based on Heimler A, Zanko A. Huntington disease: a case study describing the complexities and nuances of predictive testing of monozygotic twins. *J Genet Counsel* 1995;4(2):125–137.

26. Gert B. Applying morality to the nine Huntington disease cases: an alternative model for genetic counseling. In: Gert B, et al., eds. *Morality and the New Genetics*. Boston: Jones and Bartlett, 1996:97–124.

27. Reilly PR. Efforts to regulate the collection and use of genetic information. *Arch Pathol Lab Med* 1999;123(11):1066–1070.

28. Knowles LP. Reprogenetics: a chance for meaningful regulation. *Hastings Center Rep* 2002;32(3):13.

29. Fost N. Ethical issues in genetics. *Med Ethics* 1992;39(1):79–89.

30. Plaisance K. To test or not to test: ethical issues in genetic testing. Bioethics.net. October 19, 2001. Available at: http://www.bioethics.net/articles.php?viewCat=7&articleid=155.

31. Beeson D. Social and ethical challenges of prenatal diagnosis. *Med Ethics* 2000; Winter:1–2, 8.

32. Holm S. The expressivist objection to prenatal diagnosis: can it be laid to rest? *J Med Ethics* 2008;34:24–25.

33. Shakespeare T. Debating disability. *J Med Ethics* 2008;34:11–14. EDITORIAL ENDNOTE: The opinion of the chapter author on this point is not shared by the editors. See also editorial endnote 4 in Chapter 11.

34. Wiskott-Aldrich syndrome is an X-linked disorder of hematopoietic cells with defects of platelets and lymphocytes. Sequence analysis of the WAS gene detects mutations in ninety-nine percent of affected males.

35. Wexler N. Genetic information: its significance for patients, families, health professionals, ethics and policy development. Remarks to the President's Council on Bioethics, September 2006.

36. Parens E, Murray TH. Preimplantation genetic diagnosis: beginning a long conversation. *Med Ethics* 2002;9(2):1–2, 8.

37. Heyd D. Male or female, we will create them: the ethics of sex selection for non-medical reasons. *Ethical Perspect* 2004;11(1):84–87.

38. Caplan AL, McGee G. Reproductive medicine: issues over rights to control their body, in-vitro fertilization, preimplantation genetic diagnosis. Bioethics.net. June 7, 2004. Available at: http://www.bioethics.net/articles.php?viewCat=3&articleid=8.

39. American College of Obstetricians and Gynecologists, Committee on Ethics. ACOG committee opinion no. 360: sex selection. *Obstet Gynecol* 2007;109(2 pt 1):475–478.

40. Nuffield Council on Bioethics. *Genetic Screening: Ethical Issues*. London: Nuffield Council on Bioethics, 1993.

41. Alpha$_1$-antitrypsin deficiency is caused by homozygosity for the common deficiency allele protease inhibitor Z. It is characterized by chronic obstructive pulmonary disease (COPD) and liver disease. In nonsmokers, onset of COPD can be delayed to the sixth decade.

42. Predisposition testing for Alzheimer disease using APOE analysis is not fully specific or sensitive. APOE e4 is therefore not a good predictor of dementia.

43. Council on Ethical and Judicial Affairs, AMA. Use of genetic testing by employers. *JAMA* 1991;266(13):1827–1830.

44. Borry P, Stultiens L, Nys H, Cassiman J-J, Dierickx K. Presymptomatic and predictive genetic testing in minors: a systematic review of guidelines and position papers. *Clin Genet* 2006;70:374–381.

45. American Society of Human Genetics Board of Directors, American College of Medical Genetics Board of Directors. ASHG/ACMG report. Points to consider: ethical, legal, and psychosocial implications of genetic testing in children and adolescents. *Am J Hum Genet* 1995;57:1233–1241.

46. Familial adenomatous polyposis is a disorder that predisposes to colon cancer. Precancerous polyps can appear in the colon as early as seven years of age. Mutations in the APC gene are inherited in an autosomal dominant pattern and are detected in ninety-five percent of at-risk individuals.

47. The American Society of Human Genetics. Statement on informed consent for genetic research. *Am J Hum Genet* 1996;59:471–474.

48. Khoury MH, McCabe LL, McCabe ERB. Population screening in the age of genomic medicine. *N Engl J Med* 2003;34(81):50–58.

49. McInerney J. Behavioral genetics. Human Genome Project Information. 2007. Available at: http://www.ornl.gov.

50. Parens E. Genetic differences and human identities: on why talking about behavioral genetics is important and difficult. *Hastings Center Rep Special Suppl* 2004;34(1):S1–S36.

51. Flockhart DA, O'Kane DO, Williams MS, et al. Pharmacogenetic testing of CYP2C9 and VKORC1 alleles for warfarin. *Genet Med* 2008;10(2):139–150.

52. Greeley HT. Pharmacogenetics: promise, prospects, and potential problems. *Med Ethics* 2002;9:1–2, 8.

53. Severe combined immunodeficiency disease is an autosomal recessive purine metabolic disorder. Adenosine deaminase deficiency affects the development and function of lymphocytes, resulting in failure to thrive and opportunistic infections.

54. Ornithine transcarbamylase deficiency is an X-linked urea cycle disorder. The accumulation of ammonia and other precursor metabolites during the first few days of life associated with this disorder has led to it being included in most newborn screening programs.

55. Jaffe A, Prasad SA, Larcher V, Hart S. Gene therapy for children with cystic fibrosis—who has the right to choose? *J Med Ethics* 2006;32:361–364.

56. Berger EM. Ethics of gene therapy. In: Gert B, et al., eds. *Morality and the New Genetics*. Boston: Jones and Bartlett, 1996:209–224.

57. A proto-oncogene is a normal gene that can become an active oncogene either by mutation or by an increase in expression.

58. A tumor suppressor gene is a gene that regulates and limits cell growth. When a suppressor gene has a mutation that changes its function, overgrowth can be malignant. The BRCA1 mutations are examples.

59. Caplan A. If gene therapy is the cure, what is the disease? Bioethics.net. November 8, 2002. Available at: http://www.bioethics.net/articles.php?viewCat=6&articleid=58.

60. Juengst ET. Genetic enhancement: a conceptual and ethical challenge for gene therapy regulation. *Med Ethics* 1999;Spring:1–2.

61. Elliot C. The mixed promise of genetic medicine. *N Engl J Med* 2007;356(20):2024–2025.

62. Casey D. Cloning: from DNA molecules to Dolly. *Hum Genome News* 1998;9(1–2):17.

63. McGee G. An argument against human cloning. Bioethics.net. January 24, 2001. Available at: http://www.bioethics.net/articles.php?viewCat=2&articleid=54.

64. Blacksher E. Cloning human beings: responding to the National Bioethics Advisory Commission's report. *Hastings Cent Rep* 1997;27(5):6–9.

65. Scheuner MT, Sieverding P, Shekelle PG. Delivery of genomic medicine for common chronic adult diseases. *JAMA* 2008;299(11):1320–1334.

66. Berg C, Fryer-Edwards K. The ethical challenges of direct-to-consumer genetic testing. *J Business Ethics* 2008;77(1):17–31.

67. Watson K, Cook D, Helzlsour K. Direct-to-consumer online genetic testing and the four principles: an analysis of the ethical issues. *Ethics Med* 2006;22(2):83–91.

68. Human Genetics Society of Australasia. *Issues on Direct to Consumer Genetic Testing*. July 2007. Sydney: Human Genetics Society of Australasia.

Chapter 11

Human Reproduction and Birth

La mia vita cominciò

Come l'erba come il fiore

E mia madre mi baciò

Come fossi il primo amore

Nasce così la vita mia

Come comincia una poesia

Io credo che lassù

C'era un sorriso anche per me

La stessa luce che

Si accende quando nasce un re.

—Massimo Ranieri, *Vent'anni*

Chapter Learning Objectives

At the conclusion of this chapter the reader will be able to:

1. Distinguish between contraceptives and contragestives

2. Identify the three main positions on the abortion issue

3. Appraise the arguments for and against the conservative, liberal, and moderate views on abortion

4. Appraise the various motives for procreation and its avoidance

5. Explain the problems raised by the introduction of third parties into the procreative process

6. Explain the distinction between Robertson's procreative liberty—a negative right—and a positive right to procreate

7. Discuss the problems with the concept of a right to procreate and their implications for discussions of reproductive ethics

8. Identify morally relevant differences and similarities among procreation through sexual intercourse, through existing assisted reproductive technologies, and through futuristic means, such as cloning

9. Describe the distinction between logistical and duplicative cloning

10. Appraise the motives and assumptions underlying the use of preimplantation genetic diagnosis and prenatal screening

11. Discuss the complexities underlying pregnant women's failures to adhere to medical advice

Although procreation is common, it is not an unqualified good. Like many other human activities, whether procreation is morally permissible depends on features of the context in which it occurs. The emergence and ongoing development of reproductive and genetic technologies continue to raise new questions about the permissibility of procreation while also prompting us to examine established procreative attitudes and practices. This chapter analyzes morally controversial reproductive decisions and behaviors as well as many of the prevailing assumptions about procreation and its avoidance.

Preventing Procreation

Procreation is an important part of many people's lives, but avoiding it is also important for most people during certain stages of their lives. The desire to have sexual intercourse with another person is not identical to a desire to procreate. As Alan Goldman has pointed out, "most people engaging in sex view the prospect of reproduction as a *threat*, not a *goal* [italics added]."[1] Procreation may be undesirable for many reasons, but all of them are based on the fact that the creation of a new person imposes myriad obligations on those who bring the child into the world.

Sterilization, contraception, and abortion are all ways of preventing procreation, where procreation is understood as having children to whom one is obligated morally and legally. Although there are religious objections to the use of certain types of contraceptives (e.g., the Catholic Church's opposition to birth control pills or condoms), there are no compelling moral objections to preventing fertilization. Setting aside religious beliefs regarding reincarnation or the premortal existence of souls, it is not reasonable to construe the failure to bring people into existence by preventing fertilization as a moral wrong or harm. Although we have moral obligations to existing children, we do not have any independent moral obligation to create them. In some cases, we may have a moral obligation to *refrain* from procreation.

Long-Acting Contraception: Nonvoluntary and Involuntary Uses

Although there are no compelling *moral* arguments against the voluntary use of contraception, compulsory contraceptive use is morally controversial. In recent years, individuals who have failed in some way to fulfill their parental obligations have been told that a condition of their continued freedom from incarceration is the use of long-term contraception or sterilization or to otherwise refrain from bringing more children into the world. Such decisions have been met with outrage by those who assert that people have a "right to procreate," but there are good reasons to question the assumption that there is such a right. A right *to* procreate does not follow from a right to *refrain* from procreating (e.g., by using contraception or abortion). A detailed examination of the concept of a right to procreate is presented later in this chapter.

Many would argue that there is no controversy at all regarding compulsory contraceptive use and that it is just *wrong* to require a person to use contraception either *against* his or her will (involuntarily) or in cases where an individual is incapable of providing voluntary informed consent (nonvoluntarily), for example, because the individual is cognitively impaired. But this is an oversimplification. In cases where a person has demonstrated either unwillingness or inability to care for existing children, it may be morally justifiable to compel a person to use contraception. An appeal to John Stuart Mill's harm principle, which allows for the interference with an individual's liberty in cases where his or her exercise of liberty would cause harm to *others*, would support compulsory contraceptive use under some circumstances. Granted, these cases would be quite rare, and Mill would require the use of the least restrictive means possible to prevent harm to others, but this does not imply that compulsory contraception could never be a permissible means of preventing harm to others. Insofar as compulsory use of contraception would not interfere with the individual's liberty to continue engaging in sexual intercourse, it is less restrictive than incarcerating a person to prevent him or her from procreating.

Restricting procreative activity as a condition of parole is likely to be less common than requests for the use of nonvoluntary long-acting contraception (or, possibly, sterilization). For example, a guardian might determine that the use of long-acting contraception would promote the well-being of a cognitively impaired dependent who is sexually active but unaware of the connection between sex and pregnancy; unable to handle the stress of pregnancy, labor, and delivery; unable to comprehend the connection between pregnancy and the subsequent existence of a dependent child; or unable to care for a child given the limits of her social support system. The individual who does not understand the connections between sex, pregnancy, and the existence of children can hardly be said to possess the ability to make genuinely autonomous reproductive decisions. Hence, the claim that such an individual's "reproductive autonomy" is being violated by the nonvoluntary use of long-acting contraception lacks foundation.

Although the principle of respect for autonomy tends to be dominant in bioethical discourse, particularly in the context of reproductive ethics, this is one type of case in which the principle of beneficence should carry greater weight. It is likely that a person who lacks understanding of the processes of pregnancy, labor, and delivery will be excessively frightened and anxious about these events, and this imposes on others a duty to prevent her from having to endure such physical and psychological harms. Furthermore, the use of long-acting contraception, which allows one's reproductive capacity to be restored at a later time, allows for the possibility of procreation in the event that there is an alteration in the particulars of the case—for example, an enhanced support network or improved cognitive abilities.

The primary goal of contraception is to allow individuals to control whether or when they procreate, thereby expanding instead of limiting their freedom, and in some cases, helping individuals limit their procreative activities may promote both present and future autonomy. To assert that there are legitimate moral objections to mandating contraceptive use is not to say that it would *never* be morally permissible to require the use of contraceptives. Although there are good reasons to refrain from advocating for a public policy that mandates contraceptive use (or sterilization), we should not infer that there are *no* individual cases where requiring contraceptive use would be morally permissible. Our scandalous history, which includes state laws that permitted the forcible sterilization of those deemed "unfit" to procreate, has led many to be wary of intervening in others' procreative decision making, even where procreation is clearly morally problematic. Nonetheless, society's "past application of morally reprehensible policies designed to restrict reproduction does not entail the wrongness of all attempts to regulate procreative behavior."[2] Although we should prevent abuses of power like those that occurred during the eugenics movements of the late nineteenth and early twentieth centuries in the United States and abroad, we should make sure that our reluctance to judge others' procreative decisions does not amount to "an irresponsible compliance with demands made by people who make bad choices."[3]

Abortion

Because we do not live in an ideal world where every pregnancy is wanted, many women find themselves faced with the decision whether to continue a pregnancy.[4] For logistical reasons, a woman's ability to safely end a pregnancy depends on the assistance of a health care professional (HCP). The HCP may provide a woman with a contragestive agent to procure a *medical abortion*. Mifepristone (RU-486), methotrexate, and oral or vaginal misoprostol may be used within the first sixty-three days of pregnancy. The mifepristone or methotrexate is usually taken at the HCP's office, whereas the misoprostol may be taken at home or during a return visit to the HCP. It is important to note here that RU-486, which is more widely known as "the abortion pill," is not identical to emergency contraception or "the morning-after pill" (sold as Plan B in the United States). The latter usually works by suppressing or delaying ovulation or by interfering with sperm migration,[5] whereas RU-486 interferes with the progesterone supply and stops a pregnancy already in progress. Unlike RU-486, the morning-after pill is effective only within seventy-two hours after unprotected sexual intercourse.

The use of contragestive drugs such as RU-486, which was approved by the U.S. Food and Drug Administration (FDA) in September 2000, has been less common than the use of *surgical abortion* to end pregnancy. A surgical abortion may be done by "menstrual aspiration," also known as manual vacuum aspiration (MVA), as early as five gestational weeks; by dilation and curettage (D&C) before twelve weeks; by dilation and evacuation (D&E) between twelve and twenty-one weeks; or by induction in the later stages of pregnancy.[6]

The abortion issue continues to be one of the most contentious issues in both academic and nonacademic spheres. A great deal of discussion within the field of bioethics—especially reproductive ethics—has focused on the abortion issue over the past few decades.

Before the 1973 *Roe v. Wade* decision,[7] which relegalized abortion in the United States, the focus of discussion was on not only whether abortion was morally permissible but also whether abortion should be legal. (Abortion prior to fetal quickening—that is, the detection of fetal motion—had been legal in the United States until the end of the nineteenth century. It was outlawed out of concern for the health of women, who often died of infection following abortion procedures, not because of concerns about the moral status of the fetus.) Although the decision did alter the legal status of abortion, it did nothing to resolve the moral controversy. The debate about the moral permissibility of abortion rages on, and although many logical fallacies have been committed in attempting to defend either the pro-choice or the antiabortion (also known as pro-life) view, carefully reasoned arguments about the issue have emerged.

Although not every participant in the abortion debate dwells on the question of whether the embryo or fetus is a person with a right to life, the moral status of the embryo or fetus is one relevant consideration in the debate. There is no dispute about whether an embryo or fetus created by adult human beings is biologically human—nobody thinks that a pregnant woman is going to give birth to a buffalo—but not everyone agrees that membership in the species *Homo sapiens* is a sufficient, or even a necessary, condition for moral consideration. There is disagreement among various parties to the abortion debate about what sort of consideration is due embryos or fetuses. Opponents of abortion claim that embryos and fetuses have a right to life just like adult human beings and that to deprive them of this right to life is prima facie unjust killing. That is, according to the antiabortion view, absent the lack of a compelling justification (e.g., a threat to the life of the woman), killing an embryo or fetus is morally on a par with murder.[8] At the other end of the spectrum is the liberal view that embryos and fetuses are due no moral consideration; hence, it is morally permissible to kill an embryo or fetus at any time during the woman's pregnancy if the woman does not want to continue sustaining its life. Nevertheless, not every proponent of the pro-choice view falls into the liberal camp. A more moderate pro-choice view does not assume that abortion is always morally permissible. Unlike either the conservative view, which holds that full protection of the moral rules vests at fertilization, or the liberal view, which holds that such protection vests only at birth, this gradualist view holds that an embryo or fetus gains moral status during its journey toward birth. There is no single moderate view, but several versions of it. Defenders of the moderate pro-choice view draw the line at varying stages of embryologic or fetal development and distinguish between acceptable and unacceptable reasons for abortion.

The moral status of embryos or fetuses is not the only relevant consideration in the abortion debate. The *location* of the embryo or fetus and its relationship to the woman sustaining its existence are also relevant considerations. Some discussions of the abortion issue lack any reference to the woman or the fact of pregnancy and its transformative effects. As Margaret Olivia Little points out, the abortion controversy raises deep questions about what makes a person a parent and whether one can have parental duties toward embryos or fetuses or only toward children.[9] Parenthood is best understood as having a certain kind of relationship with one's offspring rather than having a mere genetic or biological connection to the individual, but there are questions about when that parental relationship begins and the corresponding duties take effect. One does not have the legal status of a parent until a child is delivered, but Little points out that an individual's values, including differing views about what should determine the course of one's life, may affect a person's understanding of when motherhood begins.[9(p322)] Consequently, some may view abortion as morally akin to contraception—that is, preventing the maternal–child relationship from developing—whereas others may view abortion as "exiting a parental relationship" that has already begun.[9(pp320-321)] Gestation, she points out, "turns one into a mother," but it is not clear at precisely what point this transformation occurs, nor is it clear that it occurs at the same point for every individual.[9(p321)] Let us now examine some arguments in defense of the conservative, moderate, and liberal views on abortion.

The Conservative Antiabortion View

The most extreme antiabortion view holds that abortion is never morally permissible. Most proponents of the conservative view, however, hold that in cases where continuing a pregnancy presents a threat to the life of the woman, abortion is morally permissible, though not morally required. Some opponents of abortion hold that from the point of fertilization onward, the conceived being has the same rights or interests as an adult human being, including a right to life. Others stop short of claiming that early-stage humans have rights and instead assert that human life at *any* stage has intrinsic value and that the *potentiality* of developing humans is adequate justification to refrain from killing them. That is, although zygotes, embryos, or fetuses lack the qualities that normally distinguish humans from nonhumans, killing them causes the extinction of morally significant beings whose life has already begun.

The "fertilization view" holds that the zygote (fertilized egg), as a genetically distinct entity, ought to be valued as a unique individual whose interests are distinct from its genetic parents.[10] The assumption is that once fertilization occurs, the blueprint is in place for development into an adult member of the human species. This view is problematic, however, because it assumes that everything needed to create a new person is present from the point of fertilization and contained within the genetic program of the zygote. It ignores the many factors external to the genetic code that influence whether the zygote will be able to develop into a mature human being. Whether an embryo develops from the zygote "depends on interactions with neighboring cells and other environmental cues."[10(p66)] To claim that the development of a zygote into a person is determined entirely by internal features is to misunderstand the complexity of embryologic development. Moreover, the fertilization view has some difficulty accounting for the phenomenon of twinning, which can occur up until the point of gastrulation (approximately thirteen days after fertilization). If morally significant life begins at fertilization, what of the identical twin that comes into being at a later stage? The phenomenon of twinning suggests that there is something problematic about grounding the attribution of moral status in the appearance of a unique genome.

In an attempt to avoid some of the problems with the fertilization view, some defenders of the conservative view claim that one should refrain from killing the embryo or fetus not because it is a *person* from the moment of fertilization but because it has the *potential* to become a person. Because human embryos lack the capacities that adults or children possess, they are particularly vulnerable and incapable of actualizing their potential without the help of adult humans. As such, proponents of this view hold that we should refrain from frustrating the embryo's journey toward becoming a mature member of the human species. This view escapes some of the problems with attributing rights or interests to zygotes or embryos, but it fails to provide an adequate basis for the claim that potential persons should be given the same moral consideration as actual persons. It does not follow from the claim that it is wrong to kill persons that it is also wrong to kill *potential* persons. Moreover, as Cynthia Cohen has pointed out, the concept of potential is "too broad and indiscriminating in its meaning to be helpful."[10(p69)] Many qualifying conditions are relevant in determining a being's potential, including not only the being's internal constitution but also its interactions with the surrounding environment. Finally, even if one has determined that an embryo or fetus is a person, this does not end the discussion.[11] As Little points out, "conversation usually *starts*, not stops, once we realize people's lives are at issue."[9(p314)]

Because a precise determination of the moral status of the embryo or fetus is challenging, some participants in the abortion debate attempt to defend their position on the issue without solving the question of whether the embryo or fetus is a person. A well-known defender of the conservative view is Don Marquis, who argues that killing an embryo or fetus is wrong for the same reason killing an adult human being is wrong. The wrong-making feature of killing, according to Marquis, is that it deprives a being of a "future like ours" (FLO), which includes all of the "activities, projects, experiences, and enjoyments" that would have constituted one's future.[12] Marquis assumes that a "standard fetus" has a FLO and that to interfere by killing the fetus is as morally problematic as, say, gunning down a person as she jogs through the park. Marquis argues that because it is morally wrong to deprive an adult or child of a FLO, it is equally wrong to deprive a fetus of a FLO. A fetus has no less of a FLO, according to Marquis, than does the average child or adult. Hence, to assert that it is wrong to deprive an adult or child of a FLO but morally permissible to deprive a fetus of one is as unacceptably arbitrary as asserting that whereas the wanton infliction of pain on adult humans is wrong, because it causes suffering, the wanton infliction of pain on nonhumans is all right.[12(pp31-32)] The morally relevant consideration in the latter case is whether the being in question is capable of suffering. Because suffering is a bad thing, it is wrong to inflict it unnecessarily. Likewise, Marquis argues, whether a moral agent's actions would deprive another being of a FLO depends solely on whether the being has a FLO, not on other features it may possess or lack (e.g., consciousness, sentience, or the ability to reason).

Unlike the case of pain, however, it is not clear that the loss of an adult's FLO is comparable to the loss of a fetus's FLO. As Robert Card has pointed out, it is worse to deprive an adult than a fetus of a FLO because killing the adult deprives her not only of what would have been valued in the future but also of any investment she and others had made in her future.[13] To illustrate this, Card, following Michael Tooley, presents the following thought experiment:

> Imagine that a mad scientist has created a new technology that allows him to erase your brain and reprogram it so that you have an entirely new set of memories, beliefs, hopes, desires, and so on. Card asks: "If the mad scientist reprogrammed you (reader) and also performed this procedure on a fetus, would the harm resulting from these actions be equal?"[13(p269)]

For the reason noted earlier, Card thinks that the loss to you is significantly greater than the loss to the fetus, who had yet to make any kind of investment in its future and who could not be said to have any clear relationship to its future in the way that you do. Hence, Card would argue, depriving the fetus of a FLO does not result in the same kind of loss.

Moreover, because Marquis' view permits voluntary euthanasia in cases where the individual faces "a future of pain and despair," it implies that not all futures are of equal value and that futures lacking certain features are less worthy of preservation. Given the inherently subjective nature of pain and what would propel a particular individual into a state of despair, Marquis' view seems to permit abortion in more cases than it appeared initially. If euthanasia is permissible given the projected quality of an individual's future, Marquis' view seems also to permit abortion in cases where there is a reasonable probability that the fetus's future will be of sufficiently poor quality.

The Liberal Pro-Choice View

At the other end of the spectrum is the liberal view, which holds that there are no moral limitations on abortion, that the government should not restrict access to abortion, and that to criminalize it constitutes an injustice against pregnant women. In contrast to the conservative view, the liberal view does not hold that genetic humanity is either necessary or sufficient for personhood. A being's biological features (e.g., having human DNA or looking like a human being) are not adequate bases for bestowing rights on or attributing distinctively human interests to that being. This view allows for the possibility that nonhumans on either this planet or another might qualify as persons in the morally relevant sense, but it also implies that zygotes, embryos, and fetuses, as well as more developed humans that lack morally relevant features, may not qualify as persons.

Mary Anne Warren, a main proponent of the liberal view, sets forth five criteria for personhood: (1) consciousness, (2) reasoning capacity, (3) self-motivated activity, (4) the capacity to communicate, and (5) the presence of self-concepts and self-awareness.[14] A being need not meet all five of these criteria to qualify as a person, and indeed, Warren asserts that "(1) and (2) alone may well be sufficient ... and quite probably (1)–(3) are sufficient."[14] If, however, a being fails to satisfy even a single criterion on Warren's list, it is, for her, not a candidate for personhood.

Warren claims that the fetus "may have a rudimentary form of consciousness,"[14(p69)] but that it is not fully conscious and fails to meet any of the other criteria for personhood. She concludes that if continuing to sustain the fetus's life poses a threat to any of a pregnant woman's interests—not just her interest in continuing to live—it is morally permissible for her to end the pregnancy. For example, Warren claims that it would be morally permissible for "a woman in her seventh month of pregnancy to obtain an abortion just to avoid having to postpone a trip to Europe."[14(p70)] The rights and interests of actual persons, according to Warren, should always take precedence over those we might attribute to potential persons.

The liberal view, like the conservative view, is not without its problems. Warren's view in particular has been criticized because it suggests the moral permissibility of infanticide as well as abortion, given that a late-term fetus is not significantly different from a newborn infant in terms of its ability to meet the criteria for personhood put forth by Warren. Although one critic, Michael Tooley, accepted this implication and proceeded to defend infanticide as morally permissible, most others, including Warren, find this implication of her view unacceptable. Warren's response to this objection was to focus on the significance of the location of fetuses compared with newborn infants. Whereas a pregnant woman can free herself of the burdens of sustaining fetal life only by detaching the fetus from her body, no such action is required in the case of a newborn. A woman who does not want to nurture a newborn infant can walk away, leaving the burden of child rearing to others. Comparing a newborn infant to a work of art, she claims that, although a woman may not want a newborn infant, someone else might, and because its continued existence no longer imposes a burden on her, she has no right to kill it any more than one has a right to destroy the Mona Lisa because one does not value it. Of course, not every painting is a Mona Lisa, and neither is every infant. Are we obligated to preserve only those infants whom someone else wants? What about those infants for whom nobody seems to care at all? In the end, Warren's view is rendered inconsistent by her attempt to escape this undesirable implication of her argument.

Another problem with this view is that the criteria for personhood are not entirely clear—a problem that Warren herself points out—and some criteria seem so stringent that many people whom we would normally consider persons would not make the cut. Even though many would agree that her criteria for personhood include things that separate persons from nonpersons, she does not explain why these criteria are morally relevant. Do we simply give special status to these features because they are features possessed by most normally functioning human beings? If so, how is that any less problematic than the claim by some proponents of the conservative view that mere membership in the species *Homo sapiens* (at any stage in development) endows us with special moral status?

The Moderate Pro-Choice View

The moderate pro-choice view does not treat abortion as morally unproblematic in the way that Warren's defense of the liberal view does, nor does it claim that most abortions are "seriously immoral"[12(p24)] or equivalent to murder, as does the conservative view. Although there are variations of the moderate view, they all claim that abortion is morally permissible under some circumstances and at certain points during pregnancy but not others. For example, Daniel Callahan claims that "abortion is justifiable only if there is a serious health or family reason; simply an unwanted or unplanned pregnancy is not a sufficiently grave reason."[15] He points out further that "the legalization of abortion . . . emerged as a way of helping *women* with troubled pregnancies, not that of legitimating the killing of embryos."[15(p184)] Callahan, like other moderates, views abortion as a morally grave matter, but he does not rest his case on particular attributes of the embryo or fetus; instead, he acknowledges that the death of an embryo or fetus is a morally significant loss that is offset by a benefit to the woman who terminates the pregnancy. Moderates vary regarding what counts as a sufficiently serious reason to end a pregnancy, but preventing the birth of an infant with a severe hereditary or congenital disease or impairment (e.g., Tay-Sachs disease, trisomy 18) would be a candidate. Likewise, preventing harm to the physical or psychological welfare of a woman or her existing dependents would count as serious reasons.

For some moderates, however, whether such weighty reasons are required depends on the point in pregnancy at which one decides to end it. A moderate who would accept a relatively trivial reason for a first trimester or early second-trimester abortion may not accept the same reason for a late-term (i.e., twenty gestational weeks and beyond) abortion because the fetus has arguably accrued moral status during its development. Some have suggested brain development, or its beginnings, as a reasonable criterion for determining a developing human's moral status. For example, some have suggested drawing the line at the appearance of the primitive streak (approximately fifteen days after fertilization), insofar as we can be confident that until then—without even the beginning of a nervous system—the embryo lacks the capacity to sense pain and therefore cannot be said to have an interest in avoiding painful stimuli. Because most women do not learn that they are pregnant until after this point, using this as the line of demarcation would permit very few abortions. Those who appeal to neurologic criteria in determining the moral permissibility of abortion look at not only whether certain organs are present but also whether and to what extent the brain and nervous system are functioning at different stages of embryologic and fetal development.

L. W. Sumner, for example, criticizes both the conservative and liberal views for attributing the same moral status to all stages of prenatal development and for ignoring the obvious differences between zygotes and forty-week fetuses. Unlike either the conservative or the liberal, Sumner holds that sentience—the capacity to experience pain or pleasure—is an appropriate threshold prior to which abortion is morally permissible and after which abortion is morally similar to infanticide.[16] Based on his understanding of neuroembryology and neuromaturation—"the functional development of the central nervous system . . . [which] is the result of continuous interactions between the environment and the genome of the fetus, infant, and child"[17]—Sumner is reasonably confident that a third-trimester fetus is sentient and equally confident that the first-trimester fetus is not. Hence, Sumner claims that a woman's autonomy is absolute in the first and early second trimesters but that a compelling justification is required for abortions in the late second trimester or third trimester. If a fetus (or any other being) is capable of experiencing pain, we ought to assume that it has an interest in not experiencing pain and act accordingly—that is, avoid causing that being unnecessary pain. Under this view, ending the life of a presentient fetus does not harm it even if others might be wronged or harmed by its destruction. One relevant consideration is whether aborting a sentient fetus would cause it more or less harm overall than allowing it to develop into an infant.

Still other moderates draw the line at the point of viability, which is defined as the "capability of living; usually connot[ing] a fetus that has reached 500 grams [approximately 1 pound, 2 ounces] in weight and 20 gestational weeks,"[18] or "capable of living, especially outside the womb."[19] Although the *Roe v. Wade* decision asserts that the state has a legitimate interest in restricting abortions after the end of the first trimester to protect the health of the woman, the state is not said to have a legitimate interest in intervening on behalf of the fetus until after the point of viability, which is when the fetus is "potentially able to live outside the mother's womb, albeit with artificial aid."[20] Although *Roe v. Wade* placed the point of viability at twenty-eight weeks, noting that it may be as early as twenty-four weeks, this conflicts with the foregoing medical definition of viability. Moreover, the legal definition of viability is inherently slippery, insofar as technological developments have and will continue to affect the viability of fetuses. It is believed that ectogenesis—artificial womb technology that would allow the gestation of the fetus outside a woman's body—will eventually move out of the world of science fiction into our local medical centers. Dr. Hung-Ching Liu of Cornell University has already grown a human embryo for six days in an artificial womb, and Dr. Yoshinori Kuwabara has been growing goat fetuses in artificial wombs since the 1990s.[21] Because eighty-nine percent of abortions are performed during the first trimester of pregnancy,[22] the viability of the fetus is not usually an issue, but if ectogenesis becomes a reality, it will probably further complicate rather than quell the abortion debate.

Some have cited the abortion issue as an example of an intractable or unresolvable issue,[23,24] and perhaps the foregoing analysis has led you to agree with this assessment. Reasonable people do disagree about this issue, but as Gert and colleagues point out, the unresolvable nature of this problem "should promote moral humility or tolerance on both sides of the issue."[23(p74)]

Making Babies

In the United States nearly half of all pregnancies are unplanned, and a significant portion of those pregnancies are carried to term.[25] It is therefore a bit of a stretch to speak of procreative decision making in many cases, because there may have been no decision at all to become pregnant. And if one's circumstances are such that ending a pregnancy is not a real option, the continuation of a pregnancy cannot be construed as genuinely autonomous, much less autonomy-enhancing. A woman and her partner may decide either quite readily or somewhat grudgingly to carry an unplanned pregnancy to term, depending on their particular circumstances as well as their beliefs about the moral status of the embryo they have created through consensual sexual intercourse. In other cases, procreation is an intentional act, or at least the *attempt* to procreate is intentional, given that once the sperm is inside a woman's reproductive tract there is very little she or her partner can do to ensure that fertilization will definitely occur. Focusing for a moment only on cases of intentional procreation, one might wonder *why* an individual or couple would procreate on purpose. What motivates people to procreate? Do any of those motives raise questions about the moral permissibility of procreation?

Usually, the motives for procreation go unquestioned unless there is something unconventional about either the stated purpose for creating a child (e.g., to save an existing child), the means of creating a child, or the prospective child's family structure. Questions are also raised when a child is born in what Joel Feinberg has called a "harmful condition" (i.e., a condition such that the child's future interests are doomed)[26] or when we are confronted with news of a child who is abused, neglected, or killed by his or her parents. Aside from tragic or atypical procreative means or contexts, the prevailing assumption is that as long as people are making babies, there is no cause for concern and certainly no need to question people's procreative actions. This laissez faire attitude has been reflected in the United States' public policy regarding assisted reproductive technologies (ARTs). The problems with this approach have been brought into sharp relief through some of the events that have occurred in the context of ART use.

Assisted Reproductive Technologies

It is important to talk about ARTs because of the relative novelty of these means of creating children. As the use of ARTs has become more widespread since the July 25, 1978, birth of Louise Brown, who was created through in vitro fertilization (IVF), the types of ARTs available and the expansion of procreative ability that they allow have raised questions about procreation outside of the ART context as well. Although some of the issues raised by the use of ARTs are not new, analysis of the motives and contexts for procreation were largely absent until ARTs brought procreation out into the light. Owing to people's myopia or resistance to change, the focus is often on a particular technological intervention and not its implications for deeply entrenched practices. In fact, prior to the introduction of ARTs, questions surrounding procreation most frequently arose when people wanted to *avoid* this "natural" outcome of sex through the use of contraception, sterilization, or abortion.

The emergence of ARTs made possible procreation under conditions that nature had never allowed and has led some people to raise questions about the permissibility of procreation under certain circumstances. Not only are heterosexual couples with blocked tubes, poor-quality sperm, and other problems with their reproductive systems rendered capable of procreation, but also homosexual couples, postmenopausal women, and even dead people. Ironically, the emergence and development of new ARTs has simultaneously reinforced and challenged traditional beliefs about the importance of genetic connections between parents and children and the structure of the family.

Procreative Liberty
The emergence of ARTs has also raised new issues about the meaning of the supposed right to procreate. Whereas respecting people's reproductive freedom had previously required only that we not interfere with other people's attempts to procreate or refrain from doing so, the use of ARTs actually requires intervention into people's procreative endeavors. Although several court decisions have effectively prescribed a policy of noninterference with people's procreative actions (e.g., *Skinner v. Oklahoma* [1942], *Griswold v. Connecticut* [1965], *Eisenstadt v. Baird* [1972], and *Roe v. Wade* [1973]), this is not adequate for dealing with cases in which procreation requires the intervention of third parties. A right *to* procreate does not clearly follow from a right to refrain from procreation, and a negative right—that is, a right against interference by others—does not entail a positive right to assistance in procreation.

John Robertson claims that reproduction is central to "personal identity, meaning, and dignity" and that the moral right to reproduce is "widely recognized as a prima facie moral right that cannot be limited except for very good reason."[24(p30)] In addition to the central role of procreation in the lives of many, Robertson and others who defend "procreative liberty" or a "right to procreate" appeal to individual autonomy as a basis for such a right. Often individuals look to the right to refrain from procreation, which is grounded in the idea that individuals have a right of *self*-determination. It is important to understand that a decision to procreate, as opposed to a decision to refrain from doing so, is not a mere exercise of one's individual autonomy because, as Onora O'Neill reminds us, "successful reproduction always affects others, and in particular it affects any child who is brought into existence."[27] Procreation always involves at least one other person and will affect the welfare of others; hence, it is clearly a moral matter regardless of the context in which procreation is attempted.

Questioning whether there really is a right to procreate is unpopular, but it is important to examine briefly why it is problematic to *assume* that there is a right to procreate. If a right to procreate is taken to be a *positive* right—that is, a right to assistance in procreation—the moral implications are repugnant. For it is possible that an individual who desires to procreate might be unable to find any person willing to help him or her in the quest to have children. Although this is a sad situation, it would be morally unacceptable to attempt to ameliorate it by overriding another's individual autonomy and forcing him or her to provide assistance in procreation. Robertson agrees that asserting a positive right to procreate is morally indefensible, and so he provides a more plausible account of a *negative* right—a "right against public or private interference."[24(p29)] Robertson's "procreative liberty" is defined as "the freedom to reproduce or not to reproduce in the genetic sense, which may also include rearing or not, as intended by the parties . . . includ[ing] female gestation whether or not there is a genetic connection to the resulting child."[24(p23)] Those who think that the permissibility of procreation should be more closely tied to the willingness to rear offspring might view Robertson's procreative liberty as overly inclusive and wonder why, for example, selling one's sperm or eggs for others' use in procreation should be considered deserving of special protection. Problematically, however, Robertson ends up invoking a *positive* right to procreate when it comes to those for whom procreation is impossible without medical assistance and leaves it unclear why only this subset of the population should have this entitlement and what specific obligations it might impose on others.[2(p113)]

Third-Party Involvement in Procreative Endeavors: Donor Gametes and Surrogacy
The first uses of IVF were aimed at circumventing the fertility problems of heterosexual couples. IVF that uses only genetic material from the couple who intends to rear the child is known as the "simple case" of IVF. Often, however, gametes from third parties are used, and in a few cases—fewer than one percent of ART births—a third party's uterus is used to gestate the child. Because the use of ARTs means that a child may have far more than two people involved in bringing him or her into the world, this has raised questions about the definition of parenthood. For example, the 1998 *Buzzanca* case[28] involved a couple, Mr. and Mrs. Buzzanca, who had contracted with a surrogate to gestate an embryo created using donor gametes. However, a few weeks before the surrogate gave birth, Mr. Buzzanca filed for divorce and claimed no responsibility for the child that was eventually born. During the first trial the judge determined that Mr. Buzzanca was not the father, but this implied that Mrs. Buzzanca was not the mother. Furthermore, since the gestational surrogate had waived her parental rights, she was not the child's mother either. Hence, according to this first ruling, even though there were at least five people involved in bringing the child into existence, she had no legal parents. Upon appeal, however, it was determined that Mr. and Mrs. Buzzanca were the legal parents, based on the fact that their intentions had set in motion the processes that brought the child into the world. So, instead of genetic or even gestational connections determining parenthood, *intention* was taken to be the relevant factor in determining legal parentage.

Although the emphasis on intention is relevant from both a legal and moral standpoint, it raises questions about other sorts of cases in which parental rights or duties are called into question. Consider two different kinds of cases. First, a man sells his sperm to a sperm bank and specifies that he wants his genetic material to be used to help other people create a child. Because the Uniform Parentage Act assumes that a married woman's husband is the legal father of the child so long as he has agreed to the fertility clinic's assisted insemination of his wife, and the sperm donor has no parental rights, the sperm donor has no legal duties toward the resultant offspring. In a second kind of case, a man and a woman meet in a bar and have a one-night stand that results in a pregnancy that the woman takes to term. In this case, it is reasonably safe to assume that the goal of the sexual encounter was not procreation but pleasure. There was no intention to create offspring, as in the case of the sperm donor; however, if the man's genetic connection to the child is confirmed, the law will require him to contribute to the child's welfare.

The intentional use of one's gametes to create children for whom one will bear no responsibility has troubled some people. In discussing the phenomenon of anonymous sperm donation, Callahan made the following remark: "It is as if everyone argued: Look, males have always been fathering children anonymously and irresponsibly; why not put this otherwise noxious trait to good use?"[29] Herbert Krimmel has expressed similar concerns about *full* surrogacy, which involves not only the use of the surrogate's uterus but also her egg. He distinguishes full surrogacy from *gestational* surrogacy, or "womb rental," which he takes to be morally unproblematic and akin to a nanny or teacher facilitating a child's development.[30]

As the use of ARTs proceeds in the United States, there is no assurance that the resultant offspring will be protected properly, in contrast to cases in which an unplanned pregnancy results in a child being put up for adoption, a system in which prospective adoptive parents are put through a rigorous screening process. Our current procreative practices reflect conflicting attitudes about the relative importance of intentions and genetic connections, and child welfare might be compromised if we insist that genetic connections matter only when adults say they matter—something we are beginning to see among certain men's rights groups who are campaigning for a right to a "financial abortion" in cases where women bring children to term whom the men do not want. Among other things, we want to make sure that our policies and practices do not further compromise the welfare of children who did not ask to be brought into existence.

Designer Children

Although many people were happy about the birth of Louise Brown, the prospect of more widespread use of IVF raised many ethical questions. There were concerns about whether IVF was safe for women and offspring, whether moving fertilization from a woman's reproductive tract into a lab would compromise women's control over procreation or their bodies, and whether people would view children differently—for example, as commodities—if they were created in a lab instead of through the process of sexual intercourse. The fact that Ms. Brown's birth was a byproduct of research that involved the destruction of embryos was not lost on anyone and was viewed as problematic by those who believed that fertilization is morally significant.

Regardless of one's conclusions about the moral status of embryos or fetuses, the moral (and legal) status of children is unambiguous. Whether a child's life story begins in a woman's reproductive tract or a petri dish in a laboratory has no bearing on either the child's parents' or society's moral obligations toward the child. Although we should avoid using procreative techniques that are likely to increase the risk of harm to prospective offspring, rejecting a method of creating a child on the ground that people might mistreat children created in that manner reflects a failure to understand that how one ought to treat a child has nothing to do with how the child came to be among us.

Motives for procreation are sometimes questioned when parents attempt to bring "savior siblings" or "designer children" into the world. Although the creation of a savior sibling to provide tissue for an existing child has occurred without using preimplantation genetic diagnosis (PGD)—for example, the Ayala family in 1990[31]—some parents have used PGD to create offspring whose tissue will be a match for an existing child suffering from a life-threatening or seriously debilitating condition. Like the Ayala case, the 2000 case of Molly and Adam Nash[32] was highly publicized and led to public debate about the moral permissibility of creating savior siblings. One question was whether the child would be welcomed by the family even if she failed to save her sibling. In the Ayala case, this consideration was more relevant because they did not use PGD and did not know until the child was born whether she would be a good match for their first child. It turned out that Marissa, their second child, was a match for their ailing child, but what if things had turned out differently? Would they have given up the child for adoption or mistreated the child in some way if she had not been a good match for her older sister? What if the older sibling required more than just cord blood or a single bone marrow transplant, as depicted in the novel *My Sister's Keeper*,[33] in which the parents required significant sacrifices of the savior sibling to promote the welfare of her ailing older sister? It would be particularly troubling to know that a couple had intentionally created a child only to relinquish it because the child failed to meet certain parental expectations or specifications, but it would be equally troubling if remaining with the biological family meant that the child would suffer significant psychological or physical harms associated with feeling like a failure for his or her inability to save an older sibling or being burdened with medical interventions aimed at keeping an ailing sibling alive.

In some cases prospective parents may not be attempting to save an existing child, but they may want to ensure to the best of their ability that their child will possess a certain trait or be free of an undesirable hereditary condition. In many cases, parents will use PGD and implant only those embryos that are free of the undesired condition. For example, if a couple knew that they were at risk of having a child with an autosomal recessive disease such as Tay-Sachs disease or cystic fibrosis, they would reject those embryos that were homozygous for the relevant trait. In the case of an X-linked (i.e., sex-linked) recessive condition, such as Duchenne muscular dystrophy or hemophilia, the parents might choose to implant only female (XX) embryos. Selecting against embryos solely on the basis of sex has caused greater moral controversy than using PGD to avoid having a child who will develop a serious disease; there is some concern that this practice, like selective abortion, which is aimed at avoiding having a particular type of child rather than a more general desire to avoid taking *any* pregnancy to term at a specific time in one's life, will negatively affect attitudes or behavior toward impaired individuals who are part of our communities.

Although there are legitimate moral concerns about using PGD to select against embryos predisposed to developing maladies, the desire to refrain from creating a child who will be afflicted with a disease may be morally defensible, especially if the disease is likely to cut off the child's opportunity to flourish despite modifications made to accommodate impairments associated with the condition (e.g., Tay-Sachs disease). Greater controversy arises, however, when prospective parents select *for* particular traits that they deem desirable. For example, there has been significant publicity surrounding cases of prospective parents selecting gamete donors or using PGD in order to improve their odds of having a deaf child.[34] The case of selecting for deafness is particularly problematic because it is viewed as a "disability" by some and a "culture" by others. Members of the Deaf community do not view themselves as having "broken ears"; instead, they view themselves as a "linguistic minority" that should not be discriminated against by the hearing population.

Cloning

Although it is unlikely that somatic cell nuclear transfer, or cloning, will become a popular means of creating children, it is worth exploring ethical issues related to cloning insofar as it requires us to "reflect deeply on our basic conceptions of individual identity" and longstanding assumptions about how procreation should occur.[35] Moreover, such an analysis can help dispel misconceptions that some popular films (e.g., *Boys from Brazil*, *Multiplicity*, *The 6th Day*, *The Island*) perpetuate about the cloning process and characteristics of clones.

An important distinction made by Dena Davis is between *duplicative* and *logistical* cloning.[36] The goal of the former is to duplicate a particular genome, whereas the latter is aimed at finding a way around barriers to creating a genetically related child through sexual intercourse or through the use of other ARTs. Whereas logistical cloning may be justifiable, Davis is critical of duplicative cloning, as are many other people. One of the main problems with duplicative cloning is that the desire to duplicate a genome frequently rests on erroneous assumptions. For example, an individual who claims that he wants to clone himself to achieve immortality or the grieving parents who want to clone their recently deceased child are operating under the assumption that the clone would be an exact copy of its progenitor. This is inaccurate. In addition to the fact that there would likely be a genetic difference between the clone and his or her progenitor because of the mitochondrial DNA (mDNA) in the cytoplasm of the donor egg (assuming the egg donor is not the same person who created the progenitor as well), the phenomenon of *developmental plasticity* means that "there is no one-to-one relationship between a particular genome and a particular phenotype; a single genome may be associated with any number of phenotypic variants."[37] Even though a clone and his or her progenitor would share a genotype, they would not necessarily be identical in appearance, much less share the same interests, beliefs, or personality. If the goal is to duplicate some particular individual because of his or her endearing or admirable qualities, cloning will not deliver. Stated otherwise, cloning will be *futile* with regard to this goal.

If, however, the goal is merely to create a child who is genetically connected to at least one of the parents, this may, in principle, be as morally defensible as procreation via more conventional ARTs. A clone is not a mere copy of another person; instead, as is true of those of us created via fertilization, a clone would forge a unique identity and relationships with other people. At present, however, the attempt to create a child via cloning would violate the requirement that prospective parents refrain from bringing an individual into an avoidable harmful condition.[38] On the topic of obligations toward fetuses destined to become children, Joel Feinberg asserts that "a duty of care is owed toward *anyone* who is likely to be harmed as a consequence of his conduct, and this includes persons not yet born nor even conceived."[39]

Setting aside serious questions about whether the risks of human cloning will ever be low enough to make cloning morally permissible, consider the following hypothetical scenario offered by Grant Gillett:

> [A] couple after a long period of fertility treatment finally manages to conceive a child, who tragically threatens to miscarry early in the pregnancy because of some transient disorder. What would we say if they wanted to clone their developing fetus so that after the miscarriage they could still have their own genetic child (which had cost them, in every way, so much to produce)?[35(p278)]

In this paradigmatic case of logistical cloning, the couple merely desires to have a genetically related child and has no expectation or desire to copy a particular, identifiable individual with whom they had developed a relationship. *If* creating a genetically related child is a legitimate goal, and assuming for the sake of argument that cloning does not increase a prospective child's risk of being born in a harmful condition, the claim that logistical cloning is necessarily immoral requires further defense.

Ethical Issues in Pregnancy Management and Birth

The availability and expansion of various medical technologies mean that women can learn more about their fetuses and do so earlier in their pregnancies than ever before. Admittedly, "knowledge is power," but it may also inspire significant fear in a pregnant woman if she finds out that there is something seriously wrong with her developing fetus, especially as she approaches labor and delivery. The ability to detect problems may allow for intervention (e.g., fetal surgery, early delivery, or caesarean delivery), which may decrease infant morbidity or mortality. Unfortunately, however, patients and HCPs do not always agree regarding the best course of action in cases where a prenatal test indicates that the fetus has a disease or malformation. There may also be disagreements regarding general pregnancy management or preferred methods of delivery. In some cases these disagreements are the result of a patient's failure to understand the importance of following medical advice or the HCP's failure to understand certain details about the patient's situation, but in other cases the patient's refusal to adhere to medical advice may be deliberate and not based on ignorance or misunderstanding.

Prenatal Screening and Testing

Although technologies such as PGD allow people to determine whether the embryo is male or female and whether it carries a hereditary or congenital malady, most people still procreate through sexual intercourse and thus are not able to avail themselves of PGD. Hence, in order to determine whether a fetus carries a malady, a woman may undergo prenatal screening and subsequent diagnostic testing during the first or second trimester of pregnancy. The HCP may conduct prenatal testing through blood tests, ultrasound, chorionic villus sampling (CVS), or amniocentesis. The HCP will recommend CVS or an amniocentesis only if the initial screening or the woman's medical history indicates that there is a high risk of fetal anomaly, especially because both of these procedures may put the woman at risk of losing the pregnancy.

Prenatal screening of pregnant women has become routine, and although such testing is not legally mandated, it is often strongly encouraged by HCPs and other members of society. Even though it may benefit some prospective parents, one should not view it as an unqualified good. Although prenatal screening has been presented as a way to reassure women or expand their control over reproductive decision making, it is unclear whether prenatal screening achieves either end or that it is the best way to achieve them.[40] Women may feel pressured to undergo genetic testing to avoid being labeled as an uncaring or irresponsible prospective parent or a "noncompliant" patient. Mary Mahowald points out that "unlike genetic counselors . . . obstetricians are trained to be directive rather than nondirective with patients. The goal . . . is to ensure that the woman and her potential child are both healthy."[41] Lippman has also observed that "rates of induced abortion are higher when obstetricians relate the results of testing than when geneticists do."[40(p361)] Although some people suggest that prenatal screening and genetic testing are aimed at helping prospective parents prepare to meet a child's special needs, some women have reported that they have been "encouraged to terminate when the result is positive."[41(p233)] Whereas the birth of an impaired child used to be accepted as merely a tragic roll of the dice, the birth of such a child in contemporary society is more likely to be viewed as something that should have been prevented.

Under such conditions, a woman's "choice" to undergo prenatal screening may not be genuinely free and may limit rather than expand her individual autonomy. In a case in which a woman is presented with a positive test result, she must then face the decision whether to continue the pregnancy—a burden she may not have wanted. Furthermore, although it would not be morally permissible to force a woman to end a pregnancy, she may be under significant pressure from her HCP, her insurance company, the prospective father, or other family members to end a pregnancy she wants to continue or to continue a pregnancy she no longer wants. She may find herself in a position where she is considered either irresponsible for bringing an impaired child into the world or callous if she decides to have an abortion. Because prenatal screening results are usually negative, a woman might be caught off guard by a positive test result and unprepared to address the issue of whether to continue the pregnancy. Furthermore, a woman's choice may be constrained by her social circumstances. For example, she may not have access to an abortion provider, abortion may be against her religious or cultural code of conduct, or she may lack the financial and social resources to rear a child with special needs. Ultimately, "whether prenatal testing is truly . . . an option depends on the parties involved, the quality of the relationship between the woman and her physician, the adequacy and accuracy of the information provided, and on the availability of social and economic supports for continuing or discontinuing an affected pregnancy."[41(p234, n53)]

Despite the pressure that both women and their HCPs feel to bring forth healthy infants, some have pointed out that it is necessary to keep our society's "ableist" bias in check. Although there are some maladies that are so severe as to be incompatible with a "minimally decent life" (e.g., trisomy 18, Tay-Sachs disease), we should not assume that any particular malady necessarily precludes a life worth living. Whether an impaired individual is capable of flourishing depends to some extent on whether the available accommodations allow them to interact successfully with their environment. Although it might seem too obvious to mention, access to a wheelchair greatly expands the opportunities afforded a person whose legs do not function normally. Along these lines, Martha Nussbaum reminds us that normally functioning individuals would be disabled relative to their environment if certain specific accommodations were not made, such as elevators and properly spaced stairs to reach the upper levels of buildings.[42] Impairments *do* place limitations on people's ability to function, but the degree of disability caused by certain types of impairments depends to some degree on society's ability and willingness to look beyond preconceived notions and accommodate people with impairments. Regarding the latter, Nussbaum provides the following observation:

> Many problems of children with Down syndrome that had been taken to be unalterable cognitive limitations are actually treatable bodily limitations: the weak muscles of the neck, especially, which prevent exploration of the environment at a crucial time; the weak muscles of the tongue, which prevent speech from developing. The prejudice that these children were just "dumb" and ineducable prevented an accurate understanding of what they could achieve.[42(p189)]

Just as it is important to limit the influence of biases about impaired individuals, it is also important to reject genetic determinism and genetic reductionism, beliefs that are quite prevalent in our society. *Genetic reductionism* assumes that everything about a person is grounded in that person's genotype, and *genetic determinism* assumes that a person's destiny—at least in terms of his or her health—is determined entirely by the person's genes.

These erroneous assumptions should not guide decisions about whether to continue a pregnancy, nor should individual biases about the quality of life with a particular impairment. Furthermore, HCPs should be clear about what a genetic test does and does not reveal; for example, it may tell a person that her child will have cystic fibrosis, but because there are over 1,200 mutations of the CFTR gene, HCPs cannot be certain about how severe the disease will be for a particular individual. Additionally, HCPs should prepare their patients for the possibility that they may learn something surprising about either their own genetic makeup or that of their fetus. Through testing the fetus, a woman may unexpectedly discover that she carries a gene for a hereditary disease or that she is mistaken about the identity of the child's genetic father.

Maternal–Fetal Conflict

It is important to guard against misapplication of the *maternal–fetal conflict* label, because it may worsen rather than ameliorate problems that arise in caring for pregnant women. Conflicts arising in the care of pregnant women are not necessarily between a woman and her fetus, and describing a situation as a case of maternal-fetal conflict may obscure the actual nature of the conflict and therefore preclude resolution of the problems at hand. As Baylis and colleagues point out, the conflict may be between women and "others [e.g., HCPs] who believe they know best how to protect the fetus."[43] There are some cases of genuine maternal-fetal conflict, in which the woman's interests are at odds with promoting the life or health of the fetus. In many such cases, the woman will terminate the pregnancy. However, when a woman decides to carry a pregnancy to term, her interests and those of her fetus (or the child the fetus will become) overlap significantly, given that a primary goal is *usually* to deliver a healthy baby with whom the mother will be able to establish a parent-child relationship. Although a pregnant woman is advised to alter her life in many ways to benefit the fetus, many things that are good for the fetus are also good for the woman. Likewise, certain things, such as drug and alcohol abuse, exposure to environmental toxins, and intimate partner violence, are bad for both the woman and the fetus.

Still, there are some cases in which the patient's actions are at odds with what both she and her HCP agree is good for the fetus or in which the patient and the HCP simply disagree about what is best for the fetus. An example of the former would be a woman who is addicted to drugs, alcohol, or cigarettes and does not stop using these substances despite her understanding that they are bad for the developing child. However, the HCP should not assume that the pregnant woman who fails to shake her addiction is a malevolent person; she may very desperately want to be free of addiction yet find herself unable to stop for a number of reasons. One problem is that many drug treatment programs refuse to admit pregnant women due to concerns about legal liability.[44] Another problem is that treatment facilities rarely offer coordinated services that include, among other things, prenatal care and child care.[44,45] In the face of such obstacles to overcoming addiction, the HCP should continue to encourage the patient to discontinue drug use, further educate the patient about the harms of substance abuse, and increase awareness of treatment options.[44] The HCP should also encourage dietary changes or the use of additional nutritional supplements that might counteract the effects of drug use.

Additionally, while discussing the dangers of drug use during pregnancy, the HCP should inquire and determine whether intimate partner violence is a contributing factor to the woman's abuse, because some women turn to drugs in order to numb the pain associated with an abusive relationship. Even if a woman's partner is not abusive, he may also be addicted to drugs and encouraging her to use them. Despite the almost exclusive focus on *women's* behavior where reproductive matters are concerned, it is important to note that *men's* use of drugs, alcohol, or tobacco, or exposure to certain environmental toxins (e.g., lead) before conception or during pregnancy can negatively affect the fetus as well. Understanding the complexity of the situation should encourage the HCP to foster a relationship of trust with troubled patients so as to maximize the HCP's ability to help pregnant patients overcome serious problems and bring about the best possible outcome for the child who will be born under less than optimal circumstances. Ultimately, because neither women nor fetuses benefit from drug and alcohol abuse, such cases are not genuine cases of maternal–fetal conflict. Overcoming the addiction is a shared interest of the woman and her fetus.

More frequently, the phrase *maternal–fetal conflict* refers to cases in which a woman refuses the HCP's medical advice, such as a recommendation to deliver via caesarean section (c-section). Some complications (e.g., placenta previa or preeclampsia) carry an increased risk of maternal morbidity or mortality, but concern about a woman's health or overall well-being may not be a motive for recommending a c-section delivery. If the HCP believes that a vaginal delivery at any time would increase fetal morbidity or mortality, or that waiting for the woman to go into labor on her own would increase her odds of delivering a stillborn or a severely impaired infant, the HCP may recommend a c-section. In addition to medical reasons for recommending a c-section, the HCP may recommend a c-section for nonmedical reasons, including concerns about legal liability or a desire for more control over the timing of delivery.

Although patients have a moral and legal right to refuse treatment, court orders have been issued to force women to undergo c-sections. In one tragic U.S. case (*In re A.C.*),[46] a dying pregnant woman was court ordered to undergo a c-section in an attempt to save her twenty-six-week fetus. The infant died within two hours of delivery, and the mother died two days later. Although the mother's death was imminent prior to delivery, overriding her refusal to undergo a c-section was not only an egregious breach of her right of self-determination, but also defeated an important goal of end-of-life care, which is to promote "the fullest, best possible living of the last moments of life."[47]

In light of the fact that some women who had been court ordered to undergo c-sections ultimately gave birth vaginally to healthy babies, coupled with the high c-section rate in the United States (30.1 percent),[48] women may doubt the evidentiary basis for the HCP's claim that a c-section is necessary. Along these lines, Baylis and Sherwin point out that a woman may *deliberately* refuse to follow the HCP's medical advice for different types of reasons: differing values, distrust, or epistemologic conflict.[49] She and her HCP may value fetal life differently, thus influencing the patient's willingness or unwillingness to terminate a pregnancy. A woman may distrust either a particular HCP or the medical establishment in general. In addition to a woman's concerns about the evidentiary basis for her HCP's medical advice, she may view her lived experience as a more reliable source of knowledge, because it includes an intimate understanding of how her body responded during previous pregnancies and deliveries.[49] One case that combined all of these factors was the case of a woman with nine children who refused a c-section, not only because she prioritized her ability to continue caring for her existing children, something recovering from a c-section would have made impossible, but also because she trusted her own experience more than the physician's medical judgment.[50]

Speaking from her thirty-five years of obstetric experience, Wendy Savage shares the only two cases of c-section refusal she has experienced and their outcomes:

> The first, a woman in Nigeria, told me at 5:00 a.m. that she did not want a CS [c-section], which I had recommended because she appeared to be in obstructed labour in her fifth pregnancy, as she always delivered when the sun rose. I told her that I thought this baby was bigger and that she would not do so this time. When the sun rose at 6:45 a.m. and she was still not delivered, she agreed to a CS. . . . The second woman was only 16 years old and did not speak English; her husband, who was a devout Muslim, would not agree to a CS. When it became apparent that she was not going to deliver after several hours of full dilation, he agreed, but sadly the baby died. However, when she returned the next year, he accepted our advice and she went on to have six more children by CS because she had a small pelvis. . . . If we had gone to court would he have tried to have his wife deliver at home . . . and perhaps die from a ruptured uterus?[50(p178)]

In both of these cases, Savage had been correct in her estimation that without a c-section, things were not going to end well. These cases demonstrate the importance of resisting the temptation on the part of the HCP to allow strong views about the appropriate course of action to cause her to be dismissive of the patient's reasons for refusal. Trivializing the views of a patient instead of trying to understand them and work with them would result in alienation of the patient and a breakdown of the patient–HCP relationship, which would solve nothing and possibly lead to outcomes that are tragic for both the patient and the physician.

Chapter Summary

Reproductive ethics inquires into the moral permissibility of various means of procreation and its prevention. This chapter analyzed three main views on abortion—the conservative anti-abortion (pro-life) view and the liberal and moderate pro-choice views—and the challenges faced by each view. The moral status of the zygote, embryo, or fetus is one focal point of the abortion debate, and considerations raised in the abortion debate are relevant to debates about the moral permissibility of in vitro fertilization and other assisted reproductive technologies (ARTs), preimplantation genetic diagnosis, prenatal screening and genetic testing, and refusals to follow certain medical advice. Moving away from preventing procreation, the chapter also explored issues that the emergence of ARTs brought to light, including questions about motives for procreation, the meaning of a "right to procreate," and what our attitudes toward unconventional procreative means, motives, and contexts tell us about our assumptions regarding "natural" procreation. The concept of a right to procreate, understood as either a positive right (i.e., an entitlement to assistance in procreation) or a negative right (i.e., a right to noninterference by third parties; Robertson's "procreative liberty") remains problematic. Also explored was the influence of technological and medical interventions during pregnancy and near birth and how these may give rise to disagreements between patients and health care professionals regarding the best way to manage pregnancy, labor, and delivery. Although there are genuine cases of maternal–fetal conflict, not all cases of conflict in pregnancy management are properly identified by that label.

Review Questions

1. How do contraceptives differ from contragestives?

2. According to the pro-life view described in the chapter, who do the moral rules (including the rule against killing) protect? Moral agents? Potential moral agents? Sentient beings? Potential sentient beings? Persons?

3. According to the more liberal pro-choice view described in the chapter, who do the moral rules (including the rule against killing) protect? Moral agents? Potential moral agents? Sentient beings? Potential sentient beings? Persons?

4. According to the more moderate pro-choice view described in the chapter, who do the moral rules (including the rule against killing) protect? Moral agents? Potential moral agents? Sentient beings? Potential sentient beings? Persons?

5. Of what moral importance is the location of the fetus (vis-à-vis the mother) in the abortion debate?

6. What did the U.S. Supreme Court decide in *Roe v. Wade*?

7. Regarding the case (discussed in this chapter) of Marissa and Anissa Ayala, what would Aristotle say about the decision to conceive Marissa? What would Aquinas say? Kant? Mill? Would any of their opinions be different on the facts of the Nash case? (Review Chapter 1.)

8. What is duplicative cloning? Logistical cloning?

Endnotes

1. Goldman AH. Sexual ethics. In: Frey RG, Wellman CH, eds. *A Companion to Applied Ethics.* Malden, MA: Blackwell Publishing, 2005:180.
2. Pearson YE. Storks, cabbage patches, and the right to procreate. *J Bioethical Inquiry* 2007;4:105–115, p. 106.
3. Shanner L. The right to procreate: when rights claims have gone wrong. *McGill Law J* 1995;40:823–874, p. 867.
4. EDITORIAL ENDNOTE: "The ethics of abortion are, and probably will remain, a matter of intense debate." So wrote Jonsen, Siegler, and Winslade in the third edition of their text *Clinical Ethics* in 1992 (New York: McGraw-Hill, 1992:175). The sixth edition of the same text does not discuss ethical issues in reproductive medicine and obstetrics "because the presence of the fetus presents special problems that do not fit well into [their] form of analysis" (New York: McGraw-Hill, 2006:4). Gert has written that "there is an unresolvable disagreement about the moral acceptability of abortion" (Gert B, Berger EM, Cahill GF, et al. *Morality and the New Genetics.* Sudbury, MA: Jones and Bartlett, 1996:117). It is the opinion of the editors that notwithstanding the disagreement about the general moral acceptability of abortion, physician participation in *elective* abortion falls outside the scope of legitimate medical practice and is a violation of the internal morality of medicine. (See Chapter 5 for a discussion of the internal morality of medicine. See also Paola F. Abortions provide medical anathema. *Tampa Tribune,* October 14, 2000, p. 15.) We believe that it is possible for a physician to be pro-choice and yet opposed to physician involvement in abortion, just as it is possible for a physician to be in favor of capital punishment and yet opposed to physician involvement in the same.
5. Davidoff F, Trussel J. Plan B and the politics of doubt. *JAMA* 2006;296(14):1775–1778.
6. American College of Obstetricians and Gynecologists. Induced abortion. *ACOG Education Pamphlet.* Available at: http://www.acog.org/publications/patient_education/bp043.cfm. Accessed May 12, 2008.
7. *Roe v. Wade,* 410 U.S. 113 (1973).
8. EDITORIAL ENDNOTE: Indeed, even Justice Blackmun, who authored the opinion of the Court in *Roe v. Wade,* wrote, "If this suggestion of [fetal] personhood is established, the [mother's right to terminate her pregnancy] collapses, for the fetus' right to life would then be guaranteed specifically by the [Fourteenth] Amendment." See *Roe v. Wade,* 410 U.S. 113 (1973).
9. Little MO. Abortion. In: Frey RG, Wellman CH, eds. *A Companion to Applied Ethics.* Malden, MA: Blackwell Publishing, 2005:316–317.
10. Cohen CB. *Renewing the Stuff of Life: Stem Cells, Ethics, and Public Policy.* New York: Oxford University Press, 2007.
11. EDITORIAL ENDNOTE: But see endnote 8.
12. Marquis D. Why abortion is immoral. In: Dwyer S, Feinberg J, eds. *The Problem of Abortion.* New York: Wadsworth Publishing, 1997:24–39, p. 29.
13. Card RF. Two puzzles for Marquis' conservative view on abortion. *Bioethics* 2006;20(5):264–277.
14. Warren MA. On the moral and legal status of abortion. In: Dwyer S, Feinberg J, eds. *The Problem of Abortion.* New York: Wadsworth Publishing, 1997:59–74, p. 67.
15. Callahan D. *What Price Better Health?* Berkeley: University of California Press, 2003:181.
16. Sumner LW. A third way. In: Dwyer S, Feinberg J, eds. *The Problem of Abortion.* New York: Wadsworth Publishing, 1997:98–117.

17. Allen MC. Assessment of gestational age and neuromaturation. *Ment Health Res Dev Disabil Res Rev* 2005;11:21–33, p. 21.
18. *Stedman's Medical Dictionary.* 26th ed. Baltimore: Williams and Wilkins, 1995.
19. *Black's Law Dictionary.* 8th edition. St. Paul, MN: Thomson-West, 2004.
20. Blackman HA. Majority opinion in *Roe v. Wade.* In: Mappes TA, Zembaty JS, eds. *Social Ethics: Morality and Social Policy.* 6th ed. New York: McGraw-Hill, 2002:39–44, p. 43.
21. Pence G. What's so good about natural motherhood? (In praise of unnatural gestation). In: Gelfand S, Shook JR, eds. *Ectogenesis: Artificial Womb Technology and the Future of Human Reproduction.* New York: Rodopi, 2006:77–88.
22. Guttmacher Institute. *Facts on Induced Abortion in the United States.* January 2008. Available at: http://www.guttmacher.org/pubs/fb_induced_abortion.html. Accessed May 13, 2008.
23. Gert B, Culver CM, Clouser KD. *Bioethics: A Systematic Approach.* New York: Oxford University Press, 2006.
24. Robertson JA. *Children of Choice: Freedom and the New Reproductive Technologies.* Princeton, NJ: Princeton University Press, 1994.
25. Finer LB, Henshaw SK. Disparities in rates of unintended pregnancy in the United States, 1994 and 2001. *Perspect Sex Reprod Health* 2006;38(2):90–96.
26. Feinberg J. *Harm to Others.* New York: Oxford University Press, 1984:98.
27. O'Neill O. "Reproductive autonomy" *versus* public good? *Prenatal Diagnosis* 2006;26:646–647.
28. *Buzzanca v. Buzzanca,* 72 Cal. Rptr. 2d 280 (Cal. App. 1998).
29. Callahan D. Bioethics and fatherhood. *Utah Law Rev* 1992;735(3):735–746, p. 741.
30. Krimmel H. The case against surrogate parenting. In: Pence GE, ed. *Classic Works in Medical Ethics.* New York: McGraw-Hill, 1998:127–137.
31. In 1989, Marissa Ayala was conceived "in part to be a bone marrow donor for [her sister] Anissa, who would likely have died without Marissa's bone marrow. The Ayalas claim they love little Marissa just as much as Anissa, and both children now seem fine." See Pence G. *The Elements of Bioethics.* Boston: McGraw-Hill, 2007:68.
32. CBS News. A genetically screened baby saved the life of his sister. Available at: http://www.cbsnews.com/stories/2002/01/31/health/main326728.shtml. Accessed May 18, 2008.
33. Picoult J. *My Sister's Keeper.* New York: Atria Books, 2004.
34. BBC Online. Couple "choose" to have deaf baby. April 8, 2002. Available at: http://news.bbc.co.uk/2/hi/health/1916462.stm. Accessed May 12, 2008.
35. Gillett G. *Bioethics in the Clinic: Hippocratic Reflections.* Baltimore: Johns Hopkins University Press, 2004:279.
36. Green RM. Much ado about mutton: an ethical review of the cloning controversy. In: Lauritzen P, ed. *Cloning and the Future of Human Embryo Research.* New York: Oxford University Press, 2001:114–131, p. 126.
37. Robert JS. *Embryology, Epigenesis, and Evolution: Taking Development Seriously.* New York: Cambridge University Press, 2004:79.
38. Indeed, in its July 2002 report, *Human Cloning and Human Dignity: An Ethical Inquiry* (available at http://bioethics.gov/reports/cloningreport/pcbe_cloning_report.pdf), the President's Council on Bioethics wrote, "The Council is in full agreement that cloning-to-produce-children is not only unsafe but also morally unacceptable, and ought not to be attempted." The council held unanimously that cloning to produce children is unethical, ought not to be attempted, and should be *indefinitely* banned by federal law, regardless of who performs the act or whether federal funds are involved.

39. Feinberg J. Wrongful life and the counterfactual element in harming. *Soc Phil Policy* 1986;4(1):145–178, p. 154.

40. Lippman A. Prenatal genetic testing and screening: constructing needs and reinforcing inequities. In: Beauchamp DE, Steinbock B, eds. *New Ethics for the Public's Health.* New York: Oxford University Press, 1999.

41. Mahowald M. Aren't we all eugenicists? Commentary on Paul Lombardo's "Taking Eugenics Seriously." *Florida State Univ Law Rev* 2003;30:219–235, pp. 233–234.

42. Nussbaum M. *Frontiers of Justice.* Cambridge, MA: Belknap Press of Harvard University Press, 2006.

43. Baylis F, Rodgers S, Young D. Ethical dilemmas in the care of pregnant women: rethinking "maternal-fetal conflicts." In: Singer PA, Viens AM, eds. *The Cambridge Textbook of Bioethics.* New York: Cambridge University Press, 2008:97–103, p. 97.

44. Sikich K. Peeling back the layers of substance abuse during pregnancy. *DePaul J Health Care Law* 2005;8:369–401.

45. Dailard C, Nash E. State responses to substance abuse among pregnant women. *Guttmacher Rep Public Policy* 2000;December:3–6.

46. *In re A.C.*, 573 A.2d (D.C. App. 1990) (en banc).

47. Battin MP. Dying in 559 beds: efficiency, "best buys," and the ethics of standardization in national health care. In: Baergen R, ed. *Ethics at the End of Life.* Belmont: Wadsworth, 2001:285–296, p. 294.

48. Centers for Disease Control and Prevention. Teen birth rate rises for the first time in 14 years [press release]. December 5, 2007. Available at: http://www.cdc.gov/od/oc/media/press-rel/2007/r071205.htm. Accessed May 15, 2008.

49. Baylis F, Sherwin S. Judgements of non-compliance in pregnancy. In: Dickenson DL, ed. *Ethical Issues in Maternal-Fetal Medicine.* New York: Cambridge University Press, 2002:285–301.

50. Savage W. Caesarean section: who chooses—the woman or her doctor? In: Dickenson DL, ed. *Ethical Issues in Maternal-Fetal Medicine.* New York: Cambridge University Press, 2002:263–283.

Chapter 12

The Landscape of Ethical Issues in Pediatrics

Humans have a longer childhood relative to our lifespan than any other species. This provides immense plasticity—ability to learn from their environment and their culture. Most organisms on Earth depend on their genetic information which is prewired into their nervous system. While our behavior is still significantly controlled by our genetic inheritance, we have, through our brains, a much richer opportunity to blaze new behavioral and cultural pathways on short time scales. We have made a bargain with nature; our children will be difficult to raise, but their capacity for new learning will greatly enhance the chances of survival of the human species.

—Carl Sagan, *The Dragons of Eden*

Chapter Learning Objectives
At the conclusion of this chapter the reader will be able to:

1. Understand the ethical issues involved in caring for infants, children, and adolescents

2. Be familiar with classic pediatric ethical cases such as the Willowbrook School, Baby Doe, Baby K, and the Kennedy-Krieger lead abatement studies

3. Discuss issues regarding practicing procedures on children, refusal of treatment, pediatric assent, and futility

Pediatrics encompasses vast changes in physiology, growth and development, and psychological and social maturation. Accompanying these changes are a number of ethical issues that pertain only to infants, children, and adolescents. This chapter focuses on ethical dilemmas and conundrums unique to pediatrics. A *dilemma* is a situation in which there are two or more competing and potentially satisfactory solutions. A *conundrum* is a problem for which there is, at present, no satisfactory solution or answer. This chapter presents an overview of ethical issues in pediatrics based on developmental stages.

Fetus and Newborn

Abortion is an issue that has divided this nation politically and philosophically for many decades, and easily qualifies as a conundrum from the ethical standpoint. From a scientific and physiologic standpoint, the question of when life begins is easily answered.

Human life begins with the union of egg and sperm. But the question of when an individual becomes or ceases to be a person is much more difficult philosophically. If an individual ceases to be a person when he or she loses brain waves and brain function, then it would seem logical to assume that he or she becomes a person when brain waves first appear. But our technology for detecting brain waves in the fetus may be limited, such that we may fail to detect brain waves that might be there.[1] If an individual ceases to be a person when he or she can no longer ever interact with others or the environment, then a logical corollary would be that an individual becomes a person when he or she develops the ability to interact with others and the environment. But then many newborn infants, who spend the vast majority of their time eating, sleeping, and crying, would not qualify as persons, which flies in the face of public and professional opinion.

Fetal Viability

The limits of fetal viability are another contentious issue when it comes to abortion. When *Roe v. Wade* was decided, the limits of fetal viability were approximately twenty-six weeks of gestation, and therefore states used that limit to establish when abortions could or could not be done. Since that time, however, neonatology has continually pushed back the limits of fetal viability,[2,3] to the point that nowadays one can be resuscitating and stabilizing in the neonatal intensive care unit (NICU) an infant younger in gestational age than an infant being aborted in the Obstetrics/Gynecology department. The law has clearly not kept pace with advances in neonatology.

The pushing back of the limits of fetal viability has created its own ethical issues. As neonatologists compete to see who can salvage the most premature infant, more and more infants are being "saved" who end up with devastating, life-long handicaps, some of whom will require custodial care for the rest of their lives.

Fetuses and Pain

Another hotly debated issue with obvious ramifications for abortion is whether fetuses can feel pain.[4-6] Some experts have data suggesting that fetuses can feel pain by twenty weeks of gestation, and possibly earlier. They have demonstrated that pain receptors are present in the human fetus's perioral area at seven weeks of gestation, and encompass the entire face, palms of the hands, and soles of the feet by eleven weeks. The trunk, arms, and legs develop pain receptors by fifteen weeks of gestation. What is uncertain is whether the anatomic presence of pain receptors is equivalent to the capacity to sense or feel pain. Other experts argue that the capacity to truly feel pain does not appear until twenty-nine to thirty weeks of gestational age when pain pathways to the brainstem and thalamus are completely myelinated, and that the placenta produces certain chemicals that prevent the fetus from actually sensing pain. The latter data come from impressions gained from performing fetal surgeries, where the fetus is removed from the uterus but still attached to the placenta, a surgical procedure is performed to alleviate obstruction of cerebrospinal fluid flow, or urine flow from the kidney, and then the fetus is returned to the uterus to complete development.

Babies and Pain

Until recently, clinicians assumed that babies did not feel pain or recognize pain. This assumption was based on the belief that the neurologic system of babies was immature and poorly myelinated. This premise was supported by observations that a neonate or infant could be calmed and would stop crying after a painful procedure if given a pacifier soaked in sugar water[7] or a bottle to drink. This barbaric belief was perpetuated by an anesthetic technique called the "Liverpool technique," which was widely used for major surgical procedures in newborns and infants.[8] The Liverpool technique consisted of completely paralyzing the infant with neuromuscular blocking agents and then operating on the infant without analgesics or with very small, clearly subtherapeutic doses of analgesics. The proponents of this technique believed they were protecting the infants from the adverse hemodynamic effects of opiate analgesics. The Liverpool technique was widely employed for open-heart and abdominal surgeries on infants in this country as well as abroad. It wasn't until the early 1990s that studies demonstrated a significantly increased mortality and morbidity when infants underwent cardiac surgical procedures without complete and deep anesthesia.[9] The natural stress response to surgery in conscious or only partially anesthetized patients adversely affects surgical outcome.

Lack of myelination has been invoked to support the argument that neonates are not capable of pain perception. However, even in adults nociceptive impulses are carried by unmyelinated or poorly myelinated nerve fibers. All that incomplete myelination implies is a slower conduction of pain impulses in the neonate, which is usually offset by the shorter distances traveled by the impulses.

Another example of the belief that babies do not feel pain is the current practice of performing circumcisions on male neonates without anesthesia or analgesia.[10] Despite overwhelming evidence that babies feel pain, and the existence of effective means of anesthetizing the infant, including penile nerve blocks or topical local anesthetics, circumcision is still performed on many male infants without pain relief.

We now know conclusively that newborns and infants feel pain and that, although their expression of pain is different from that of older children or adults, their perception of pain is not. Much work still needs to be done to determine the most effective analgesics and their doses in pediatric patients. Unfortunately, much work also needs to be done to educate health care providers that babies and children feel pain, are adversely affected by pain, and deserve to be pain free.

Fetal Research

Fetal research is another area of controversy. Especially when it was thought that fetal adrenal tissue transplants might benefit patients with Parkinson disease,[11] a number of ethical issues surfaced. One of the most important was the question of who was authorized to donate fetal tissues. The tissues were obtained from aborted fetuses, and some assumed that the mother was the appropriate individual to consent to donation of fetal tissue. Others, however, asked whether a mother who had decided to abort the fetus had a conflict of interest in deciding to donate fetal tissue for research and transplantation. This issue came to a head when a woman conceived a child expressly for the purpose of aborting the fetus in order to obtain adrenal tissue for transplantation into her father, who had advanced Parkinson disease.

Some of the most egregious examples of unethical research have involved fetuses. In a famous 1966 study of the ethics of human experimentation, Henry Beecher examined twenty-two studies he identified as unethical that had been published in prestigious medical journals.[12] Two of those studies involved research on fetuses. In one study, researchers from Western Reserve University and the University of Helsinki decapitated eight fetuses of twelve to twenty weeks' gestation to examine whether the fetal brain could metabolize ketones. The severed heads continued to function metabolically for hours. In another study, U.S. scientists immersed fifteen fetuses in oxygenated salt solutions to determine whether they could absorb oxygen through their skin. One fetus survived for twenty-three hours.

Baby Doe and Baby K

In 1973 Raymond Duff and A. G. M. Campbell published an article in the *New England Journal of Medicine* discussing the ethical issues involved in deciding to forgo life-sustaining therapy in defective newborns.[13] This was the first time that such decisions were made public. Subsequently two high-profile cases involving Down syndrome infants with duodenal atresia resulted in government intrusion into what had traditionally been a decision between parents and their babies' physicians.[14] The first case involved a baby born with trisomy 21 and duodenal atresia at Johns Hopkins University. The parents and physician decided to forgo surgery to correct the duodenal atresia, and the baby was left unfed until it died fifteen days later. A similar case, referred to as the Baby Jane Doe case, involved a baby with multiple congenital anomalies on Long Island, New York. The parents were well-educated professionals, and decided in concert with their pediatrician not to surgically correct any of the anomalies and to allow the baby to die.[15] At that time, C. Everett Koop, a pediatric surgeon, was surgeon general of the United States. When he heard of these cases, which were easily correctable from a surgical standpoint and with a good prognosis, he convinced Congress to enact the Baby Doe regulations. These regulations defined any withholding of life-sustaining measures from newborn infants as a violation of child abuse and neglect statutes, and required state child protection teams to intervene. Unfortunately, the regulations were so broad that neonatologists were required to continue to maintain and resuscitate hopelessly ill, severely deformed, and comatose or dying newborns. The American Academy of Pediatrics challenged these regulations in court, and the regulations were eventually overturned, but not before a large number of neonates were subjected to repeated surgeries and resuscitations for hopeless and futile conditions.[16]

Baby K (see also Chapters 5 and 15) was an anencephalic infant born at Fairfax Hospital in Virginia. Her mother insisted that everything be done, including cardiopulmonary resuscitation (CPR) and mechanical ventilation, arguing that only God could take a life. At first, the hospital complied with the mother's wishes. After a few months, the baby was transferred to a chronic care facility. Hospital physicians and nurses began to question the appropriateness of repeatedly admitting and ventilating the baby whenever respiratory problems or apnea developed. The hospital sought judicial validation of its claim that continually resuscitating and ventilating this anencephalic infant was futile, based on the prognosis. The mother countered that she believed that physicians have an obligation to do whatever is possible to maintain biologic life. The mother's lawyer cited the Emergency Medical Treatment and Active Labor Act (EMTALA) to support their case. The case was heard at the federal level and appealed to the Federal Appeals Court. The judges ruled in favor of the mother, citing EMTALA and the Consolidated Omnibus Budget Reconciliation Act (COBRA) regulations. However, the judge stated in his written opinion that he did not believe that this was what Congress had in mind when it wrote EMTALA. He stated that his job was only to interpret the law, and that it was up to Congress to right the wrongs they had created in the way they wrote the law.[17]

At one time anencephalic infants were considered a source of transplantable organs, especially hearts, for infants in need of new organs. Loma Linda University in California had a number of anencephalic infants, which had been flown in from all over the world, being maintained on ventilators in the NICU, so that Dr. Leonard Bailey could transplant their hearts into babies with hypoplastic left heart syndrome.[18] (This is the same Leonard Bailey who transplanted a chimpanzee heart into Baby Fae.[19])

Anencephalic babies lack cerebral hemispheres, but may have varying degrees of brainstem present (Fig. 12-1). Most anencephalic infants die in utero, and with modern diagnostic techniques of uterine ultrasounds and alpha-fetoprotein levels from amniocentesis, the vast majority are diagnosed in the early stages of pregnancy. Most parents elect to terminate such pregnancies when informed of the lethal anomaly. Only the rare mother would agree to carry an anencephalic infant to term. Because of the lack of a skull, the anencephalic infant cannot be born by vaginal delivery, but must be delivered by cesarean section.

The problem with obtaining organs for transplantation from anencephalic infants is the requirement that the donor be dead, either from cardiopulmonary criteria or brain death (see also Chapter 13). Brain death requires the absence of all brain function, including the brainstem. As stated previously, anencephalic infants that are born alive have functioning brainstems and breathe, nurse, and cry. In fact, they behave like normal newborns, who also only breathe, nurse, cry, and sleep. Born-alive anencephalic neonates have only a limited life span of days to weeks before the exposed brainstem ceases to function, but as was learned from the Loma Linda experience, the brainstem loses function gradually,

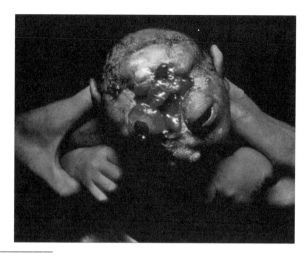

Figure 12-1 An anencephalic infant, born alive, with a lack of top of skull and absence of brain hemispheres.

with periods of apnea, cyanosis, and poor perfusion before the heart and lungs stop functioning. During this period of stepwise loss of function, the organs are irreversibly damaged and rendered unfit for use in transplantation. Loma Linda attempted to avert this progressive damage to the organs by intubating and ventilating some of the anencephalic infants, but if their breathing and circulation were supported artificially, they never progressed to brain death or cardiopulmonary death.

A different attempt to solve this dilemma, supported by the American Medical Association's Council on Ethical and Judicial Affairs,[20] was to declare anencephalic infants "brain absent," a new category that would permit organs to be harvested from these infants without the necessity for them to be declared brain dead or dead by cardiopulmonary criteria. This suggestion met with a great deal of resistance from the public and the ethics community, and was subsequently abandoned when it became clear that no members of Congress would introduce such legislation. Another problem with using anencephalic infants for organ donation was that the anomaly of anencephaly is often associated with anomalies in other organs, such that the deformed organs could not be used for transplantation. In the end, Loma Linda and other transplant programs abandoned the use of anencephalic infants as organ donors.

Extremely Preterm Birth and the Parental Right to Refuse Therapy

The case of *Miller vs. HCA* involved a severely premature infant born in 1990, but the Supreme Court of Texas did not decide the case until the fall of 2003.[21] The infant, Sidney

Miller, was born at twenty-three weeks' gestation and weighed 615 grams. Her mother had gone into premature labor, and although attempts were made to stop her labor, her obstetrician and a neonatologist told her and her husband that the fetus had little chance of being born alive, and that if it did survive it would probably suffer severe impairments, including brain hemorrhage, blindness, lung disease, and mental retardation. The doctors asked the parents to decide whether or not the baby should be treated at birth, and the parents requested that no heroic measures be employed. Hospital administrators informed the father that the hospital had a policy that any baby born alive and weighing more than 500 grams had to be resuscitated and asked him to sign a consent form allowing resuscitation, but he refused. The mother developed an infection that necessitated delivering the baby, and when born the baby had a heartbeat, cried spontaneously, and gasped for air. Another neonatologist, who was not present at the original meeting, attended the delivery and determined that the baby had to be resuscitated, including being intubated and ventilated. A few days later, the baby suffered a grade IV intraventricular hemorrhage, and when the case went to trial seven years later, Sidney was blind and severely mentally retarded, with cerebral palsy, seizures, and spastic quadriparesis.

The parents sued the hospital and its parent company (HCA), but not the doctors because they felt that the doctors were just doing what they were told to do by the hospital administrators. The jury concluded that the resuscitation had been performed without consent and was the proximate cause of the child's injuries, and awarded the family sixty million dollars. The Texas Court of Appeals reversed the jury verdict and ordered that the Miller family get nothing. The Texas Supreme Court ultimately ruled that a physician, confronted with an emergency situation, may provide lifesaving treatment to a child without first obtaining consent from the parents. The court concluded that physicians in emergencies are permitted to err on the side of the preservation of life. The court held that the best practice was to obtain parental consent before birth to make an evaluation and render warranted medical treatment, but declined to impose liability on a physician solely for providing life-sustaining treatment under emergent circumstances to a newborn infant without that consent. The Supreme Court of Texas made clear that, after the initial emergency assessment and treatment, subsequent treatment decisions in the NICU require parental consent, and that if such consent is not forthcoming, a court order must be obtained before treatment proceeds.

Based on an outcome calculator available from the National Institute of Child Health and Human Development (NICHD),[22] Sidney Miller had only a nine percent chance of surviving without moderate to severe neurodevelopmental impairment, and an eighty-six to ninety-one percent chance of death or moderate to severe impairment. According to this calculator, babies born at twenty-two weeks or less and weighing less than 500 grams have only a one percent chance or less of survival without profound neurodevelopmental impairment. Today, babies at twenty-three weeks gestation can be saved, whereas a decade ago the threshold was twenty-five weeks.

Children and Adolescents

For many years, dwarfism was treated with growth hormone procured from cadavers. However, cases of Creutzfeldt-Jakob disease began to be reported in children being treated with cadaver-derived human growth hormone (hGH). Poised to take advantage of this unfortunate situation was a pharmaceutical/genetic engineering company that could manufacture hGH by recombinant DNA technology. Not satisfied with the thousands of dollars per month per patient with growth hormone–deficient dwarfism, the company sponsored studies of short stature in children, which showed that recombinant hGH could provide one to two inches of increased height in children whose parents were short. Suddenly short stature, which had been considered a normal variant, was now considered a disease that could be treated with monthly injections of hGH at a cost of thousands of dollars per child.[23] (See Chapter 5's discussion of the goals of medicine.)

An area where the law and ethics vary considerably is pediatric consent and assent to therapeutic procedures and research. The law requires the attainment of the legal age of majority, typically eighteen years, before an individual can consent to medical procedures or participation in research. If the patient is under eighteen years of age, consent must come from one or both parents. Ethically, it is held that children of sufficient maturity and understanding should participate in the informed consent process, should be encouraged to ask questions, and should provide their assent. Typically, children older than seven years have the ability to comprehend information sufficiently to participate in the informed consent process and medical decision making and to provide their assent to procedures, treatment, or research. Depending on their maturity, knowledge base, and experience, adolescents aged thirteen or fourteen may have comprehension sufficient to require their ethical consent to medical procedures or research.

Differences exist even within the legal system on the issue of pediatric consent. Two recent cases underscore the differences between legal jurisdictions in the approach to the issue of consent in pediatrics. In Florida, a fifteen-year-old boy who had undergone two liver transplants at the University of Pittsburgh was in the process of rejecting his second transplant. He decided that he could no longer tolerate the side effects of his anti-rejection medications and was adamant that he did not want to undergo another liver transplant. With the support of his parents, he stopped taking his immunosuppressant medications. When the transplant team at the University of Pittsburgh became aware of what he was doing, they had the Florida child protective team take the boy into custody, hospitalize him against his will, and force him to take his medications. The case came before a judge, who ruled in favor of the boy and his decision-making rights, stating that this young man probably understood better than even his transplant physicians the adverse effects of the medicines he had to take and the consequences of his decision.[24] At about the same time, a young man in New York, only days short of his eighteenth birthday, decided to stop taking his chemotherapy drugs for cancer because he found the side effects intolerable. A judge in New York ruled in favor of the physicians, and the young man was forced to be hospitalized and receive chemotherapy drugs against his will.

What if the parents or child dissent or refuse to consent to obviously beneficial medical procedures or treatment? Children or adolescents may refuse a procedure or therapy for reasons that adults might consider inconsequential, immature, lacking in perspective, or short-sighted. Such reasons might include fear of needles, fear of pain, loss of bodily integrity, or an unwillingness to be perceived as different from their peers. Rather than seeking a court order, health care providers and parents should work with the pediatric patient to gain the patient's confidence and cooperation. When parents refuse clearly beneficial or lifesaving therapies for their child, health care providers should attempt to reason with and convince the parents of the importance of the therapy. If reason fails, the health care team should seek legal guidance and a court order.[25]

Research Involving Children

Research involving children is becoming increasingly common. At one time, children were specifically excluded from research studies, with most new drug development and testing excluding pregnant women and children. This approach has been reversed in recent years. Children are now being routinely entered into research studies, especially in oncology. In fact, the Children's Oncology Group (the largest consortium of pediatric oncologists in the United States) will not make experimental agents available to a patient unless the family agrees to the patient's participation in a research study, with the chance that the patient may not even receive the experimental agent as a result of randomization. Pharmaceutical companies are being enticed by the Food and Drug Administration (FDA) with the promise of a patent extension if they perform pediatric trials, even if the trials fail to demonstrate an effect in children. On the one hand, pediatric research studies may be a good thing. It is estimated that seventy-five percent of all drugs used in children have never been evaluated scientifically in children. On the other hand, there remain serious concerns about the ethics of research in children, especially research involving healthy children and the potential of greater than minimal risk to the child.[26]

In the past, children were excluded from research studies because they were recognized as a vulnerable population that needed protection, and because they were unable to consent directly to participation in research studies. The fear that children might be exploited was not totally unfounded. Some of the most egregious examples of unethical research studies were conducted on children, such as the infamous Willowbrook School hepatitis studies[27] and the Kennedy-Kreiger lead abatement studies.[28]

The Willowbrook School was a residential institution for retarded children in New York State. Hepatitis was endemic at Willowbrook, as it was in many other state institutions, and children admitted to the school inevitably developed clinical hepatitis within a year. Dr. Saul Krugman, the medical director of the facility, desired to understand the epidemiology and pathophysiology of this infectious disease, including its transmission, latency, contagiousness, and clinical course. Krugman devised a series of studies that included feeding filtered stool samples from infected residents to new inmates, following the course of the disease, and testing the ability of gamma globulin to ameliorate the disease. Although Krugman claims to have obtained consent for the research studies from parents, in fact the parents were coerced. The Willowbrook School, like most other state institutions, was seriously overcrowded. The school had only rare openings for admission, and only children whose parents agreed to allow their participation in the research studies were admitted to the institution. Although much knowledge of infectious hepatitis was gained from these studies, some children died of viral hepatitis. Ironically, Krugman was honored by the American Academy of Pediatrics for his pioneering research into viral hepatitis, with no mention of the ethics of the research. If a study is unethical, it is not justifiable simply because it produces useful results. The ends do not justify the means.

The Kennedy-Krieger lead abatement studies are an example of a recent unethical research study involving the exposure of healthy children to greater than minimal risk. The study, conducted out of Johns Hopkins University's Kennedy-Kreiger Institute, compared various methods of removing lead paint, including grinding with the generation of lead dust, from inner city housing projects in downtown Baltimore. Families with young children were then given preferential, reduced-cost access to these apartments, and lead levels were followed in the children. The intent was to determine whether certain methods of lead paint removal were better than others in terms of reduced exposure of children to toxic lead levels. The study had been approved by the institutional review board (IRB) at Johns Hopkins, but subsequently some families sued when they discovered that their children had potentially harmful levels of lead from exposure resulting from the lead abatement studies. A judge ruled that even though parental informed consent had been obtained, the studies were unethical, and that parents did not have the right to expose otherwise healthy children to research that posed greater than minimal risk to their children. The judge also opined that the study should never have been approved by the IRB, because it was unethical and dangerous.

Cancer patients are one of the most heavily represented groups in clinical research studies, and are especially vulnerable as research subjects. Many cancer patients are willing to participate in research studies because they want to try all of their options, and many are trying to hold on in the hope that a cure will be found. A few patients participate for altruistic reasons of helping others and furthering scientific knowledge. Some patients participate to reduce the cost of their medical care, and still others become research subjects for the social interaction or because they fear abandonment.

Harth and colleagues examined the psychological profile of parents who volunteered their children for clinical research studies and compared their results with the profile of parents who had refused to allow their children to be research subjects.[29] Volunteering parents tended to place more value on beneficence, whereas nonvolunteering parents were more concerned with power and prestige. The self-esteem of volunteering parents was much lower than that of nonvolunteering parents. Volunteering parents were more introverted and exhibited greater anxiety and low superego; nonvolunteering parents appeared to have greater social confidence and emotional stability.

Another area of recent concern in research ethics has been the use of placebo controls. The Declaration of Helsinki states, "In any medical study, every patient—including those of a control group—should be assured of the best proven diagnosis and therapeutics method." Unfortunately, the FDA considers placebo-controlled studies to be the gold standard of research studies to evaluate new drugs or therapies. The FDA requires placebo-controlled studies as part of the process of approval for an investigational new drug. As long as the control group receives standard therapy for their disease plus a placebo, this is not a problem. But if the control group is deprived of standard therapy and receives only placebo therapy, then the research study violates the Declaration of Helsinki. This distinction is especially important in research studies involving critically ill children or involving diseases for which placebo therapy would cause unacceptable progression of disease or harm to patients.

The important caveat in research ethics is that if a conflict between a research protocol and a patient's care develops, the ethical obligation is to protect the patient.

Secondhand Smoke

Secondhand smoke is a cause of a large number of potentially preventable illnesses in children. Now that the Back-to-Sleep campaign has significantly affected the incidence of sudden infant death syndrome (SIDS), smoking (maternal smoking during pregnancy and after birth and paternal smoking or secondhand smoke from other people residing in the same home) has become the number one associated factor in cases of SIDS.[30] Exposure to secondhand smoke is a major factor in the development and severity of asthma, the incidence of ear infections and respiratory infections, allergies, viral colds, impaired immunity to infection, growth retardation, and even some cancers, such as leukemia, in children.

Pediatric Organ Donation and Organ Transplantation

Quite apart from the issue of organ procurement from anencephalic infants addressed earlier in this chapter is the question of whether children can or should be organ or tissue donors for siblings or parents. The term *organ donation* was deliberately avoided in the discussion of anencephalic infants because the anencephalic infant cannot assent or consent to any donation. The parents are the ones who would be making the "donation"; in any event, it would be unethical to "donate" a vital organ, because the donation would cause the death of the anencephalic infant, unless such infants were brain dead, or "brain absent," as discussed earlier.

At times children end up being the only acceptable match for organ or tissue donation, and the issue arises of whether such a donation should ever come from a child. Two factors come into play in making a decision about the ethical propriety of organ or tissue donation by a child: (1) the particular organ or tissue involved and the risks of the donation, and (2) the child's comprehension of the donation and the ties to the family member in terms of benefits to the donor.[31] In essence, we are balancing benefits and risks. For example, donation of bone marrow is a relatively minimal risk procedure to the donor, whereas donation of a kidney is moderate risk, and donation of a partial liver is high risk. The child's comprehension of the risks and benefits, and his or her assent in the absence of coercion, are important factors, as discussed earlier regarding assenting for medical procedures or research. The benefits to the child may be more theoretical, but if a child's sibling or parent is at risk of dying without a transplant, then one can generally assume that donating an organ or tissue can benefit the donor. Such decision making and balancing of risk versus benefit has been employed in some court cases allowing kidney donation between twins, to siblings, or even to a parent.

In the field of pediatric transplantation, a severe disparity exists between supply and demand. There are far fewer acceptable organ donors for children both because of the limited number of brain dead donors (which is why anencephalic infants were once considered as sources of pediatric organs for transplantation) or living-related donors and because of the need to size-match the transplanted organ.

Another major problem in organ transplantation in children is the adolescent rebellion stage of development. A not uncommon problem is for pediatric patients who received transplants as infants or children to suddenly decide to stop taking their antirejection medicines when they become an adolescent (see the discussion earlier in this chapter about adolescent consent or refusal of treatment). Adolescents go through a normal stage of development in which they do not want to appear to be or feel that they are different from their peers, and having an organ transplant and taking daily medications to prevent rejection makes them very different. The ramifications of stopping their immunosuppressive medications can range from sudden illness to organ rejection and to death.

Practicing Procedures in Children

An ethical issue that faces health care providers-in-training, including medical students, physician assistant students, and nursing students, is learning invasive procedures on children. To become competent to care for children, a student must learn procedures such as blood drawing, intravenous catheter placement, Foley catheter placement, lumbar puncture, and so on, and at some time must perform his or her first procedure on a child.[32] Parents are obviously protective of their children, and would prefer that the most experienced or most talented individual perform the procedure. But if all procedures were left to the most skilled, the less skilled would never improve and the novices would never learn. Many students wrestle with the ethical dilemma of learning procedures on their pediatric patients versus not doing so and (seemingly) avoiding harming their patients; however, forgoing procedures on child patients in the present will also harm patients—future patients.

The ethical approach to this dilemma is to learn about the procedure in textbooks, practice the procedure on manikins and/or adults (unfortunately, good models or manikins do not exist for practicing many pediatric procedures), and then finally performing the procedure on a child. This will help to minimize risks while maximizing the chance of success. It is also appropriate to explain to the patient or the family, or both, that this is the student's first attempt on a real person, or that the student is just learning, and to seek the assent of the child and the permission of the parents. Procedures should be limited or restricted to a need-to-know basis. Thus, most nurses will not need to learn how to perform a lumbar puncture, but respiratory therapists may need to be proficient in arterial sticks. The other relevant issue is the number of attempts allowed to the student to perform a procedure. Even a very skilled individual may have a bad day. Most pediatric programs limit an individual's attempts to three, after which someone else is brought in to perform the procedure.

Refusal of Treatment

It is an accepted tenet of medical ethics, supported by numerous court decisions over the past century, that a mature adult of sound mind can refuse any medical therapy, even if the therapy is potentially lifesaving. On the other hand, courts have consistently ruled, and medical ethics dictates, that parents cannot deprive their children of medical treatment or lifesaving therapy, no matter what their beliefs. Adults can refuse medical therapy or lifesaving therapy based on religious beliefs, idiosyncratic beliefs, or no beliefs at all, but they are not free to impose their beliefs on their children. The theory is that children should be allowed to grow and develop and then make their own decisions about what they believe.

Classic examples of religion-based refusal of treatment have included Jehovah's Witnesses' refusal of blood and blood products, and Christian Scientists' refusal of medical and surgical treatment. The American Academy of Pediatrics has been campaigning in the last few years to reverse state laws that exempt parents who refuse treatment on religious grounds from prosecution under child abuse and neglect laws.[33] This opposition to religious exemptions has been fueled by well-publicized cases of children with easily treatable conditions such as appendicitis or meningitis who have died because their parents refused medical care and instead relied on religious healers.

On occasion, a child or adolescent strongly professes religious beliefs or opinions that may or may not coincide with his or her parents' beliefs and may affect the child's willingness to accept recommended medical therapy. Intelligence, experience, and the relationship between the child and parents can all influence the maturity and decision-making capability of the child. The limited empirical information that exists regarding the development of the mature medical decision-making ability of children generally suggests that the decision-making ability of minors by the age of fourteen years cannot be distinguished from that of adults. Of course, we all know even adults who do not have mature decision-making capability.

Although courts routinely grant court orders to treat infants or children when parents refuse treatment on religious or other grounds, courts should assess (and are assessing) the maturity and decision-making capacity of adolescents before ruling on treatment. Obviously, if the adolescent is critically ill, his or her participation may not be possible. Another factor to be considered in deciding on a petition for court-ordered medical treatment is the prognosis. In a Delaware case involving a child with non-Hodgkin lymphoma, a cancer with an exceptionally poor prognosis, the court sided with the Christian Scientist parents who refused treatment.[34] This decision was based on the difficult course of treatment being recommended, the less than forty percent probability of one-year survival, and the considerably smaller likelihood of long-term survival. Similarly, a recent law passed in Virginia, as a result of the case of a fifteen-year-old boy named Starchild Abraham Cheerix, states that parents of a child at least fourteen years old with a life-threatening condition can refuse medically recommended treatment provided (1) the parents and child made the decision jointly, (2) the child is sufficiently mature to have an informed opinion on the treatment, (3) other treatments have been considered, and (4) they believe in good faith that their choice is in the child's best interest.[25]

Most pediatricians and ethicists now agree that children who can experience and enjoy life, including the vast majority of patients with Down syndrome (see the earlier discussion on the Baby Doe cases in this chapter), have legitimate, independent moral and legal claims to lifesaving therapy, including intensive care and surgery, even if the parents prefer the child to die. Inherent in this moral consensus is the notion that the quality of life of these patients is sufficiently high to justify complex, difficult, or expensive treatments, despite the views of the parents, who would be the ordinary decision makers. Most of the time, communication with and counseling of parents lead to parental understanding and acceptance of the proposed treatment. When these measures fail, foster-care arrangements may be necessary.

More problematic are the situations in which health care providers are uncertain about survival, neurologic outcome, or other major medical prognoses, and in which the proposed treatment may have a profound impact on the family. Such situations might require the parents to give up employment to care for the child (e.g., in cases where continued dependence on technology will demand twenty-four-hour vigilance) or might require parental attention that significantly detracts from the time and care available for other siblings or dependents. Fortunately, with the growth of home care, respite and assistance for parents is often available; however, we should not lose sight of the tremendous demand and drain that a medically needy and technology-dependent child can place on a family.

Forgoing Life-Sustaining Therapy

Although foregoing life support is a major source of angst for any critical care physician, this anguish is magnified manyfold when the patient is a child. Several points are important for a discussion of foregoing life support in pediatric patients. The first concern is that many physicians, including pediatric intensivists and pediatric neurologists, are reluctant to make predictions about outcomes, especially in children with neurologic trauma or anoxic-ischemic injuries. Part of this reluctance may stem from the remarkable recoveries that have occurred in children after traumatic injuries or anoxic injuries associated with hypothermia. Nevertheless, despite the occasional amazing recovery, the likelihood of good neurologic outcome following global hypoxic-ischemic brain injury in children remains low, especially if no recovery has occurred following a suitable period of observation.[35] It is important for clinicians to address the likelihood of a poor outcome and to allow families to prepare for the worst, because the result is often a neurologically devastated child in a permanent vegetative state (PVS). For most of us, PVS is a fate worse than death.

Clinicians often use the lack of statistical or clinical certainty as an excuse to avoid discussing probable poor outcomes. Clinical uncertainty should not be used as a means of forestalling disclosure of reasonably available alternative courses, including withholding further treatment or withdrawing therapies already in use. We are told that ethically and legally there is no difference between withholding a therapy and withdrawing that therapy. Any therapy that can be withheld can be withdrawn, and vice versa. But in reality, there are tremendous psychological and social differences between withholding a therapy and withdrawing it. For many physicians, nurses, and even the public, it is easier to never start a therapy than to withdraw it, for once a therapy has been commenced it is often felt that there is an obligation of sorts to continue it. But in fact the opposite should be true. Because of the uniqueness of each individual and the difficulty in predicting a response to therapy, it is generally preferable to try a therapy and to withdraw it if it does not attain its desired goal, rather than to never try it at all.[36] Clinical uncertainty also should not preclude decisions to forego life support. Except in unusual circumstances, the patient's or family's values should largely dictate the direction of medical care. Health care professionals should not impose their personal beliefs concerning life with mental or physical handicaps on others.

Another point about foregoing life support concerns family guilt. Many health care professionals feel that parents are unable to handle the emotional distress and guilt attendant with making the decision to allow a child to die. However, one study reported that families who had endured such a painful experience later expressed appreciation for their involvement in the decision. These families had no demonstrable adverse psychological sequelae compared with families who did not participate in the decision to limit respiratory support for their child.[37] Families not wishing to bear this responsibility usually find ways of making their views known, and families with strong feelings or beliefs favoring continued treatment usually make their desires clear.

Futility

A number of authors have suggested that *futility* is too vague and undefinable a concept to be of value in medicine, or that futility is a medical attempt to counteract patient autonomy. These authors claim that the concept of futility should be abandoned and not employed as a reason for withholding medical therapy. However, anyone who has practiced clinical medicine realizes that clear-cut examples of futility are encountered routinely in intensive care units and clinical practice (see Chapters 5 and 14 for a fuller discussion of medical futility).

A treatment is futile, for example, when it will offer no physiologic benefit to the patient. An example of such physiologic futility in pediatrics is the use of CPR in patients who are brain dead.[38] CPR is also futile in the instance of an ongoing chemical code—the situation in which a patient is on the maximal concentrations of vasopressors (pharmacologic agents to increase or maintain blood pressure) and/or inotropes (pharmacologic agents to increase or maintain heart muscle contractions) and yet remains hypotensive and unresponsive to therapy.[38] CPR and the use of advanced life-support drugs will not work if the patient is already receiving suprapharmacologic doses of these drugs. This situation is also referred to as refractory shock.

Another example of clinical futility would be a patient with refractory hypoxemia and respiratory failure. If the patient cannot be oxygenated and ventilated and he or she progresses to cardiac arrest, CPR is simply not going to work. CPR is also futile in patients in a persistent or permanent vegetative state. A treatment is futile when it cannot, within reasonable medical probability, cure, ameliorate, improve, or restore a quality of life that would be satisfactory to or for the patient.

Other examples of situations in which the use of CPR is futile include the failure to respond to CPR and pediatric advanced life support in thirty minutes; decapitation; and putrefaction (criteria commonly employed by emergency medical services). Many emergency medical services also use being charred or burned beyond recognition as a futility criterion for not employing CPR.

A number of other examples of futility in pediatrics exist. Most intensive care clinicians consider the use of mechanical ventilation and CPR to be inappropriate and futile in anencephalic infants (see the earlier discussion on anencephalic neonates in this chapter). Likewise, for patients in a persistent vegetative state, mechanical ventilation, admission to the intensive care unit, and CPR are all considered inappropriate and futile. Other examples of futile therapy in pediatrics include the use of antibiotics for viral illnesses and the use of antipyretics for febrile seizures.[38]

One of the reasons that the concept of medical futility has fostered so much debate is that *futility* means different things to different people. To some, continued existence, no matter how poor the quality of that existence, means that the therapy is not futile. To others, therapy is futile if a sentient, functional existence cannot be achieved. To some, any therapy is worth a try; to others, a therapy must offer a reasonable chance of success. Because the principle of autonomy has gained such preeminence in Western ethics, many ethicists believe that any patient request that stands even a remote chance of working must be honored; however, autonomy is not a trump card and does not overrule all other principles and factors.

Conflicts over the issue of medical futility often signal a breakdown in communication. In cases in which the family makes inappropriate demands and the health care team insists that continued treatment is futile, the two sides are often not communicating effectively. Two factors will usually resolve such conflicts. First, it is necessary to reestablish good communication, using clear and understandable language to help the family fully appreciate the situation. At times, the use of a neutral third party or family advocate can facilitate the reestablishment of effective communication. A great deal of empathy is necessary to understand the family's reluctance to see their hopes and dreams for their child destroyed. Likewise, it must be understood that the heroic efforts of the health care team have been unsuccessful, engendering a feeling of failure and remorse. The second factor is time. Families may need hours or even days to come to grips with the reality of the situation, and patience and understanding on the part of the health care team can do a lot to resolve conflict.

Another factor that fuels the futility debate is the fact that medicine is not an exact science. What has worked or not worked in previous patients may have a completely different effect on the patient at hand. As the public becomes more medically sophisticated and knowledgeable, families may appreciate these subtleties. Medical predictions of outcome may be based more on assumptions or hunches than facts. A solid statistical basis for prediction is usually lacking because the appropriate studies have never been performed (the NICHD prediction model for premature infants mentioned earlier in this chapter is an exception). An individual health care professional is unlikely to have seen a large enough number of similar patients to form a statistically relevant basis for predictions. Further, each patient is sufficiently unique as an individual that even large databases cannot be used to predict the outcome in individual cases accurately (again, the NICHD prediction model for premature infants mentioned earlier in the chapter is an exception). Even an experienced health care professional backed by statistically relevant studies cannot predict individual outcome with a high degree of accuracy. A health care professional can state that a therapy is highly unlikely to work, but he or she can never state conclusively that it will not work.

Health care professionals can and should refuse to provide a therapy that violates professional, ethical, or moral tenets. A unilateral decision to stop medical treatment based on futility arguments may require ethics committee, and perhaps judicial, backing. The best approach is to work with the family and gain their concurrence.

Case 12-A may help elucidate some of the issues surrounding medical futility.

Case 12-A

Theresa Hamilton was a fourteen-year-old diabetic patient who presented to a hospital in Sarasota, Florida, in severe diabetic coma, and her condition rapidly progressed to brain death. The parents, partly out of guilt over having waited too long to seek medical attention, refused to

(continues)

Case 12-A (*continued*)

accept the diagnosis of brain death. Numerous consultants and experts were brought in, all of whom confirmed the diagnosis of brain death and recommended discontinuing ventilatory support. The parents continued to refuse. The case was brought to the institutional ethics committee, which also recommended disconnecting the ventilator. The parents sought support from the news media, and a number of well-meaning but misinformed people came forward with stories that they or a loved one had been pronounced brain dead by the medical profession and were now living a normal life. Meanwhile, the hospital sought legal guidance from the state attorney general's office, who offered the opinion that there was really no issue and that because the patient was brain dead, artificial support could be withdrawn. At the same time, the hospital's own legal counsel waffled and recommended that the hospital do whatever the family demanded. The hospital acquiesced and arranged for the patient to be sent home on mechanical ventilation. This corpse was ventilated at home for five months before cardiac arrest ensued.[39]

Increasingly, our society has come to believe that the maintenance of insentient, non-interactive biologic life with artificial, mechanical means represents a technologic intrusion and indignity, and that such individuals should be permitted to die without such an assault and insult. There is also increasing societal sentiment that the scarce resources consumed in the maintenance of these lives could be better used for other purposes.

Chapter Summary

The ethical conundrum presented by abortion implicates issues of fetal personhood, fetal viability, and fetal sentience. Erroneous assumptions that pediatric patients do not feel pain are not limited to fetuses, however; they underlie, as well, discredited practices such as the Liverpool technique and the performance of circumcision on unanesthetized infants. The Baby Doe regulations and EMTALA are illustrations of the law of unintended consequences. The management of anencephalic infants raises questions of medical futility, and their potential as organ donors forces us to revisit current definitions of death. The availability of recombinant hGH and its use in children with short stature implicates the goals of medicine. Although under the law an individual must attain the age of majority (typically eighteen years) before he or she can consent to medical procedures or to participation in research, ethicists typically hold that children over the age of seven years may provide their assent to procedures or research, and that at about fourteen years of age, adolescents may have sufficient comprehension to require their ethical consent to medical procedures or research. Research in children and their involvement as organ and tissue donors require us to consider their decisional capacity and to weigh benefits and burdens. Ethical concerns regarding the practicing of medical procedures on and the foregoing of life-sustaining treatment in children, and medical futility as it pertains to pediatrics, were discussed as well.

Review Questions

1. What is the difference between an ethical dilemma and an ethical conundrum?
2. When can fetuses first sense pain?
3. Should babies be anesthetized for circumcision?
4. Should Baby K have been repeatedly resuscitated?
5. Should anencephalic infants be declared brain absent?
6. Can healthy children be subjected to research that involves greater than minimal risk?

Endnotes

1. Eswaran H, Haddad NI, Shihabuddin BS, et al. Non-invasive detection and identification of brain activity patterns in the developing fetus. *Clin Neurophysiol* 2007;118:1940–1946.
2. Hernandez JA, Hall DM, Goldson EJ, et al. Impact of infants born at the threshold of viability on the neonatal mortality rate in Colorado. *J Perinatol* 2000;20:21–26.
3. Chervenak FA, McCullough LB, Levene MI. An ethically justified, clinically comprehensive approach to peri-viability: gynaecological, obstetric, perinatal and neonatal dimensions. *J Obset Gynecol* 2007;27:3–7.
4. Anand KJS, Hickey PR. Pain and its effects in the human neonate and fetus. *New Engl J Med* 1987;317:1321–1329.
5. Lowery CL, Hardman MP, Manning N, et al. Neurodevelopmental changes of fetal pain. *Semin Perinatol* 2007;31:275–282.
6. Derbyshire SWG. Can fetuses feel pain? *BMJ* 2006;332:909–912.
7. Blass EM, Hoffmeyer LB. Sucrose as an analgesic for newborn infants. *Pediatrics* 1991;87:215–218.
8. Davidson AJ, Huang GH, Czarnecki C, et al. Awareness during anesthesia in children: a prospective cohort study. *Anesth Analg* 2005;100:653–661.
9. Anand KJS, Hickey PR. Halothane-morphine compared with high-dose sufentanil for anesthesia and postoperative analgesia in neonatal cardiac surgery. *New Engl J Med* 1992;326:1–9.
10. Brady-Fryer B, Wiebe N, Lander JA. Pain relief for neonatal circumcision. *Cochrane Database Syst Rev* 2004;(4):CD004217.
11. Freed CR, Greene PE, Breeze RE, et al. Transplantation of embryonic dopamine neurons for severe Parkinson's disease. *New Engl J Med* 2001;344:710–719.
12. Beecher HK. Ethics and clinical research. *New Engl J Med* 1966;274:1354–1360.
13. Duff RS, Campbell AGM. Moral and ethical dilemmas in the special-care nursery. *New Engl J Med* 1973;289:890–894.
14. Gustafson JM. Mongolism, parental desires, and the right to life. *Perspect Biol Med* 1973;292:529–557.

15. Klaidman S, Beauchamp TL. Baby Jane Doe in the media. *J Health Politics Policy Law* 1986; 11:271–284.

16. Annas GJ. The Baby Doe regulations: governmental intervention in neonatal rescue medicine. *Am J Public Health* 1984;74:618–620.

17. Annas GJ. Asking the courts to set the standard of emergency care—the case of Baby K. *New Engl J Med* 1994;330:1542–1545.

18. Bailey LL. Donor organs from human anencephalics: a salutary resource for infant heart transplantation. *Transplant Proc* 1988;20(4 suppl 5):35–41.

19. Bailey LL. Another look at cardiac xenotransplantation. *J Cardiac Surg* 1990;5:210–218.

20. Council on Ethical and Judicial Affairs, American Medical Association. The use of anencephalic neonates as organ donors. *JAMA* 1995;273:1614–1618.

21. Annas GJ. Extremely preterm birth and parental authority to refuse treatment—the case of Sidney Miller. *New Engl J Med* 2004;351:2118–2123.

22. National Institute of Child Health and Human Development Neonatal Research Network. Extremely preterm birth outcome data. Available at: http://www.nichd.nih.gov/about/org/cdbpm/pp/prog_epbo/epbo_case.cfm. Accessed 4/18/2008.

23. Allen DB, Fost N. hGH for short stature: ethical issues raised by expanded access. *J Pediatr* 2004;144:648–652.

24. Traugott I, Alpers A. In their own hands: adolescents' refusal of medical treatment. *Arch Pediatr Adol Med* 1997;151:922–927.

25. Mercurio MR. An adolescent's refusal of medical treatment: implications of the Abraham Cheerix case. *Pediatrics* 2007;120:1357–1358.

26. Committee on Drugs, American Academy of Pediatrics. Guidelines for the ethical conduct of studies to evaluate drugs in pediatric populations. *Pediatrics* 1995;95:286–294.

27. Krugman S. The Willowbrook hepatitis studies revisited: ethical aspects. *Rev Infect Dis* 1986;8:157–162.

28. Wendler D. Risk standards for pediatric research: rethinking the *Grimes* ruling. *Kennedy Inst Ethics J* 2004;14:187–198.

29. Harth SC, Johnstone RR, Thong YH. The psychological profile of parents who volunteer their children for clinical research: a controlled study. *J Med Ethics* 1992;18:86–93.

30. Fleming P, Blair PS. Sudden infant death syndrome and parental smoking. *Early Hum Develop* 2007;83:721–725.

31. Committee on Hospital Care and Section on Surgery, American Academy of Pediatrics. Pediatric organ donation and transplantation: policy statement: organizational principles to guide and define the child health care system and/or improve the health of all children. *Pediatrics* 2002;109:982–984.

32. Williams CT, Fost N. Ethical considerations surrounding first time procedures: a study and analysis of patient attitudes toward spinal taps by students. *Kennedy Inst Ethics J* 1992;2:217–231.

33. Committee on Bioethics, American Academy of Pediatrics. Religious exemptions from child abuse statutes. *Pediatrics* 1988;81:169–171.

34. *Newmark v. Williams,* 588 A.2d 1108 (Del. 1991).

35. Perkins RM, Ashwal S. Hypoxic ischemic encephalopathy in infants and older children. In: Swaiman KF, Ashwal S, eds. *Pediatric Neurology: Principles and Practice.* St. Louis: Mosby, 1999:916–921.

36. President's Commission for the Study of Ethical Problems in Medicine and Biomedical and Behavioral Research. *Deciding to Forgo Life-Sustaining Treatment—A Report on the Ethical, Medical*

and Legal Issues in Treatment Decisions. Washington, DC: U.S. Government Printing Office, 1983:73–77.

37. Benfield DG, Leib SA, Vollman JH. Grief response of parents to neonatal death and parent participation in deciding care. *Pediatrics* 1978;62:171–177.

38. Orlowski JP. Ethical issues in pediatric intensive care. In: Orlowski JP, ed. *Ethics in Critical Care Medicine.* Hagerstown, MD, University Publishing Group, 1999:466–470.

39. Lack of futile care policy compromises hospital's authority. *Medical Ethics Advisor* 1994;10: 51–53.

Chapter 13

Death

They are not long, the weeping and the laughter,

Love and desire and hate;

I think they have no portion in us after

We pass the gate.

They are not long, the days of wine and roses:

Out of a misty dream

Our path emerges for a while, then closes

Within a dream.

— Ernest Dowson, "Vitae Summa Brevis Spem Nos Vetat Inco"

Chapter Learning Objectives

At the conclusion of this chapter the reader will be able to:

1. Understand the bedside diagnosis of death

2. Define *le coma dépassé*

3. List the Harvard criteria

4. Explain the reasoning underlying the contention that patients who have suffered irreversible loss of function of the whole brain are dead

5. Understand and apply the Uniform Determination of Death Act

6. Discuss how organ transplantation and the medical determination of death affect each other

7. Explain and apply the dead donor rule

8. Compare and contrast the whole-brain and higher brain (neocortical) formulations of brain death

9. List the characteristics of, and be able to recognize the patient in, permanent vegetative state (PVS)

10. Distinguish among brain death, anencephaly, and PVS

11. Explain the meaning of a non-heart-beating donation

The current chapter deals with death, the final domain of ethics across the lifespan. Although there is much that could be said on this topic, the chapter is limited to the concepts and ethical issues surrounding the diagnosis of death. In particular, it covers brain death and related concepts. Also discussed is the relationship between the diagnosis of death and the practice of harvesting vital organs for purposes of transplantation. It is hoped that by the end of the chapter the reader will have gained a solid grasp of the brain death concept and how it differs from similar concepts such as neocortical death.

Why Redefine Death?

From a medical point of view, death is fundamentally a physiologic phenomenon. It is the final sequence of psycho-physical collapse that transitions a person from the state of being alive to that of being dead. Associated with this transition are the immediate and classic bedside physical signs of unresponsiveness, fixed and dilated pupils, and absence of pulse and respiration. In the days that follow, one observes further postdeath signs such as rigor mortis,[1] algor mortis,[2] and livor mortis,[3] followed by putrefaction, and finally advanced decomposition. For the health care professionals of the early twentieth century, the presence of the classic clinical signs of death made the bedside diagnosis of death an easy and unproblematic affair. Matters became difficult only when new resuscitative technology was developed and deployed in the 1950s. This marked the first time in human history that a person could simultaneously exhibit some of the classic signs of death and some of the classic signs of life. With the advent of effective cardiopulmonary resuscitation (CPR) techniques and mechanical ventilation, a person could be resuscitated and ventilated successfully, maintaining a heartbeat while yet exhibiting complete unresponsiveness, absence of spontaneous respirations, and fixed and dilated pupils. This posed a dilemma: were such patients to be regarded as dead because they exhibited many of the classic signs of death? Or were they to be regarded as alive, because they had a beating heart? This dilemma was described in a French paper in 1959 entitled *"Le coma dépassé."*[4]

Coma dépassé was particularly problematic for medical practitioners. Because medicine has special expertise in diagnosing illness and death, and because society looks to medicine to certify that death has occurred, it was legitimate for medicine to examine and clarify the status of this unprecedented phenomenon, in which resuscitated and ventilated patients simultaneously exhibit classic signs of life and classic signs of death. Two principal issues needed to be addressed: (1) were patients in *coma dépassé* alive or were they dead? and (2) if they were dead, what conditions must exist in order to declare a person to be dead?

Are Patients with Coma Dépassé Alive or Dead?

Although this question was first raised in 1959, it would be ten years before an answer was given by U.S. medicine.[5] In 1968, a group at Harvard promulgated guidelines for the diagnosis of death in patients with *coma dépassé*. They did not, however, use the French term. Instead, they referred to such patients as being in *irreversible coma*, noting as well that the condition was already being referred to as *brain death syndrome*. The criteria for diagnosing brain death came to be widely known as the Harvard criteria.

The Harvard criteria included the following:

1. *Unreceptivity and unresponsivity:* a total unawareness of externally applied stimuli and inner need and complete unresponsiveness, despite application of intensely painful stimuli.

2. *No spontaneous movements or breathing:* absence of all spontaneous muscular movement or breathing, as well as absence of response to stimuli such as pain, touch, sound, or light.

3. *No reflexes:* fixed, dilated pupils; lack of eye movement despite turning the head or ice-water stimulus; lack of response to noxious stimuli; and generally, lack of elicitable deep tendon reflexes.

Additionally, the committee recommended that the preceding observations be confirmed by two electroencephalograms (EEGs), taken at least 24 hours apart, documenting the absence of cortical electrical activity above baseline. It was also deemed necessary to exclude the presence of any metabolic state, hypothermia, or drug intoxication that might cause or contribute to a reversible loss of brain activity or function.[6]

The Harvard criteria detail specific findings on the neurologic exam that, if present, lead to the presumptive conclusion that the patient is brain dead. Once reversible causes have been excluded and the person has been determined to have had an illness or injury consistent with lethality, the exam must be repeated after the passage of sufficient time to justify the conclusion that the condition is irreversible. After all of the conditions are met, and the second exam remains unchanged, the person is declared to be dead.

The physiologic basis for the neurologic diagnosis of death was explored in detail in a publication produced by the President's Commission for the Study of Ethical Problems in Medicine and Biomedical and Behavioral Research.[7] The reasoning underlying the conclusion that such patients are dead is complex but important to understand.

Step 1: Three core systems are involved in the final physiologic pathway of death. These are the central nervous system (specifically the brain), the circulatory system (specifically the heart), and the respiratory system. Primary critical failure of any one of these systems necessarily results in the failure of the other two. For example, if the circulatory system fails due to myocardial infarction and cardiac arrest, the brain will soon fail to function due to lack of blood flow; the impulses from the brainstem will then no longer propagate down the phrenic nerves, and therefore no further breaths will be taken. If the respiratory system fails due to bilateral pneumonia that is severe enough to prevent vital air exchange, the brain will fail due to hypoxia, and the heart will eventually stop due to a combination of hypoxia and acidemia. If the nervous system fails due to primary brain disease or injury (such as hypoxic encephalopathy), respiration will soon cease because phrenic nerve impulses will no longer be transmitted from the brain to the diaphragm; the heart will finally stop due to resulting hypoxia and acidemia.

Step 2: Of the three core systems, brain failure is the only condition where function cannot be augmented, replaced, or restored by medical intervention. When the respiratory system fails, mechanical ventilation can often be used to force oxygen into the lungs. When the circulatory system fails because of the critical failure of the heart, the heart's function can often be augmented via assistive devices, restored through resuscitation, or replaced altogether with transplantation. In some cases, both the heart and the lungs can be transplanted together. The brain, however, cannot be augmented in any way; once lost, its function cannot be restored, and it certainly cannot be replaced.

Step 3: When the brain has been damaged to the point at which brain signs of death (unresponsiveness and fixed, dilated pupils) are irreversibly manifest, the patient can legitimately be regarded as dead, because unlike lung or heart function, nothing can be done to restore or replace brain function. When lung signs of death (absent respiratory movement and breath sounds) are detected in time (e.g., when a patient has a sudden, witnessed respiratory arrest), this can often be treated using mechanical ventilation or other interventions, with the result that independent respiratory function may be restored. Similarly, when heart signs of death (absent pulse and heart sounds) are detected in time, (e.g., when a person has a sudden, witnessed cardiac arrest), this can often be treated with resuscitative measures including electrical countershock or defibrillation. The result is often a restoration of the heartbeat.

Step 4: Because complete brain failure will necessarily result in respiratory and circulatory failure, if we intervene in such a case with cardiopulmonary resuscitative techniques and support, we will at best have restored the circulation of oxygenated blood to no avail, because the patient will remain in complete brain failure no matter what we do. That patient will continue to manifest the brain signs of death. Such patients will have breathed their last breath because no nerve impulse will ever again travel down their phrenic nerves to trigger diaphragmatic contraction. Although the chest moves up and down, the patient is not breathing; air is being pumped into the chest by a mechanical ventilator. The heart has been restarted and can remain beating only because the ventilator is pumping air into the chest so that passive air exchange can take place. Such a patient will thus manifest classic signs of death (complete unresponsiveness, fixed and dilated pupils, absence of spontaneous respiration) and classic signs of life (respiratory sounds, pulse, and heart sounds). Nevertheless, such a person can rightly be regarded as dead because irreversible brain signs of death are present, and those signs of life that are present are only present because of ongoing medical intervention. If that intervention is removed—for example, if the ventilator is stopped—continuation of the classic cascade of psycho-physical collapse will immediately ensue.

Because of this understanding, it is appropriate to see cardiopulmonary resuscitative interventions in patients with irreversible complete brain failure as restoring the circulation of oxygenated blood in a corpse.

Brain Death

Because of the primacy of brain signs in the neurologic diagnosis of death in ventilated patients, the phenomenon that was initially called *coma dépassé* by French physicians is now commonly called *brain death*. Brain death is an unfortunate term, because it leads people to think that only the *brain* has died, but that in some way the *person* is still alive. In actuality, based on the multistep reasoning described previously, from a medical standpoint brain death is rightly regarded as the death of the person.

It is rightly so regarded from a legal standpoint as well. In 1980, the National Conference of Commissioners approved and recommended for enactment in all the states the so-called Uniform Determination of Death Act, which read in part as follows:

> **§ 1. [Determination of Death].** An individual who has sustained either (1) irreversible cessation of circulatory and respiratory functions, or (2) irreversible cessation of all functions of the entire brain, including the brain stem, is dead. A determination of death must be made in accordance with accepted medical standards.[8]

"The Uniform Determination of Death Act [UDDA] has been enacted by statute in a majority of states as well as the District of Columbia. Several states . . . have adopted brain death by court decision, and the remainder have enacted brain death legislation without relying on the [UDDA]."[9] All fifty states and the District of Columbia have accepted brain death as a legal standard.[10]

Problems with the UDDA's Definition of Death

The main problem with the UDDA definition is that it sets up a false dichotomy between the bedside diagnosis of death and the neurologic diagnosis of death.

The first part of the definition has often been labeled "heart-lung death," with the idea being that death is diagnosed at the bedside by heart signs of death and lung signs of death. This overlooks the fact that the brain signs of death—specifically, complete unresponsiveness and fixed and dilated pupils—have traditionally been a part of the bedside diagnosis of death. The UDDA creates the impression that these brain signs are not a part of the classic bedside diagnosis of death, when in actuality these are among the first signs of which a health care professional will take note.

The second part of the definition is labeled "brain death" because it relies not on heart and lung signs, but on brain signs. The definition fails to make clear that this diagnostic approach is only applied to patients on mechanical ventilators. As it stands, the UDDA creates the impression that there are two ways to diagnose death and that these two ways are dissociated from each other. The reality is that the core physiology is the same. In some dead patients—those in whom medical interventions have arrested the cascade of psychophysical collapse and prevented the expression of the heart and lung signs of death—other criteria (brain death criteria) must be employed to distinguish between the living and the dead.

It is also unfortunate that the UDDA definition was framed in terms of "functions" as opposed to the physical signs upon which health care professionals have traditionally relied. Function, or the lack thereof, is inferred from clinical findings or signs. A better definition might have been as follows: (1) Any person who manifests the classic signs of death associated with the brain (complete unresponsiveness, fixed and dilated pupils), the heart (absent pulse and heart sounds), and the lungs (absent respiratory movements and breath sounds) for a duration sufficient to regard the presence of such signs as permanent, is dead. (2) Any person supported by a mechanical ventilator who manifests the classic signs of death associated with the brain (complete unresponsiveness, fixed and dilated pupils) and whose neurologic exam is consistent with complete brain failure shall be considered dead when these exam findings are present for a duration sufficient to regard them as irreversible.

Critiques of the Brain Death Concept

Although medicine and law have by and large concluded that patients in *coma dépassé* are dead and have accepted the UDDA's definition of death, not everyone is in agreement. A number of critiques have been launched against the idea that *coma dépassé,* or brain death, should be regarded as the death of the person.

Some, for example, have criticized brain death because the patients simply do not look dead, even though they have some of the classic signs. That is, they exhibit signs not seen in patients traditionally diagnosed as dead at the bedside. Thus, brain dead patients sweat, their hearts beat, and in cases of pregnancy, they can give birth to babies. All of these things suggest to some that our inference about the (dead) status of these unfortunate individuals is wrong. Although the juxtaposition of signs of death with signs associated with life is certainly disorienting, it must be kept in mind that it is modern resuscitative and supportive technology that has made it possible for one to pass the point of no return in the physiologic cascade of death, interrupting and arresting a process that cannot be reversed. Although the process is arrested, other things—such as giving birth to babies—can still go on.

Others critics of brain death have focused on the presence of a beating heart as the sine qua non of life, and conversely would dismiss any concept of death—such as brain death—that would allow persons with beating hearts to be declared dead. However, it should be pointed out that focusing solely on the heart, although simple, is not unproblematic. What are we to say regarding the status of patients undergoing heart transplantation? There is a time during such surgery when the patient has no heart in his or her body. If the presence of a beating heart is an absolute requirement for being regarded as alive, how should we classify persons who, for a short time, have no heart?

Still other critics would say that although we have interrupted the process of psychophysical collapse that results in death, and have done so past the point of no return in terms of brain function, the fact that the process is not complete in the domains of respiratory and cardiac function means that the person in such a situation should not be considered dead. This criticism gets to the very crux of the brain death inference. Does the process have to be complete? Or is it enough to know that there has been complete failure of the one component that cannot be augmented or replaced, and that the other two components would necessarily fail as well but for our intervention to arrest and suspend this process with resuscitative and supportive interventions? Medicine and the law have decided that actual completion of the process, either via the withdrawal of medical interventions or despite such interventions, is not necessary—that such patients are dead because they have the classic brain signs of death and other neurologic signs that indicate complete brain failure. In other words, the presence of signs of complete and irreversible brain death is sufficient to establish the death of the patient.

Brain Death and Organ Donation

A full discussion of the ethics of organ donation and transplantation is beyond the scope of this chapter. Herein, we shall limit ourselves to discussing the connection between organ donation and the determination of death.

Some critics of brain death have voiced the suspicion that the concept of brain death was simply a ruse to increase the supply of organs available for transplantation. This impression is strengthened by the fact that it took almost ten years for American medicine to address the status of *coma dépassé* patients, and it did so at a time when transplantation of scarce vital organs had become a viable therapy.

Although it is true that the Harvard criteria emerged at a time when organ transplantation had become a medical reality, it does not follow that the potential for organ harvest was the sole reason for adopting the concept of brain death. Remember that as far back as 1959 the question of whether *coma dépassé* patients were alive or dead was a real and legitimate question that medicine had to answer. This was a question that arose long before organ transplantation was considered feasible. Nevertheless, there was no great practical need to answer the question at that time. Sufficient interest in the question only emerged when organ donation became a reality, for it was then that it was realized that if such patients were dead, they would in many cases be ideal candidates for organ harvesting.

In some ways, the situation existing in the early days of organ transplantation was analogous to the situation that existed in major cities in the eighteenth century. In those days, the reality creating the great practical need to make a determination of death as quickly as possible was the public health interest in interring the dead as soon as possible to prevent the spread of disease. Unfortunately, at the time there was no such reliable method; this led to the practice of keeping bodies in charnel houses until signs of decomposition began to appear. When the widespread use of the stethoscope allowed physicians to make a more reliable early determination of death, bodies could be interred earlier, prior to the onset of putrefaction, thus allowing a public health benefit to be realized. In a similar way, the ability to reliably diagnose death in mechanically ventilated patients manifesting irreversible cerebral signs of death allowed a different health benefit to be realized—the timely (i.e., before the onset of organ deterioration) harvesting of vital organs capable of being transplanted into other patients. In both cases, a compelling public health need provided the impetus for the medical profession to make a determination of death as early as possible.

The Dead Donor Rule

Acting as a check or balance against these impetuses to make a determination of death as early as possible was a countervailing need to avoid making an erroneous determination of death prematurely. An erroneous determination of death in the eighteenth century might have led to burial of the living, the stuff of nightmares and horror stories. In the era of organ transplantation, the importance of determining the occurrence of death before harvesting vital organs derives from the fact that removing such organs from a person who is not dead would rightly be regarded as a homicide (see Chapter 14). The reason for this is simple: the removal of a vital organ from a person not yet dead causes the death of the person. The requirement that a person be dead before vital organs are removed is known as the *dead donor rule*.[11]

This rule became an issue in cases dealing with the harvesting of organs from babies born with anencephaly,[12] because these babies are born with severe cranial defects and are destined to live for only a short period of time. Because these babies were not seen as viable, the question arose about the propriety of harvesting vital organs from them so that they could be used to help other babies who might be given a longer life. The problem is that, under current brain death criteria (requiring the death of the whole brain), anencephalic babies are not dead. They are born alive, and are therefore persons under the law. One cannot simply remove vital organs from them because, in the process, the physician removing the organs will cause the death of the baby. This became an issue in a noteworthy Florida case in 1992, the case of T.A.C.P. (Case 13-A).[13]

Case 13-A

In or about the eighth month of pregnancy, the parents of the child T.A.C.P. were told that she would be born with anencephaly. Anencephalic infants typically are born with only a brainstem, with the cerebral hemispheres—and hence the substrate for consciousness—lacking. In T.A.C.P.'s case, the back of her skull was entirely missing and her brainstem was exposed to the air, except for the presence of a dressing. Anencephaly is invariably fatal.[14] (In this case, T.A.C.P. would die a few days after birth.)

Case 13-A (*continued*)

On the advice of physicians, T.A.C.P.'s parents continued the pregnancy to term and agreed that the mother would undergo caesarean section, with the hope that the infant's organs could be transplanted into other sick children. However, when they requested that T.A.C.P. be declared legally dead for this purpose, her health care providers refused out of concern that they thereby might incur civil or criminal liability.

The parents then filed a petition in court asking for a judicial determination of whether an anencephalic newborn is considered dead for the purposes of organ donation. At the time of the hearing, the child was breathing unaided.

Analysis

First, the court looked to applicable Florida statutory law, which provided that "where respiratory and circulatory functions are maintained by artificial means of support so as to preclude a determination that these functions have ceased, the occurrence of death may be determined where there is irreversible cessation of functioning of the entire brain."[15] The court reasoned that, because T.A.C.P.'s respiratory and circulatory functions were not being maintained artificially, the statute was not applicable to the infant. Therefore, under Florida common law, T.A.C.P. would be considered dead only if she had sustained irreversible cessation of circulatory and respiratory functions. Because she had in fact not sustained irreversible cessation of those functions, she was not dead under cardiopulmonary criteria. Finally, the court considered whether there was a good reason in public policy for the court to expand the common law definition of death to include anencephaly. The court, in deciding not to do so, cited a number of reasons, including the lack of any consensus regarding whether the definition of death should be so expanded and the lack of consensus regarding the number and utility of organs that could be harvested from anencephalic infants. Accordingly, T.A.C.P was not an appropriate donor of vital organs.

In this case, an attempt was made to have the baby declared dead for the purposes of transplantation, even though the baby, albeit doomed to a short life, was not dead. It illustrates the desire to decouple the diagnosis of death from the underlying physiology of death and link it instead to human purposes, altruistic though they may be. T.A.C.P. had none of the classic signs of death at birth, nor at the time of the hearing was she on a ventilator; thus, the concept of brain death could not be applied. Without any of the classic signs of death, T.A.C.P. had yet to enter the final common physiologic pathway of death, and so should not have been labeled "dead" for this or any other purpose.

Neocortical Brain Death (Higher Brain Death) and Permanent Vegetative State

Some have argued that the whole-brain formulation of brain death is underinclusive. They find fault with the whole-brain formulation because it allows patients who have brainstem function but no cortical function to be regarded as alive. These neocorticalists believe that a person should be considered dead if he or she has lost those higher brain (cortical) functions—including consciousness, self-awareness, reasoning, and the capacity to communicate or interact with others—that are essential to personhood.[16-19] Under this higher brain or neocortical definition of death, anencephalic newborns, for example, would be regarded as dead and so could serve as organ donors without having suffered irreversible cessation of cardiopulmonary function. So, too, would patients in permanent (or persistent) vegetative state (PVS).

What is PVS? As you will see momentarily, anencephaly may be thought of as a form of congenital PVS in which the very neocortical substrate that underlies consciousness is missing. There have been a number of famous cases involving patients in PVS, including Karen Quinlan,[20] Nancy Cruzan,[21] and most recently Terri Schiavo.[22]

> Patients in a persistent vegetative state . . . represent a subgroup of patients who suffer severe anoxic brain injury and progress to a state of wakefulness without awareness. PVS may represent a transition between coma and recovery or between coma and death. The term . . . is defined as:
>
> - No evidence of awareness of self or environment and an inability to interact with others
> - No evidence of sustained, reproducible, purposeful, or voluntary behavioral responses to visual, auditory, tactile, or noxious stimuli
> - No evidence of language comprehension or expression
> - Intermittent wakefulness manifested by the presence of sleep-wake cycles
> - Sufficiently preserved hypothalamic and brain stem autonomic function to permit survival with medical and nursing care
> - Bowel and bladder incontinence
> - Variably preserved cranial nerve reflexes and spinal reflexes[23]

Because they retain brainstem functions, PVS patients are, like anencephalic infants, *not* brain dead. They can usually breathe air, digest their food, and void without assistance. They experience cycles of waking (eyes open) and sleeping (eyes closed).

> They may smile, utter unintelligible sounds, or move their eyes, arms and legs sporadically. PVS patients also manifest a range of reflex reactions to different stimuli; they will grimace, cough, gag and move their arms and legs. While all of this activity gives the appearance of consciousness, there is none.[9(p530)]

Although the higher brain formulation of death has a certain appeal, there are some problems associated with it. First, "reliable clinical tests for higher brain death are not available."[24] Although PVS patients lack awareness of their internal and external environments, they do not manifest the classic signs of brain failure (unresponsiveness and fixed, dilated pupils).

Second, the higher brain death formulation seems to conflate the concepts of personhood and life.

> The concept of higher brain death seems to confuse what it means to be a *person* with what it means to be *alive*. It might be appropriate to say that individuals without cortical function are no longer persons in the philosophic sense of having rights and interests. However, it does not follow logically that they should be considered dead.[24] (Italics added)

Finally, "higher brain criteria contradict deeply held beliefs about death. Burying or cremating individuals . . . who have no cortical function but who are still breathing [on their own] and have a pulse seems intuitively wrong."[24] As of yet, no state has adopted the higher brain death formulation.

Non-Heart-Beating Donation of Organs

Non-heart-beating donation (NHBD) refers to the harvesting of organs for transplantation from individuals who are declared dead according to the circulatory-respiratory criteria as opposed to neurologic (brain death) criteria. Prior to the acceptance of brain death criteria, all vital organ transplants came from NHBD. Following the medical and legal adoption of brain death criteria, brain dead donors largely supplanted non-heart-beating (NHB) donors as a source of vital organs, because the organs of brain dead patients (whose cardiopulmonary status is being maintained artificially) continue to be perfused up until the very moment of harvesting; in contrast, the vital organs of NHB donors begin to deteriorate the moment cardiopulmonary functions cease.

Recall from previous discussion that some critics of the brain death concept argued that a person whose heart continued to beat could not be declared dead—that in order for death to be declared, there must be irreversible cessation of circulatory and respiratory function, as well as of all functions of the brain. Some have taken that argument and reversed it in their criticism of NHBD. Thus, it has been argued that the death of the brain is a sine qua non for the death of a person.

> According to [this way of] thinking, [circulatory-respiratory] criteria should not be used to declare death but only to infer brain death. A significant problem with this approach is that the inference of brain death from [circulatory-respiratory] criteria requires at least a ten-minute wait. The ramification is that most of the body's organs would be unusable for transplantation by the time the declaration of death is made, which is required under the dead-donor rule.[25]

Because most NHBD protocols do not require a ten-minute wait, some have argued that not all NHB organ donors are truly dead when vital organ harvesting begins—a violation of the dead donor rule. Others, however, have argued that the practice of NHBD is ethically legitimate:

> [I]t is legitimate to declare death when it is established: (1) that circulation and respiration have ceased; (2) that these functions will not resume spontaneously; and (3) that the physician should not resuscitate.... [T]o provide a concrete frame of reference, it should be noted that the Pittsburgh protocol for NHBDs uses tests that seem to satisfy these criteria. The patient is weaned from the ventilator and apnea is determined; pulselessness is verified using a femoral arterial catheter; ventricular fibrillation, electrical asystole, or electromechanical dissociation is determined using an electrocardiogram. Death is declared after verifying that [circulatory-respiratory] functions have been lost for two minutes—the time period currently believed sufficient to rule out autoresuscitation. That the physician should not resuscitate—even were this possible—is known by the fact that all of the patients in question or their proxies made a decision to withdraw life support because it was deemed excessively burdensome or futile.[26]

Recall what we wrote earlier about how the following question has been answered: Is a person with irreversible loss of function of the whole brain who is maintained on a ventilator dead, or must a declaration of death await the withdrawal of ventilatory support?

> Medicine and the law have decided that actual completion of the process, either via the withdrawal of medical interventions or despite such interventions, is not necessary—that such patients are dead because they have the classic brain signs of death and other neurologic signs that indicate complete brain failure. In other words, the presence of signs of complete and irreversible brain death is sufficient to establish the death of the patient.[27]

Similarly, defendants of NHBD argue that "brain death is not essential to death—it provides, at most, one set of criteria for meeting the definition of death."[26] They point to the report of the President's Commission, *Defining Death*, which offered two concepts or definitions of death.[7] The first was death as the irreversible loss of "the integrated functioning of the organism as a whole"; the second was death "as a single phenomenon—the collapse of psycho-physical integrity."[7(p73)] Once it is clear that cardiopulmonary functions have ceased, that they will not resume spontaneously, and that CPR is not an option, "the integrated functioning of the organism as a whole" may be said to have been irreversibly lost, its "psycho-physical integrity" to have collapsed.

Some Exceptions to the Rules

As should be clear from the previous discussion, a patient who is declared dead under the second clause of the UDDA (irreversible cessation of all functions of the entire brain, including the brainstem) is just as dead as a patient who is declared dead under the first clause of the UDDA (irreversible cessation of circulatory and respiratory functions). In general, in both cases the patient is medically and legally dead, and should be declared so in the chart. The use of medical equipment should be discontinued, because no longer are any of the goals of medicine achievable.

With almost any rule, however, there are exceptions. Here, too, there are exceptions to the rule that brain death is treated the same as cardiopulmonary death. First, as we have already mentioned, ventilatory support of the brain dead patient is continued in those instances in which the patient is to serve as an organ donor. Continued medical support of the brain dead patient preserves the organs to be donated and is justifiable on at least two counts: (1) it allows the brain dead patient's wishes to serve as an organ donor to be effectuated, demonstrating (posthumously) respect for his or her autonomy, and (2) by preserving organs for transplantation, it maximizes our opportunity to confer medical benefits on other (recipient) patients.

Second, ventilatory support of a brain dead pregnant patient might be continued in order to save the life of the fetus she is carrying. Thus, there was a 2005 case in which ventilatory support was continued for this reason for three months after the declaration of death by brain criteria.[28]

Third, in certain jurisdictions there are religious exceptions to the determination of death by brain death criteria. In New Jersey, for example, a person who suffers irreversible cessation of either cardiopulmonary or brain function is dead. However, New Jersey law also provides that

> [t]he death of an individual shall not be declared upon the basis of neurological criteria . . . when the licensed physician authorized to declare death, has reason to believe, on the basis of information in the individual's available medical records, or information provided by a member of the individual's family or any other person knowledgeable about the individual's personal religious beliefs that such a declaration would violate the personal religious beliefs of the individual. In these cases, death shall be declared, and the time of death fixed, solely upon the basis of cardio-respiratory criteria.[29]

Similarly, New York State Department of Health regulations provide that hospitals shall establish "a procedure for the reasonable accommodation of the individual's religious or moral objection" to the determination of death by neurologic (brain death) criteria.[30]

Chapter Summary

Death is the irreversible loss of "the integrated functioning of the organism as a whole," "the collapse of [individual] psycho-physical integrity." The immediate and classic bedside physical signs of death include unresponsiveness, fixed and dilated pupils, and absence of pulse and respiration. With the advent of effective CPR techniques and mechanical ventilation, a person could be resuscitated and ventilated successfully, maintaining a heartbeat while yet exhibiting complete unresponsiveness, absence of spontaneous respirations, and fixed and dilated pupils. This condition, initially labeled *le coma dépassé*, later came to be known as *brain death*.

The Harvard criteria are guidelines for the diagnosis of brain death. All fifty states and the District of Columbia have accepted brain death as a legal standard. The majority have done so by enacting the Uniform Determination of Death Act, which provides, "An individual who has sustained either (1) irreversible cessation of circulatory and respiratory functions, or (2) irreversible cessation of all functions of the *entire* brain, including the brain stem, is dead." Neocorticalists have criticized the whole-brain formulation of death, arguing that a person should be considered dead if he or she has lost those higher brain (cortical) functions—including consciousness, self-awareness, reasoning, and the capacity to communicate or interact with others—that are essential to personhood. Under this higher brain or neocortical formulation of death, anencephalic newborns and patients in PVS—neither of whom are dead under the whole-brain formulation—would be regarded as dead.

How death is defined and determined has implications for organ donation, because the dead donor rule requires that a person be dead before vital organs may be harvested from him or her. Currently, vital organs are harvested from brain dead patients and from non-heart-beating donors; use of the latter as sources of vital organs is ethically more controversial.

Review Questions

1. What are the classic bedside signs of death?

2. Under the Uniform Determination of Death Act, when is a person dead? When is he or she dead by neurologic criteria? By cardiopulmonary criteria?

3. May vital organs be harvested from a brain dead patient? An anencephalic infant? A patient in PVS? Why or why not?

4. May vital organs be harvested from a non-heart-beating donor? If so, when?

5. State the dead donor rule.

6. What are some of the problems associated with the higher brain (neocortical) formulation of death?

7. Describe the neurologic examination of a patient in PVS. How does it differ from the patient who is brain dead? Of what moral significance are the differences?

8. List three circumstances under which health care professionals might choose to continue ventilator support of brain dead patients.

Endnotes

1. Refers to "stiffening of the body, from 1 to 7 hours after death." *Stedman's Medical Dictionary*. 23rd ed. Baltimore: Williams and Wilkins, 1976:1238.

2. Refers to "the chill of death." *Stedman's Medical Dictionary*. 23rd ed. Baltimore: Williams and Wilkins, 1976:41.

3. Refers to the "livid discoloration of the skin on the dependent parts of a corpse." *Stedman's Medical Dictionary*. 23rd ed. Baltimore: Williams and Wilkins, 1976:802.

4. Mollaret P, Goulon M. Le coma dépassé. *Rev Neurol* 1959;101:5–15.

5. A definition of irreversible coma. Report of the Ad Hoc Committee of the Harvard Medical School to examine the definition of brain death. *JAMA* 1968;205(6):337–340.

6. Paola FA, Anderson JA. The process of dying. In: Sanbar SS, Gibofsky A, Firestone MH, LeBlang TR, eds. *Legal Medicine*. 3rd ed. St. Louis: Mosby, 1995:404–423, p. 405. See also the 1968 *JAMA* article cited in endnote 5.

7. President's Commission for the Study of Ethical Problems in Medicine and Biomedical and Behavioral Research. *Defining Death: Medical, Legal and Ethical Issues in the Determination of Death*. Washington, DC: U.S. Government Printing Office, 1981.

8. Uniform Determination of Death Act. Available at: http://www.law.upenn.edu/bll/archives/ulc/fnact99/1980s/udda80.htm. Accessed July 10, 2008.

9. Hall MA, Bobinski MA, Orentlicher D. *Health Care Law and Ethics*. 7th ed. Austin, TX: Aspen Publishers, 2007:638.

10. Meisel A, Cerminara KL. Section 6.04[A]. In: *The Right to Die: The Law of End-of-Life Decision-making*. 3rd ed., 2007 suppl. New York: Aspen Publishers, 2007.

11. "According to the law of every state, organs necessary for life (e.g., the heart or an entire liver) cannot be removed for transplantation unless the person is dead (the "dead donor" rule). See, e.g., Ind. Code Ann. Section 29-2-16-2." Hall MA, Bobinski MA, Orentlicher D. *Health Care Law and Ethics*. 7th ed. Austin, TX: Aspen Publishers, 2007:655.

12. Anencephaly refers to the "markedly defective development of the brain, together with absence of the bones of the cranial vault. The cerebral and cerebellar hemispheres are usually wanting, with only a rudimentary brain stem and some traces of basal ganglia present. Colloquially, individuals with this malformation [were] sometimes called 'frog babies.' The condition is incompatible with life." *Stedman's Medical Dictionary* 23rd ed. Baltimore: Williams and Wilkins, 1976:71.

13. *In re T.A.C.P.*, 609 So. 2d 588 (Fla. 1992).

14. The court wrote, "Two months was the longest confirmed survival of an anencephalic, although there are unconfirmed reports of one surviving three months and another surviving fourteen months." See *In re T.A.C.P.* The decision in *In re T.A.C.P.* preceded the Baby K case, in which an anencephalic child lived for about thirty months.

15. Section 382.009(1), Fla. Stat. (1991).

16. For a discussion of personhood, see Moeschler JM. Abortion and the new genetics. In: Gert B, Berger EM, Cahill GF, et al., eds. *Morality and the New Genetics*. Sudbury, MA: Jones and Bartlett, 1996:189–208, p. 196. See also Warren MA. On the moral and legal status of abortion. *The Monist* 1973;57(1):43–61.

17. Veatch R. The whole-brain-oriented concept of death: an outmoded philosophical foundation. *J Thanatology* 1975;3:13–30.

18. Capron AM. Brain death—well settled yet still unresolved. *N Engl J Med* 2001;344:1244–1246.

19. Youngner SJ, Bartlett ET. Human death and high technology: the failure of whole-brain formulations. *Ann Intern Med* 1983;99:252–258.

20. *In the Matter of Karen Quinlan*, 355 A.2d 647 (N.J. 1976).

21. *Cruzan v. Director, Missouri Department of Health*, 497 U.S. 261 (1990).

22. Pence GE. Terri Schiavo: when does personhood end? In: *The Elements of Bioethics*. New York: McGraw-Hill, 2007:137–171.

23. Weinhouse GL, Young GB. Anoxic-ischemic brain injury: assessment and treatment. UpToDate. Available at: http://www.uptodate.com. Accessed July 13, 2008.

24. Lo B. *Resolving Ethical Dilemmas: A Guide for Clinicians*. 3rd ed. Philadelphia: Lippincott Williams & Wilkins, 2005:144.

25. Non-heart-beating donor (NHBD). Available at: http://www.ascensionhealth.org/ethics/public/issues/NHBD.asp. Accessed July 12, 2008.

26. DuBois, James M. Non-heart-beating organ donation: a defense of the required determination of death. *J Law Med Ethics* 1999;27(2):126.

27. See this chapter, p. 295.

28. Willing R. Brain-dead woman dies after baby born. *USA Today*, August 4, 2005, p. 3A.

29. N.J. Stat. Ann. 26:6A-5.

30. N.Y. Comp. Codes R. & Regs. Tit. 10, section 400.16(e)(3).

Chapter 14

End-of-Life Decision Making

The hour of departure has arrived, and we go our ways—I to die, and you to live. Which is better only the god knows.

—Plato, *Apology*

Chapter Learning Objectives
At the conclusion of this chapter the reader will be able to:

1. Understand how the four ethical principles of beneficence, nonmaleficence, respect for autonomy, and justice apply in the context of end-of-life decision making

2. Understand how the right to refuse life-sustaining treatment arguably implicates two traditions—the traditional right to control one's body and the antisuicide tradition

3. Understand and recognize the competing interests in cases involving life-sustaining treatment, including the four societal or state interests commonly cited by courts that have ruled on cases involving the right to refuse treatment

4. Understand and apply the approach to end-of-life decision making in patients with current decisional capacity, in patients with previous decisional capacity, and in patients who have never had decisional capacity

5. Understand and distinguish among the subjective, substituted judgment, and best interest decision-making standards

6. Understand and distinguish between the evidentiary standards of *clear and convincing* and *preponderance of the evidence*

7. Distinguish between a health care surrogate and a proxy, and describe the role of each in end-of-life decision making

8. Understand and distinguish among the various types of advance directives

9. Be familiar with the key legal cases in end-of-life decision making as discussed in this chapter

10. Define and distinguish the various types of homicide

11. Define, distinguish, and recognize the various types of physician aid in dying

12. Be familiar with the arguments for and against physician aid in dying

311

13. Be familiar with the U.S. Supreme Court cases dealing with physician aid in dying

14. Understand the Oregon Death with Dignity Act

15. Understand and apply the rule of the double effect

Medicine's rapid technical advances have obscured its long-held ethic of compassionate care at the end of life. Before medicine had any significant ability to extend the life of the dying patient, its chief activities lay in the realms of prognostication, symptom relief, and providing comfort. A doctor would typically take care of a patient in the patient's home until that patient succumbed to his or her disease. With the advent of medical technology in the twentieth century, the focus shifted to applying medical technology to patients, regardless of their prognosis. The location of care was also shifted to hospitals, where such technology could be more conveniently applied. In many cases, patients near the end of life were supported using life-sustaining technology simply because they could be. Concern for comfort and symptom management receded into the background. As a result, more and more patients died high-tech deaths in hospital settings, until this eventually became the norm.

Technology was not the only force driving high-tech care at the end of life. The increase in medical malpractice litigation led to a strategy of defensive medicine on the part of physicians, one that viewed doing everything medically possible as the best way to minimize legal risk. The physician who "did everything possible" could not easily be accused of negligence, or so the thinking went.

Still another force driving the high-tech approach was the culture of medicine, which had changed, coming to view patient death not as part of the natural order of things, but rather as a discrete medical failure. Under this new view, whatever the end result might be, patients should not die without physicians at least trying to save them. Coupled with this medical cultural shift was a desire on the part of families of incapacitated patients to have high-tech care provided to their loved ones. The explanation for this desire was at least twofold: (1) enamored of medicine's astonishing successes, there was the ever-present hope that the patient, no matter how dire his or her condition, might yet improve as long as medical treatment and support was continued; and (2) the difficult alternative—to actually make the hard decision to stop treatment and supportive interventions—was felt by many to be too burdensome. It is much easier to salve the conscience by authorizing physicians to "do everything" than to decide to withhold a particular intervention or, even worse, to withdraw it. In forgoing medical treatment, a person must live with the uncertainty that the wrong decision may have been made—that if only the treatment had been continued, the patient might well have recovered.

Eventually, some began to question and even challenge the status quo of high-tech death and dying, thus ushering in the age of autonomy. The first high-profile right to refuse treatment case was that of Karen Ann Quinlan, a young woman who stopped breathing after an overdose.[1] After being revived by medical personnel and transported to a hospital, Quinlan did not improve, but instead remained in a permanent vegetative state (PVS) on ventilator support. Eventually, her father, who had also become her legal guardian, asked that her ventilator be discontinued. Because it was thought that she could not survive without ventilator support, the hospital refused, forcing the matter into the courts. The New Jersey Supreme Court eventually settled the matter with its landmark decision allowing Quinlan's father to authorize the physicians to stop the ventilator.

What followed was a long line of court decisions in various states that increasingly recognized and expanded a patient's right to be free of unwanted medical intervention. Eventually, in the case of Nancy Cruzan, the United States Supreme Court ruled on the issue and suggested that the right to refuse medical treatment is grounded in the Fourteenth Amendment to the U.S. Constitution.[2] In the aftermath of the *Quinlan* decision, states gradually began passing laws that would allow persons to refuse unwanted medical treatment in advance through written documents that became known as *living wills*. States also allowed patients to designate another individual to make medical decisions should the patient enter a condition of mental incapacity. Also in the aftermath of Quinlan, hospitals began to craft policies that would allow patients to forego attempts at cardiopulmonary resuscitation (CPR). In these policies, physicians were allowed to write a do-not-resuscitate (DNR) order, since the default position was to attempt to resuscitate every person who suffered cardiopulmonary arrest.[3]

Another important development took hold well after the law established that a patient could refuse unwanted medical treatment, namely, the emergence of the field of hospice and palliative medicine. This was, in a sense, a return to medicine's pretechnological focus on prognostication, symptom relief, and providing comfort. Hospice was a way to avoid dying a high-tech death. It allowed patients to avoid transport to the hospital. They could instead die at home with the help of an interdisciplinary team of caregivers that typically included a physician, nurses, a counselor/social worker, and optionally a person with expertise in spiritual care. This movement became so successful that the Medicare program was modified to include a specific hospice benefit. Hospices are now common across the United States. Whereas hospices previously served predominantly cancer patients, the majority of hospice patients today carry noncancer diagnoses, such as end-stage chronic obstructive lung disease, congestive heart failure, dementia, end-stage renal disease, and so on.

Although hospice care is typically delivered in the patient's home, there are now some hospitals that have dedicated hospice beds, or even hospice units. For hospitals that do not have hospice beds per se, there is the option of developing a palliative care consultation service that can assist health care professionals in the care of patients who do not want a high-tech death and yet are unable to leave the hospital. The emergence of palliative care services in acute care hospitals has been rapid and widely accepted. It is as if medicine has finally started to take seriously the fact that large numbers of patients and families are willing to stop aggressive care at some point or other and shift to alternative comfort care. With the emergence of hospice care and then palliative care services in hospitals, the field of hospice and palliative medicine has matured to the point at which the American Board of Medical Sciences and the Accreditation Council on Medical Education have recognized hospice and palliative medicine as a subspecialty on par with cardiology or gastroenterology.

Despite all of these advances, the difficult problems associated with end-of-life decision making remain. When ethics committees began forming in the late 1970s to help physicians grapple with difficult end-of-life decisions, a central focus was to help the physician do his or her job. It was never the committees' role to take decisions away from the primary physician at the bedside; it was instead to inform, to advise, and to assist by providing knowledge of law, policy, and the wisdom gained by a study of past cases. Armed with this assistance, it was felt that the physician would be in a better position to counsel patients and families as they engaged in a process of shared decision making that would culminate in decisions that were informed and reflected the patient's desires for forms of care.

It is significant that ethics committees were formed to address end-of-life decisions, rather than mere prognosis committees (as was suggested by the *Quinlan* court), risk management committees, or resource utilization committees. For the questions at hand were typically ethical in nature. Are we overtreating? Should ventilators be used on everyone, regardless of the likelihood of successful outcome or of the burdens it might impose? Must we always use CPR? If not, what ethical parameters should guide its use and nonuse? Are we obligated to provide treatment we think is futile? Is there a difference between stopping a treatment and not starting it in the first place? Is the physician who withdraws a life-sustaining treatment killing the patient, or is the physician merely allowing the patient to die a natural death?

These questions are most acute at the end of life because the burdens of intervention are often high, the benefits marginal, and the quality of life markedly diminished. The remainder of this chapter reviews the ethical principles that inform and guide medical decision making in general and then looks at how these principles play out in end-of-life decisions. It also examines a number of issues that commonly arise in end-of-life decision making, including the right to refuse life-sustaining therapy, medical futility, the distinction between killing and letting die, and physician-assisted suicide.

Ethical Principles in End-of-Life Care

The core principles of medical ethics date from antiquity and are commonly labeled *beneficence* and *nonmaleficence*. The principle of beneficence holds that health care professionals should aim to "benefit the sick," whereas nonmaleficence means that they should "do no harm" in the process. These principles are reflected in medicine's chief goal, which is to help the sick by endeavoring to return them to health while working to prevent or at least minimize any suffering that may be associated with the disease and also with the treatment itself. Minimizing treatment harm is accomplished first by educating the patient regarding the potential for adverse effects of treatment so that adverse effects might be recognized early, when there is greatest opportunity to reverse them or at least minimize their magnitude. Second, there must be a good communication channel between the patient and the physician, as well as others who may be involved in the care. Third, once an adverse effect is suspected or recognized, quick and appropriate action must be taken by the health care professional to address the problem. Medicine is a double-edged sword, employed in an attempt to help the sick, but also with the potential to harm them. Thus its ethical use is quite properly located between the poles of the two principles of beneficence and nonmaleficence.

The principle of *respect for autonomy*, as it has found expression in American medicine, boils down to patients guiding their own care by either selecting among available options for treatment or declining the treatment(s) offered. Although the principle of respect for autonomy has been considered at some length in other chapters (see, for example, Chapter 2), the essential point to grasp is that autonomy considerations stand apart from the beneficence/nonmaleficence dyad that guides health professionals. Considerations of beneficence and nonmaleficence determine what options are ethically appropriate to offer to patients from a medical point of view, with the aim being to achieve the best possible health care outcome in terms of maximum benefits and minimum harms. In contrast, autonomy is about the patient's acceptance or rejection of what is actually offered in particular cases. It is the power to choose among available choices for treatment, and the power to reject the choices altogether.

The principle of *justice* has often been seen as central to concerns about fair allocation of medical resources and access to care. The classic example is the question of fair allocation of scarce medical resources such as transplantable organs. Another example is the question of what health care needs should be addressed when fiscal resources for health care are limited. This question arose in Oregon in the 1990s when the state had to decide how to spend limited Medicaid dollars to address health care needs across its population. Rather than leaving this to the health professions to decide alone, or deciding on a haphazard first-come, first-served basis, Oregon involved its populace in deciding on health priorities and used preference data to guide spending. As a result, providing immunizations for Oregon's children, for example, was valued more highly and hence prioritized above saving a relatively small number of lives by spending funds on heart transplants.[4]

The principles of medical ethics also come into play when patients are at the end of life. As such, they can be used to frame our consideration of end-of-life decision making. In the time before the advent of technological medicine, there was relatively little that could be done to prolong any patient's life. In the days before antibiotics and anesthesia, before open-heart surgery and mechanical ventilation, people lived shorter lives and died of acute diseases that are now almost all treatable in some measure or another. There was no talk of stopping life-sustaining treatment (LST) because medicine had no ability to sustain life—in other words, LST did not exist. The doctors of the past tried to help as best they could, but with no power to lengthen a patient's days, they would focus on prognosis, comfort, and symptom relief for those who were dying. These are still vital functions for the health professions, but have taken a back seat as medicine began to achieve unimaginable scientific and technological success. Again, they have enjoyed a renaissance in the form of hospice and palliative care medicine.

As medicine achieved success in treating disease and sustaining life through illnesses that would ordinarily have been fatal, there were cases where success was limited. There were people who were successfully resuscitated, only to be left dependent on mechanical ventilation. There were people whose lives were saved by medicine but who were left in a permanent vegetative state with no realistic prospect of improving. The burdens and costs of a high-tech approach to patient care began to be seen by some as simply too high. Questions were raised. Does a prolonged stay in the intensive care unit (ICU) make sense when the best outcome that can be expected is life in a nursing home with catheters, feeding tubes, and in some cases ventilators? Does everybody have to be resuscitated? Can mechanical ventilators be stopped? Do we always have to start dialysis when kidneys fail? If treatment is started, can it be stopped? Can a Jehovah's Witness refuse a transfusion if it means that without it he or she will die?

The central question in the care of the dying is the appropriate use of life-sustaining interventions. In some cases, there is little or no benefit to be gained by these interventions, and yet the potential for significant harm commonly remains. Ordinarily, when the benefits are clearly outweighed by the potential harms of intervention, the use of that intervention is properly regarded as inappropriate. But who has the ultimate authority to decide the matter of appropriateness? Should it be the physician alone? Should inappropriateness be decided at the policy level?

From an ethics point of view, the patient is the one who should decide about forgoing life-sustaining interventions, based on the third ethical principle—patient autonomy. The principle of autonomy, or respect for persons, has its roots in analytic philosophy and has become synonymous with the concept of self-determination.[5] This concept was expressed well by Justice Cardozo in a famous medical malpractice case: "Every human being of adult years and sound mind has a right to determine what shall be done with his own body."[6] The principle of respect for autonomy lies at the root of the medical and legal doctrine of informed consent and also at the root of decisions by patients to forgo LST at the end of life.

The fourth ethical principle is that of distributive justice, which guides the fair allocation of medical resources. Justice considerations arise in end-of-life care when one compares the high cost of marginally beneficial end-of-life care to the lack of funding for the basic care of a large portion of our country's residents. Although the issues regarding medical costs and the design of just health care systems are complex and important, they are more properly approached at the social policy level and should not be left simply to the physician at the bedside. The principle of justice is mentioned to distinguish it from end-of-life ethics decisions at the bedside. In the current climate of increasing desire for a dignified death, if a better job were done of honoring patients' wishes to forgo expensive life-prolonging intervention, then both justice and autonomy would be served.[7]

In most cases, ethical treatment decisions should be shared between physician and patient. The physician has an obligation to inform the patient of established treatment options and then to recommend the treatment he or she believes is in the patient's best medical interest.[8] The patient then accepts the physician's recommendation and consents to treatment, chooses an option other than the recommended one, or chooses to forgo the treatment altogether. In each case, the physician fulfills the ethical obligation to benefit the patient while minimizing harm. The patient, in turn, exercises his or her autonomy in either choosing treatment or refusing it. Even though this shared decisional process may result in conflict, in most cases of treatment refusal the patient's autonomy should prevail. This does not mean that the physician should not attempt to persuade the patient to act in what the physician believes to be the patient's best medical interest, but it does mean that the physician should not attempt to coerce the patient.

The Right to Refuse Life-Sustaining Medical Treatment

The right to refuse medical treatment is well established in medicine and in law. The legal tradition of the right to be left alone has deep roots. Recall Justice Cardozo's oft-quoted statement in *Schloendorf v. Society of New York Hospitals:* "Every human being of adult years and sound mind has a right to determine what shall be done with his own body." When cases arose asserting that patients had a right to be free of unwanted medical intervention, the right was readily recognized and clearly affirmed.[9,10]

In the mid-twentieth century, whether the right to refuse medical treatment included a right to refuse LST posed a special problem for medicine and the law. The reason that refusal of LST was problematic was that, besides implicating the right to control one's body, it arguably also implicated the antisuicide tradition.[11] In other words, there was (and is) no legal right to suicide in the United States; does refusal of LST constitute suicide? To the extent that refusal of LST did constitute suicide, cases involving the right to refuse LST would place the two traditions—the right to control one's own body versus the antisuicide tradition—on a collision course.

In the end most courts decided that a patient's refusal of LST was not suicide. They distinguished between a patient's legitimate motive of being free of unwanted medical therapy and the illegitimate motive of self-destruction that characterizes suicide. They distinguished the two scenarios as well in terms of cause of death. Thus, the patient who refused LST (and the health care providers who went along with his or her wishes) was simply allowing nature to take its course (with the cause of death being his or her underlying disease), as opposed to the suicide situation, in which a person actively causes his or her own death.[12]

Limitations on the Right to Refuse Life-Sustaining Treatment

A patient's right to refuse LST is not absolute. Whether the individual's interest is framed as a right to privacy, as a common law right to refuse medical treatment, or more modernly as a Fourteenth Amendment liberty interest, courts have identified four societal or state interests that must be balanced against a person's right to be free of unwanted medical intervention. These are the preservation of life, the prevention of suicide, the protection of innocent third parties, and the safeguarding of the ethical integrity of the medical profession.[13] In most treatment refusal cases, these state interests are found not to outweigh a competent adult's right to refuse unwanted medical intervention. However, in some cases, the right to refuse treatment is overridden. One example of this is a court-ordered blood transfusion to save the life of a single-parent Jehovah's Witness who would leave minor children as wards of the state if lifesaving transfusion were withheld. In cases such as this, some courts have held that the state's interest in protecting the children (protection of innocent third parties) outweighs the parent's right to refuse unwanted transfusion, even though the reason for refusing is based on a deeply held religious belief. (See Chapter 4.)

The right to refuse LST seems to have evolved with time. In the *Quinlan* case, the court wrote,

> We think that the state's interest [in opposing the individual's refusal of LST] weakens and the individual's right ... grows as the degree of bodily invasion increases and the [individual patient's] prognosis dims. Ultimately there comes a point at which the individual's [right] overcomes the state interest[s].[1]

Of course, this statement suggests that in cases involving treatments requiring lesser degrees of bodily invasion, and in patients with more favorable prognoses, the state interests should prevail over the asserted individual right. But modern "courts have seemingly abandoned any effort to balance the individual's right to refuse treatment with the state's interest in preserving life, almost without exception permitting competent patients to refuse life-sustaining treatment."[14]

Approaching End-of-Life Decisions

Legal cases involving end-of-life decision making can be divided into three categories: (1) the patient possessing decisional capacity (or *competency;* see Chapter 7) in the present, (2) the patient without decisional capacity in the present but who possessed decisional capacity in the past, and (3) the patient who never possessed decisional capacity. The second category may be further subdivided into those patients with prior decisional capacity who had expressed treatment preferences for end-of-life care either verbally or in a written advance directive prior to losing decisional capacity, and those patients with prior decisional capacity who had made no prior expression of treatment preferences before losing decisional capacity. We deal with each of these scenarios in turn (Fig. 14-1).

The Patient with Current Decisional Capacity

In cases of patients with intact decision-making capacity, courts have ruled that such patients have the right to refuse medical interventions even when those interventions are

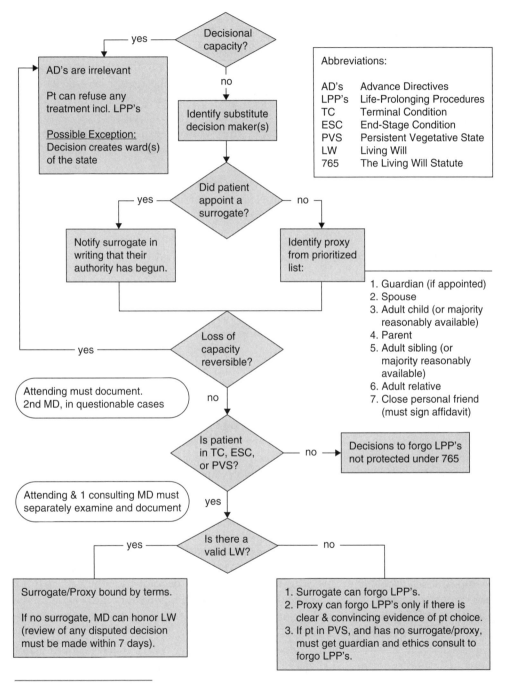

Figure 14-1 Advance Directives Algorithm.

life sustaining. *Bouvia v. Superior Court* involved Elizabeth Bouvia, a twenty-eight-year-old woman who was quadriplegic as a result of severe cerebral palsy.[15] In 1983 she sought and was denied the legal right to be cared for in a public hospital while she starved herself to death. Doctors determined that she was not eating enough and feared she was trying to starve herself to death slowly. They inserted a nasogastric tube against her will. The trial court found that, with feeding, she could live another fifteen to twenty years, and held that the state's interest in preserving her life outweighed her decisional right. Reframing her claim as the right to refuse unwanted LST, three years later the court held that Bouvia had the right to refuse any medical treatment including artificial hydration and nutrition, *even where such treatment would be lifesaving.*

Likewise, in *Satz v. Perlmutter,* a competent ventilator-dependent patient with amyotrophic lateral sclerosis (ALS) wanted his ventilator discontinued and was allowed by the court to direct physicians to remove the ventilator.[16]

The Patient with Prior—but Not Current—Decisional Capacity

As alluded to earlier, this category of patients may be further subdivided, depending on whether or not the patient executed a formal advance directive prior to losing decisional capacity. Let us discuss each of these subcategories in turn. Each state has its own body of law dealing with end-of-life decision making. For the sake of simplicity and coherence, herein we will largely focus on Florida law.[17]

The Patient with Prior Capacity Who Has Not Executed a Formal Advance Directive

In situations in which there is no written advance directive (no formal instructions about what to do) and the patient lacks decision-making capacity, courts have reasoned that the patient's loss of decisional capacity should not entail the loss of the right to refuse medical treatment. The courts have further reasoned that in order to prevent the right from being extinguished in a practical sense, another person must exercise the right on the patient's behalf.

Health Care Proxy
The first question to be answered is, Who is to exercise the right on the patient's behalf? Under Florida law, the decision is to be made by a *proxy,* where a proxy is defined as a competent adult *not expressly designated* to make health care decisions for the principal *but authorized to do so by statute.*[18] Note the difference between a *proxy* (not designated by the patient to make decisions but rather authorized to do so by statute) and a health care *surrogate* (designated by the patient himself or herself).

How does the statute authorize proxy decision making? It sets up a prioritized list of individuals who could potentially act as proxies. The highest person on the list who is ready, willing, and able to act as a proxy does so. The partial list is as follows:

- Legally appointed guardian
- Spouse
- Adult child/majority of adult children
- Parent
- Adult sibling/majority of adult siblings
- "Close" adult relative
- "Close" adult friend[18]

Any health care decision made by the proxy must be based on the proxy's informed consent and must be the decision the proxy reasonably believes the patient would have made under the circumstances. If there is no indication as to what the patient would have chosen, then the proxy may consider the patient's best interests. Furthermore, where the proxy decides to withhold or withdraw life-prolonging procedures (LPPs),[19] that decision must be supported by clear and convincing evidence either that the decision would have been the one the patient would have chosen, or (if there is no indication of what the patient would have chosen) that it is in the patient's best interest.

Substantive Decision-Making Standards

The second question to be answered is, What substantive decision-making standard should be employed by the proxy decision maker? The courts have employed a number of different substantive decision-making standards to guide proxies in making the decision on the patient's behalf.

The *subjective standard* asks, What *did* the patient in fact decide before losing decision making capacity? This standard is employed, for example, in New York (*O'Connor*),[20] and Missouri (*Cruzan*).[21] The subjective standard is a very strict and exacting standard, because it requires the patient actually to have made the precise decision facing the proxy. Thus, if a proxy is faced with the question of whether or not to discontinue a life-sustaining feeding tube under a particular set of circumstances, the fact that the patient had stated, before losing decisional capacity, that he would not want to be mechanically ventilated under those circumstances would not justify removal of the feeding tube under the subjective standard.

A second standard is the *substituted judgment standard.* This standard asks the question, What *would* the patient decide if the patient were able to decide? It requires that the proxy stand in the shoes of the principal. This standard is employed in most states, and is the standard that was employed in the *Quinlan* case.

Finally, the *best interest standard* allows the decision maker to forgo LST if doing so is in the patient's best interests. Where permitted, this standard is often employed when the other two standards cannot be met.

Evidentiary Standards

Besides the decision-making standards just outlined, *evidentiary standards* also play a critical role in cases involving patients with prior capacity who have not executed a formal advance directive. For example, how sure does one have to be that the patient refused (subjective standard) or would refuse (substituted judgment standard) LPPs under the circumstances before implementing that decision? How sure does one have to be that the patient is actually in a condition or state that triggers his or her advance directive?[22,23] The evidentiary standard employed by most courts is *clear and convincing evidence.*

When is evidence clear and convincing? Clear and convincing proof requires more than a *preponderance of the evidence* (the standard employed in most civil trials) but less than proof *beyond a reasonable doubt* (the standard employed in criminal trials).[24] The following elements support the contention that evidence of a patient's wishes is clear and convincing:

- Solemn pronouncements by the patient were made on serious occasions.
- Those pronouncements were consistently repeated by the patient.
- Those pronouncements are consistent with the patient's life values.
- They were made shortly before the need for treatment.
- They were specific.

Not all courts subscribe to the clear and convincing evidentiary standard. Thus, a Pennsylvania court, in the case *In re Fiori,* decided that adherence to a clear and convincing evidentiary standard was overly restrictive and would tend to thwart the actual wishes of the patient.[25]

The famous *Cruzan* case that was argued before the U.S. Supreme Court was all about standards.[2] The Court took the case to consider whether the U.S. Constitution prohibits Missouri from adopting the rule of decision making that it did. As Chief Justice Rehnquist framed the question, "Missouri requires that evidence of the incompetent's wishes as to the withdrawal of treatment be proved by clear and convincing evidence. The question, then, is whether the United States Constitution forbids the establishment of this procedural requirement by the State." The Court held that it does not. The Court assumed, for the purposes of this case, that the due process clause would protect a competent person's decision to refuse lifesaving hydration and nutrition, but pointed out that it also protected an interest in life. To guard against potential abuse, Missouri could properly and legitimately employ the rule of decision making that it did.

The Patient with Prior Capacity Who Has Executed a Formal Advance Directive

Under Florida law, an *advance directive* (AD) is defined as "a witnessed written document or oral statement in which instructions are given by a principal or in which the principal's desires are expressed concerning any aspect of the principal's health care, and includes, but is not limited to, the designation of a *health care surrogate,* a *living will,* or [the making of] an anatomical gift."[26]

ADs are important legally for a number of reasons. First of all, if the AD designates a health care surrogate, it answers the question, Who is to exercise the right on the patient's behalf? Second, ADs matter because the health care decisions made by the surrogate (if one is designated) or the instructions contained in a living will constitute clear and convincing evidence of the patient's wishes.

Health Care Surrogate

A *health care surrogate* is defined as "any competent adult *expressly designated* by a principal to make health care decisions upon the principal's incapacity [italics added]."[27] In Florida, designations of health care surrogates must be signed before two witnesses, and the surrogate may not be a witness. The designation is effective until the stated time of termination or until it is revoked.

A health care surrogate has the authority to make all health care decisions for the principal during the principal's incapacity unless the surrogate's authority is expressly limited in that regard. So, for example, if my surrogate is a Jehovah's Witness, I might specify that he or she can make all health care decisions for me except the decision to refuse a blood transfusion.

A health care surrogate can only make those health care decisions that he or she believes the principal would make under the circumstances. If, however, there is no indication of what the principal would have chosen, the surrogate may consider the patient's best interests.[28]

Living Will

A living will is defined as "A witnessed written document (executed in accordance with statutory requirements) OR a witnessed oral statement made by the principal concerning life-prolonging procedures."[29] Under Florida law, any competent adult may make a living will and direct the withholding or withdrawal of LPPs in the event such person has a terminal condition, an end-stage condition, or is in a permanent vegetative state. The living will must be signed before two subscribing witnesses.[30]

As stated previously, a living will constitutes clear and convincing evidence of the patient's wishes. The health care professional may proceed as the living will directs so long as (1) there is no reasonable medical probability of the patient recovering capacity (in which case one should wait and allow the patient to make the decision himself or herself); (2) the principal has a terminal condition, end-stage condition, or is in a permanent vegetative state; and (3) all (if any) conditions or limitations imposed by the patient in the living will have been satisfied.

Revocation of Advance Directives

ADs may be revoked by a signed, dated writing; the physical destruction of the AD by the principal or in the principal's presence and at his or her direction; an oral expression of intent to revoke; execution of a subsequent AD that differs materially from the former; or dissolution or annulment of marriage. The latter operates to revoke an AD that names the spouse as a health care surrogate.[31]

The Patient Who Never Possessed Decisional Capacity

In cases in which the patient has never communicated thoughts about end-of-life care or has never had the capacity for such thoughts, the proxy cannot make a substituted judgment because no prior judgments by the patient exist upon which to base one. Despite this, one early court case strained to apply the substituted judgment standard in deciding whether to authorize chemotherapy to treat leukemia in a sixty-seven-year-old never-competent man with an approximate mental age of two.[32]

Joseph Saikewicz, a sixty-seven-year-old man with a mental age of two and a half years, suffered from acute myeloblastic leukemia. A court-appointed guardian concluded that (1) the illness was incurable and the prospects for any benefit were limited; and (2) treatment would cause significant adverse effects, the reason for which Saikewicz would not understand. Therefore, the guardian recommended that not treating Mr. Saikewicz would be in his best interests. The court decided that the decision-making standard should be the substituted judgment standard, and concluded that Saikewicz himself would have made the same decision the guardian did. The court wrote:

> In short, the decision in cases such as this should be that which would be made by the incompetent person, if that person were competent, but taking into account the present and future incompetency of the individual as one of the factors which would necessarily enter into the decision-making process of the competent person.[32]

This is clearly a legal fiction if ever there was one. Other courts, seeing the illogic of basing decisions on the imagined choices of the never-competent, have rejected this approach as misguided. Consider the approach of New York State in *In re Storar*.[33]

John Storar was a fifty-two-year-old mentally retarded man with a mental age of eighteen months. He was diagnosed with terminal bladder cancer. His mother and guardian requested that blood transfusions, which he required periodically, be discontinued. The court heard testimony that Storar's life expectancy was three to six months, and that he found the transfusions disagreeable. The court, relying on the rule that a parent may not deprive a child of LST, no matter how well intentioned, held that the application for permission to continue the transfusions should have been granted. In essence, the court employed a best interest standard and decided that prolongation of life was in Storar's best interests.

Forgoing Treatment on the Basis of Medical Futility

It is well established that there is no ethical obligation for physicians to provide treatment that is medically futile.[34,35] The difficulty, however, lies in deciding what constitutes futile treatment. Unfortunately, *medical futility* can have several meanings. Failure to clarify the term can lead to miscommunication and the masking of differing value judgments and biases, thus enabling a subtle form of paternalism.[36] For example, in explaining to a patient that CPR would be futile, it is not uncommon for the physician to mean that CPR would have a very low chance of success, whereas the patient interprets the meaning of the term *futile* to be that treatment has no possibility of success. If the patient then agrees to forgo CPR, the decision will have been based on a misunderstanding. For this reason, it is important to be explicit about these matters by using plain language instead of hiding value judgments under the cloak of medical futility.

Medical futility can be conceptualized and organized in various ways. (See Chapter 5 for a discussion of medical futility in the context of the internal morality of medicine.) Medical futility may be divided into the categories of post-hoc futility and predictive futility. In *post-hoc futility,* treatment has been tried and has failed. One sees in retrospect that a treatment that perhaps held out some hope has proven to be futile. Post-hoc futility is useless for those who want to use futility as a reason not to try a treatment in the first place. *Predictive futility,* on the other hand, involves predicting that a treatment will be futile and therefore should not be tried.

Predictive futility can be divided into several types: conceptual futility, probabilistic futility, physiologic futility, and doctor–patient goal disagreements. *Conceptual futility* is futility based on a particular concept or definition, an example being brain death. The medicolegal concept of death holds that ventilator-dependent patients who have suffered "irreversible cessation of all functions of the entire brain including the brain stem" are dead.[37] In such cases, the ventilator is by definition a futile intervention because it cannot bring the patient back to life. Although brain death has become a medicolegal standard in the United States, some have voiced religious objections to the standard. Because of this, at least two states have passed laws allowing a "religious exemption" to the brain death standard (see Chapter 13). Apart from religious reasons, cases have occurred in which family members simply do not accept that their brain dead loved one is in fact dead. In these cases, the law would allow physicians to discontinue the ventilator without family permission. In practice, however, despite the fact that continued ventilator use is conceptually futile, time is usually allotted to the family to come to terms with the patient's death before the ventilator is removed.

Probabilistic futility means that a treatment with a very low chance of success can properly be regarded as futile. For example, some would characterize as futile the resuscitation of a patient with a one percent chance of surviving CPR. This kind of futility is never absolute, and it entails making value judgments about what risks are worth taking. Health care professionals should not make unilateral probabilistic futility judgments because their values may not reflect those of the patient. Instead, the information should be communicated to the patient, and a process of shared decision making should be followed.

Physiologic futility comes in two forms. The first is called *medical nonsense;* the second is *medical impasse.* An example of medical nonsense is a patient's request for antibiotics to treat a viral upper-respiratory infection. In this case, the physician can unilaterally refuse to give antibiotics on the ground that antibiotics are a futile intervention. There is no possibility of benefit, whereas the potential for harm (e.g., antibiotic-induced diarrhea) remains. Medical impasse occurs when a person's illness makes it physiologically impossible for sensible treatments to work. An example of this is a person with AIDS and *Pneumocystis* pneumonia who develops adult respiratory distress syndrome. If such a person were to suffer cardiac arrest, ordinarily CPR would be a sensible and indicated response. However, in the case where the infection has proven refractory to all available treatments and where gas exchange has become critically impaired and is worsening, CPR cannot possibly be effective. Once acidemia and ischemia produce cardiac arrest, it is physiologically impossible for CPR and cardiac medication to restore vital air exchange. Thus, there is medical impasse and absolute physiologic futility. In such a case, a physician can unilaterally decide not to perform CPR on the ground of medical futility.

The last futility concept is *doctor–patient goal disagreement.* In the case of Helga Wanglie,[38,39] a ventilator-dependent patient in a permanent vegetative state, the physician regarded the ventilator as futile because it could not improve the patient's status and thus benefit the patient. The patient's husband, however, did not see the ventilator as futile because it was keeping his wife alive. In this case, we have a disagreement between two different goals. The ventilator could not meet the physician's goal of health improvement, but it could meet the husband's goal of life prolongation. In such cases where value differences exist about what goals are worth pursuing, the decision should be a shared one between the doctor and the patient (or the patient's surrogate or proxy). The physician would not be justified in making a unilateral decision to discontinue the ventilator. On the other hand, the physician who believes that continued ventilation would be morally objectionable is free to preserve his or her moral integrity by withdrawing from the case.

Physician Aid in Dying

Physician aid in dying implicates the principles of beneficence and nonmaleficence and the moral rules "do not kill," "do not break the law," and "do not neglect your duty." Physicians can render aid in dying in a number of ways, some of them permissible and some of them not. We shall explore some of them in this section. First we provide a brief account of the law as it relates to killing.

Homicide

Homicide is "the killing of one human being by the act . . . or omission of another."[24(p506)] Homicide can be wrongful (e.g., *criminal homicide,* which includes the offenses of murder[40] and manslaughter[41]) or not. Examples of homicide that is not wrongful include *excusable homicide* (e.g., the killing of another human being in self-defense) and *justifiable homicide* (e.g., "as where a sheriff lawfully executes a sentence of death upon a malefactor"[24(p506)]).

It is important to note here that the victim's consent is not a defense in criminal homicide. The fact that a victim consented to the act(s) of the defendant is only a defense in those crimes in which consent—or more accurately the lack thereof—is an element of the offense. Thus, proof that a female consented to sexual intercourse is a defense against a charge of forcible rape.

Voluntary Passive Euthanasia

The first type of physician aid in dying may be referred to as *voluntary passive euthanasia* (VPE). VPE is defined as the withdrawal or withholding of life-sustaining treatment in accordance with the wishes of a competent patient or duly appointed surrogate or proxy. This is a type of physician aid in dying that we have spent much of this chapter discussing already. Consider an irreversibly incapacitated, terminally ill patient who had earlier prepared an advance directive stipulating that mechanical ventilation should not be used if his or her capacity were irreversibly lost and the disease were terminal. If these criteria are met before the need for ventilation arises, then the ventilator should not be started. If the ventilator was started before the patient became terminal and irreversibly incapacitated, then the ventilator should be discontinued once these conditions have been clearly met. In withholding or withdrawing ventilatory support, the physician's aid in dying is permissible because he or she is not causing death but is appropriately removing a form of external medical support that the patient refused in advance. The natural forces of the patient's illness continue unopposed once the ventilator is removed, and quite predictably, the patient dies. The patient's death is caused by the disease rather than by the physician.

"[N]o physician has suffered civil or criminal liability for withdrawing life-sustaining treatment at the request of a patient or the patient's family."[14(p543)] Perhaps the closest anyone has come was in *Barber v. Superior Court.*[42] In that case, a patient suffered anoxic brain damage after a cardiac arrest and entered a vegetative state that was felt would be permanent. Upon the family's request that all life-sustaining treatment be stopped, physicians discontinued ventilator support and tube feedings. After the patient died, prosecutors brought murder charges against the patient's physicians. The court recognized the family's authority to refuse LST on the patient's behalf, and concluded that "the [physicians'] omission to continue treatment under the circumstances, though intentional and with knowledge that the patient would die, was not an unlawful failure to perform a legal duty."[42(p493)]

Physician-Assisted Suicide

The second type of physician aid in dying is referred to as *physician-assisted suicide* (PAS). In PAS, the physician provides the patient with the medical know-how and/or the means enabling the patient to end his or her own life. An example of PAS would be the case of

Dr. Timothy Quill, who in 1991 reported in the medical literature that he had prescribed a lethal dose of barbiturates for a terminally ill patient.[43]

In the United States there is a statutory right to PAS in Oregon. The measure ("Measure 16") was originally approved in a 1994 referendum, fifty-one percent to forty-nine percent. Following a series of unsuccessful legal challenges in the courts by the law's opponents, another referendum was held, and this time the Oregon Death with Dignity Act was reaffirmed sixty percent to forty percent.

The act allows a terminally ill patient with decisional capacity to obtain a lethal prescription from a physician. The patient must be eighteen years of age or older and a resident of Oregon. He or she must be capable of making and communicating health care decisions for himself or herself (in other words, no proxy or surrogates can request PAS) and must be diagnosed with a terminal illness that will lead to death within six months, as verified by two physicians. Additionally, there is a fifteen-day waiting period. Somewhat disingenuously, there is contained within the act a provision that reads: "Actions taken in accordance with this Act shall not for any purpose, constitute suicide, assisted suicide, mercy killing or homicide, under the law."[44]

In response, on November 6, 2001, U.S. attorney general John Ashcroft issued a new interpretation of the Controlled Substances Act that would have subjected physicians prescribing controlled substances for use in PAS to loss of their DEA licenses. (To date, all the medications prescribed under the Death with Dignity Act have been barbiturates, which are controlled substances.) The State of Oregon challenged this move in federal court, and prevailed before the U.S. District Court. Attorney General Ashcroft subsequently lost appeals before the Ninth U.S. Circuit Court of Appeals and the U.S. Supreme Court. Thus, Oregon's Death with Dignity Act remains in effect.[45] Since its enactment in 1997, some 326 lethal prescriptions have been written, and some 246 Oregonians have taken their own lives under the assisted suicide law.

In November 2008, the state of Washington became the second state to allow PAS, when Initiative 1000 was approved by Washington voters.[46]

Voluntary Active Euthanasia

The generic term *euthanasia* refers to "the act or practice of painlessly putting to death persons suffering from incurable and distressing disease as an act of mercy."[24(p384)] Thus described, euthanasia is commonly distinguished from murder because its motive is merciful rather than malicious; however, it is nevertheless a form of wrongful homicide and remains illegal in the United States. When the physician performs euthanasia with the consent of the patient, it is called *voluntary active euthanasia* (VAE). Again, the term is applied to the physician who actively, directly, and intentionally causes the death of a competent patient who requests aid in dying. For example, a physician commits VAE when he or she deliberately injects a lethal amount of potassium chloride into a patient requesting aid in dying for the express purpose of terminating that patient's life.

An example of VAE is Jack Kevorkian's videotaped killing of Thomas Youk, a fifty-two-year-old man with ALS in September 1998. On the tape, Kevorkian is seen injecting Youk with muscle relaxants followed by a lethal dose of potassium chloride. The videotape was broadcast to a national television audience in November 1998 on the CBS program *60 Minutes*, after which Kevorkian was charged by prosecutors.[47] He was convicted of second-degree murder in March 1999,[48] and paroled in 2007.

Nonvoluntary Euthanasia and Involuntary Euthanasia

When euthanasia is performed without patient choice (such as may be the case with incapacitated patients) it is called *nonvoluntary* or *nonchoice euthanasia*. This is arguably what transpired in the anonymous *JAMA* piece entitled "It's Over, Debbie." Therein, a gynecology resident purports to have administered a lethal dose of morphine to a twenty-year-old patient (whom the resident did not know) dying of ovarian cancer, in response to the patient's ambiguous supplication, "Let's get it over with."[49] *Involuntary euthanasia* involves performing euthanasia against the patient's wishes.[50]

Physician Aid in Dying: Law and Ethics

Although Oregon and Washington allow PAS, the Hippocratic Oath, to which American medicine has traditionally appealed for its moral bearings, expressly prohibits both PAS and euthanasia. The oath reads, "Neither will I administer a poison to anybody when asked to do so, nor will I suggest such a course."[51] It is telling to note that during the time of Hippocrates, when medicine's power to effectively treat disease and ameliorate suffering was far less than it is today, assisted suicide and euthanasia were regarded as radically incompatible with the role of the physician. This at least suggests that those in favor of PAS and euthanasia have very different ideas about the role of the physician and the moral limits of medicine. It is also telling that the public interest in physician aid in dying comes at a time when the palliative powers of American medicine are greater than they have ever been before. This suggests the possibility that the public might be unaware of the advances and availability of palliative medicine or that palliative care is woefully underutilized. Whereas this is no doubt the case for some portion of the public, others in our society wish to have PAS and euthanasia available as options along with the benefits of palliative care. The chief argument for this is based on autonomy, but it is an argument that begs the question of whether it is proper for a physician to play an active role in causing a person's death via lethal doses of medication.

In PAS and euthanasia, the core ethical issue for medicine is the rightfulness or wrongfulness of a physician intending and acting to cause the death of a patient. Unfortunately, this issue is easily obfuscated. An example of this occurred in *Quill v. Vacco*, one of two federal appellate court cases that argued for a right to hasten death.[52,53] The Second Circuit Court's opinion in *Quill* argued that a person has a right to hasten death but that laws prohibiting physician-assisted suicide prevent the equal exercise of this right. This can be illustrated with an example involving two similarly situated patients. Patient A has terminal lung disease and is on a ventilator, whereas patient B is terminal with AIDS and is not on a ventilator. According to the *Quill* court's logic, patient A is able to hasten his or her death by directing that the ventilator be discontinued, whereas patient B cannot hasten his or her death because the law regards PAS as a crime. The court concluded that laws prohibiting PAS were unconstitutional because the laws set up an inequality.

The reality is that courts have not traditionally recognized a right to hasten one's own death; instead, they have consistently framed the matter as a right to refuse unwanted medical intervention. In this view, patient A exercises the right to refuse unwanted intervention by directing doctors to discontinue the ventilator. Similarly, patient B exercises the right to refuse unwanted intervention by deciding not to go on a ventilator in the first place. Because both patients exercise the same right, there is no inequity in the law. The Second Circuit's notion that patient A is hastening death by discontinuing the ventilator betrays a failure to recognize the vital difference between killing and allowing to die. Furthermore, in suggesting that discontinuing the ventilator hastens death, the court implies that patient A's ventilator has somehow become intrinsic to patient A.[54] The reality is that the ventilator is a form of optional external medical support. The decision to discontinue its use is not a decision to hasten death but a decision to cease forestalling it. Failure to make careful distinctions between killing and allowing to die and between hastening and forestalling death unnecessarily adds to the confusion surrounding the physician's role in end-of-life care.

The Legal Slippery Slope

The U.S. Supreme Court overruled the decisions of the two federal appellate courts that had held state laws prohibiting PAS to be unconstitutional.[55-57] However, the Supreme Court did not say that states were obligated to prohibit the practice. This left the door open for states to follow Oregon's lead in legalizing PAS, as Washington has now done. The Oregon law was careful not to characterize PAS as a right, but if it is ever deemed to be one in future court decisions, this designation will almost certainly entail the extension of this right to incompetent patients, just as has been the case with the right to refuse treatment. In the latter cases, court after court has agreed that losing the capacity to exercise a right does not mean that the right no longer exists. Furthermore, to prevent the right from being extinguished in a practical sense, some other person must exercise the right of the incapacitated patient for that patient. Thus the process of proxy decision making came into being. This same process could take place with PAS, especially when the courts begin to see cases involving incapacitated patients who had earlier stipulated that they would want physician aid in dying in the event of terminal illness and irreversible loss of capacity. If PAS is regarded as a right, it too will very likely be extended to incapacitated patients in order to avoid the practical extinction of their rights. However, because the patient will not be able to exercise this right, proxy decision making would be employed. Also, because the incapacitated patient would not be able to participate in PAS, the act would likely fall to the physician. Thus, we will have moved to a form of voluntary euthanasia.

Consider too that if this right were extended to incapacitated terminal patients who left no past instructions regarding physician aid in dying (as it has been in the case with the right to refuse treatment), then we would have legalized nonvoluntary euthanasia. Proxies and physicians would then be making the euthanasia decision based on their belief that it is the decision that the patient would have made, or because it is deemed to be in the patient's "best interest" to be dead. The fact that such potential exists in our legal system, which judges cases and advances law by ruling on precedent, should give us pause. Alternatively, the current effectiveness of palliative care in addressing the full spectrum of end-of-life issues leaves us with no good reason to throw open the door of euthanasia that Oregon and Washington have left ajar. Efforts should instead be made to optimize the use of palliative care and to make it available to all who need it.

Issues in Hospice and Palliative Care

Even if palliative care is optimized, there are still issues that have the potential to blur the line between causing death and allowing death to take place naturally. Hospice and palliative medicine is devoted to maximizing quality of life in patients with life-limiting disease. A central focus of hospice and palliative medicine is to relieve distressing symptoms at the end of life. In doing so, physicians must use medication such as morphine and related compounds to relieve pain. A potential problem with morphine is its ability to depress respiration. If too much is given to the patient, it is possible for the patient to stop breathing and to die. For this reason, morphine and other opiates need to be used with caution. Because of fear of respiratory depression and hastening death, morphine is often underdosed by physicians, and consequently pain is inadequately addressed.

The reality is that morphine, in proper hands, is a safe medication. Although there is a possibility of respiratory depression, it is a dose-dependent early effect seen with rapid dose escalation. The effect extinguishes within a short time, and is not seen in cancer patients on chronic stable doses of morphine. With proper dosing, respiratory depression can easily be avoided altogether, and so remain a nonissue.[58] It is a myth that any use of morphine necessarily hastens death through respiratory depression. The risk of respiratory depression does exist, however, in cases of pain crisis in which morphine must be escalated quickly. In such cases, the possibility that morphine might contribute to shortening life provides us with an opportunity to revisit the rule of the double effect. (See Case 2-C on page 53.)

If we had a drug that was as effective as morphine but had no adverse effect on respiration, we would be obligated to use it instead of morphine. But no such drug yet exists. Thus we are left with drugs that have double effects. The only morally justifiable use of these medications is to use them in a way that achieves the good effect, while minimizing the risk of the bad effect. When you think about it, this approach attempts to reconcile the principle of beneficence with the principle of nonmaleficence (do no harm).

Chapter Summary

The right to refuse medical treatment is well established in medicine and in law and includes the right to refuse life-sustaining treatment. This right is not, however, absolute; whether framed as a right to privacy, as a common law right to refuse medical treatment, or more modernly as a Fourteenth Amendment liberty interest, it must be balanced against four countervailing societal or state interests: the preservation of life, the prevention of suicide, the protection of innocent third parties, and the safeguarding of the ethical integrity of the medical profession.

End-of-life decision making is facilitated by dividing patients into three categories: (1) patients possessing current decisional capacity (or competency), (2) patients without current decisional capacity but who possessed decisional capacity in the past, and (3) patients who never possessed decisional capacity. Patients in the second category may be further subdivided into patients who had expressed treatment preferences regarding end-of-life care in an advance directive prior to losing decisional capacity, and those patients who had not. Patients with current decision-making capacity are accorded broad discretion regarding refusal of even LST. The right of patients who executed an advance directive (prior to losing decisional capacity) to refuse LST may be exercised by a health care provider acting in accordance with instructions provided in a living will or by a health care surrogate. The right of patients who have not executed an advance directive (prior to losing decisional capacity) to refuse LST may be exercised by a proxy, provided that there is clear and convincing evidence either that the decision would have been the one the patient would have chosen, or (if there is no indication of what the patient would have chosen) that it is in the patient's best interests. Courts will allow LST to be withheld or withdrawn from patients who never possessed decisional capacity where doing so is in the patients' best interests.

Physician aid in dying includes voluntary passive euthanasia (morally and legally permissible), physician-assisted suicide (morally impermissible; legally permissible in the U.S. only in Oregon and Washington), and voluntary active euthanasia (morally and legally impermissible). Physician aid in dying implicates the principles of beneficence and nonmaleficence and the moral rules "do not kill," "do not break the law," and "do not neglect your duty."

Review Questions

1. List the four state interests that weigh against an individual's right to refuse life-sustaining treatment.

2. List the three decision-making standards discussed in this chapter. How do they differ from each other?

3. Who makes health care decisions for the patient with current decisional capacity? For the patient who had capacity but lost it? For the patient who never had capacity?

4. List as many of the advance directives discussed in this chapter as you can.

5. How does a health care proxy differ from a health care surrogate?

6. What legal question did the U.S. Supreme Court decide in the *Cruzan* case?

7. How are voluntary passive euthanasia, physician-aided suicide, and voluntary active euthanasia alike? How do they differ?

Endnotes

1. *In the Matter of Karen Quinlan,* 355 A.2d 647 (N.J. 1976).
2. *Cruzan v. Director, Missouri Department of Health,* 497 U.S. 261 (1990).
3. See, for example, Walker RM. DNR in the OR: resuscitation as an operative risk. *JAMA* 1991;266(17):2407–2412.
4. Prioritized list of health services. Available at: http://www.oregon.gov/OHPPR/HSC/docs/Apr08Plist.pdf. Accessed July 13, 2008.
5. Beauchamp TL, Childress JF. *Principles of Biomedical Ethics.* 4th ed. New York: Oxford University Press, 1994.
6. *Schloendorff v. The Society of New York Hospital,* 105 N.E. 92 (N.Y. 1914).
7. Jonsen AR, Siegler M, Winslade WJ. *Clinical Ethics: A Practical Approach to Ethical Decisions in Clinical Medicine.* 5th ed. New York: McGraw-Hill, 2002.
8. Ingelfinger FJ. Arrogance. *N Engl J Med* 1980;303:1507–1511.
9. Emanuel EJ. A review of the ethical and legal aspects of terminating medical care. *Am J Med* 1988;84:291–301.
10. Gostin LO. Deciding life and death in the courtroom. From Quinlan to Cruzan, Glucksberg, and Vacco: a brief history and analysis of constitutional protection of the "right to die." *JAMA* 1997;278:1523–1528.
11. Kamisar Y. Are laws against assisted suicide unconstitutional? *Hastings Center Rep* 1993; 23(3):32–4l.
12. Not everyone would agree. See, for example, Justice Scalia's concurring opinion in *Cruzan:* "There is nothing distinctive about accepting death through the refusal of 'medical treatment' as opposed to accepting it through the refusal of natural food, or through the failure to shut off the engine and get out of the car after parking in one's garage after work."
13. See, for example, *In re Conroy,* 486 A.2d 1209 (N.J. 1985).
14. Hall MA, Bobinski MA, Orentlicher D. *Health Care Law and Ethics.* 7th ed. Austin, TX: Aspen Publishers, 2007:536.
15. *Bouvia v. Superior Court,* 225 Cal. Rptr. 297, 304–305 (Ct. App. 1986).
16. *Satz v. Permutter,* 379 So 359 (1980).
17. Florida Statutes, Title XLIV, Chapter 765. Health care advance directives. Available at: http://www.leg.state.fl.us/Statutes/index.cfm?App_mode=Display_Statute&URL=Ch0765/

titl0765.htm&StatuteYear=2007&Title=%2D%3E2007%2D%3EChapter%20765. Accessed July 18, 2008.

18. Florida Statutes, Title XLIV, Chapter 765.401. Available at: http://www.leg.state.fl.us/Statutes/index.cfm?App_mode=Display_Statute&Search_String=&URL=Ch0765/SEC401.HTM&Title=->2007->Ch0765->Section%20401#0765.401. Accessed July 18, 2008.

19. Florida Statutes, Title XLIV, Chapter 765.301-765.309. Available at: http://www.leg.state.fl.us/Statutes/index.cfm?App_mode=Display_Statute&Search_String=&URL=Ch0765/PART03.HTM. Accessed July 18, 2008.

20. *Matter of Westchester County Medical Center (O'Connor),* 72 N.Y.2d 517, 523, 531 N.E.2d 607, 608–609 (1988).

21. *Cruzan v. Harmon,* 760 S.W.2d 408, 416–417 (1988) (en banc).

22. *Knight v. Beverly Health Care Bay Manor Health Care Ctr.,* 820 So. 2d 92 (Ala. 2001).

23. *Rasmussen v. Fleming,* 154 Ariz. 207, 741 P.2d 674 (1987).

24. *Black's Law Dictionary.* Abridged 6th ed. St. Paul, MN: West Publishing, 1991:172.

25. *In re Fiori,* 438 Pa. Super. 610, 652 A.2d 1350 (1995).

26. Florida Statutes, Title XLIV, Chapter 765.101(1). Available at: http://www.leg.state.fl.us/Statutes/index.cfm?App_mode=Display_Statute&Search_String=&URL=Ch0765/SEC101.HTM&Title=->2007->Ch0765->Section%20101#0765.101. Accessed July 18, 2008.

27. Florida Statutes, Title XLIV, Chapter 765.101(16). Available at: http://www.leg.state.fl.us/Statutes/index.cfm?App_mode=Display_Statute&Search_String=&URL=Ch0765/SEC101.HTM&Title=->2007->Ch0765->Section%20101#0765.101. Accessed July 18, 2008.

28. Florida Statutes, Title XLIV, Chapter 765.205. Available at: http://www.leg.state.fl.us/Statutes/index.cfm?App_mode=Display_Statute&Search_String=&URL=Ch0765/SEC205.HTM&Title=->2007->Ch0765->Section%20205#0765.205. Accessed July 18, 2008.

29. Florida Statutes, Title XLIV, Chapter 765.101(11)(a) and (b). Available at: http://www.leg.state.fl.us/Statutes/index.cfm?App_mode=Display_Statute&Search_String=&URL=Ch0765/SEC101.HTM&Title=->2007->Ch0765->Section%20101#0765.101. Accessed July 18, 2008.

30. Florida Statutes, Title XLIV, Chapter 765.302. Available at: http://www.leg.state.fl.us/Statutes/index.cfm?App_mode=Display_Statute&Search_String=&URL=Ch0765/SEC302.HTM&Title=->2007->Ch0765->Section%20302#0765.302. Accessed July 18, 2008.

31. Florida Statutes, Title XLIV, Chapter 765.104. Available at: http://www.leg.state.fl.us/Statutes/index.cfm?App_mode=Display_Statute&Search_String=&URL=Ch0765/SEC104.HTM&Title=->2007->Ch0765->Section%20104#0765.104. Accessed July 18, 2008.

32. *Superintendent of Belchertown v. Saikewicz,* 370 NE2d 417 (Mass. 1977).

33. *In re Storar,* 420 N.E.2d 64 (N.Y. 1981).

34. Hippocrates: the art. In: Reiser SJ, Dyck AJ, Curran WJ, eds. *Ethics in Medicine: Historical Perspectives and Contemporary Concerns.* Cambridge, MA: MIT Press, 1977:6–7.

35. American Medical Association, Council on Ethical and Judicial Affairs. *Code of Medical Ethics: Current Opinions with Annotations.* Chicago: American Medical Association, 1996:8.

36. Lantos JD, Singer PA, Walker RM, et al. The illusion of futility in clinical practice. *Am J Med* 1989;87:81–84.

37. President's Commission for the Study of Ethical Problems in Medicine and Biomedical and Behavioral Research. *Defining Death: A Report on the Medical, Legal, and Ethical Issues in the Determination of Death.* Washington, DC: U.S. Government Printing Office, 1981.

38. Miles SH. Informed demand for "non-beneficial" medical treatment. *N Engl J Med* 1991;325:512–515.

39. Angell M. The case of Helga Wanglie: a new kind of "right to die" case. *N Engl J Med* 1991;325:511–512.

40. In a prosecution for murder, the state must prove (1) that the defendant voluntarily committed an act (or voluntarily failed to act where there was a duty to do so) that caused the death of the defendant, (2) that the defendant had a culpable intent, and (3) that the causative act or omission was the result of the culpable intention. States of mind that satisfy the culpable intent requirement for murder include intent to kill, intent to commit grievous bodily injury, reckless indifference to the value of human life, or intent to commit a nonhomicide felony. See Emanuel S. *Criminal Law.* Larchmont, NY: Emanuel Law Outlines, 1987.

41. There are two types of manslaughter—voluntary and involuntary. A conviction for voluntary manslaughter is proper when the facts establish what would otherwise be murder, but all of the following (mitigating) conditions are met: "(1) [the defendant] acts in response to a provocation that would be sufficient to cause a reasonable man to lose his self-control; (2) he in fact acts in a 'heat of passion'; (3) the lapse of time between the provocation and the killing is not great enough that a reasonable man would have 'cooled off' . . . ; and (4) he had not in fact 'cooled off' by the time he killed." See Emanuel S. *Criminal Law.* Larchmont, NY: Emanuel Law Outlines, 1987:234. "One whose behavior is grossly negligent may be liable for *involuntary manslaughter* if his conduct results in the accidental death of another person." Ibid., p. 241.

42. *Barber v. Superior Court,* 195 Cal. Rptr. 478 (Ct. App. 1983).

43. Quill TE. Death and dignity: a case of individualized decision making. *New Engl J Med* 1991;324:691.

44. Death with Dignity Act 127.880 s.3.14. Available at: http://www.oregon.gov/DHS/ph/pas/ors.shtml. Accessed July 18, 2008.

45. Eighth Annual Report on Oregon's Death with Dignity Act. Available at: http://www.oregon.gov/DHS/ph/pas/docs/year8.pdf See pp 6–7. Accessed July 17, 2008.

46. "Death with Dignity" act passes. Available at: http://seattletimes.nwsource.com/html/nation-world/2008352350_assistedsuicide05m.html. Accessed December 8, 2008.

47. CNN.com. Kevorkian case: video of killing shown to jury. Available at: http://www.cnn.com/2007/US/law/12/17/court.archive.kevorkian5/index.html. Accessed July 17, 2008.

48. Kevorkian convicted. Available at: http://www.mult-sclerosis.org/news/Mar1999/USnews KevorkianConvicted.html. Accessed July 17, 2008.

49. It's over, Debbie. *JAMA* 1988;259(2):272.

50. Euthanasia definitions. Available at: http://www.euthanasia.com/definitions.html. Accessed July 17, 2008.

51. *Hippocrates, with an English Translation by W. H. S. Jones.* The Loeb Classical Library. Cambridge, MA: Harvard University Press, 1923.

52. *Quill v. Vacco,* 80 F3d 716 (2d Cir 1996).

53. *Compassion in Dying v. Washington,* 850 F. Supp. 1454 (D.C. 1994).

54. Paola F and Walker R. Deactivating the implantable cardioverter-defibrillator: a biofixture analysis. *South Med J* 2000;93:20–23.

55. *Washington v. Glucksberg,* 117 S Ct. 2258 (1997).

56. *Vacco v. Quill,* 117 S Ct. 2293 (1997).

57. Paola F. How dead is the federal constitutional right to assisted suicide? *Am J Med* 1998;104(6):565–568.

58. LeGrand SB, Khawam EA, Walsh D, Rivera NI. Opioids, respiratory function, and dyspnea. *Am J Hosp Palliat Care* 2003;20:57.

Section IV

Law

Chapter 15

Health Law and Medical Malpractice

Roper. So now you'd give the Devil benefit of law!

More. Yes. What would you do? Cut a great road through the law to get after the Devil?

Roper. I'd cut down every law in England to do that!

More. Oh? And when the last law was down, and the Devil turned round on you—where would you hide, Roper, the laws all being flat? This country's planted thick with laws from coast to coast—man's laws, not God's—and if you cut them down—and you're just the man to do it—d'you really think you could stand upright in the winds that would blow then? Yes, I'd give the Devil benefit of law, for my own safety's sake.

—Robert Bolt, *A Man for All Seasons*

Chapter Learning Objectives
At the conclusion of this chapter the reader will be able to:

1. Understand health law, medical liability, and medical negligence and how they relate to one another

2. Define *negligence* and know the elements of medical malpractice (also known as medical negligence)

3. Understand the legal distinction between *nonfeasance* and *malfeasance*

4. Know and recognize the exceptions to the no-duty rule

5. Understand and apply the concept of standard of care

6. Understand the relationship between medical custom and the standard of care, and know and recognize the exceptions

7. Understand and distinguish between scientific causation and legal causation

8. Apply and distinguish the various tests for scientific causation

9. Understand and apply the concepts of actual damages, future damages, and the loss of a chance

We have seen previously that law and morality are related to each other. In our discussion of ethical theories (see Chapter 1), we considered natural law, which holds that an unjust or immoral law is not a valid law (*lex injusta non est lex*). Likewise, in our discussion of the moral rules as formulated by Gert and associates (see Chapter 3), one of the moral rules was "Obey the law," meaning that there is a *moral* duty to obey *legal* rules unless disobedience can be somehow justified. Additionally, throughout the text we have cited

339

legal authority, particularly case law, in illustrating concepts important to both law and morality.

In Section IV we turn more explicitly to a discussion of the law as it pertains to the practice of medicine.

Health Law

Health law is "law as it affects the professionals and institutions that deliver health care."[1] As such, health law addresses four major concerns: the quality of health care, the cost of health care, access to health care, and respect or concern for the interests of the patient.[2] The health law universe thus encompasses a number of smaller galaxies, including (but not limited to) the regulation of health care institutions; regulation and licensure of health care professionals; professional relationships in health care (such as medical staff privileges); health care business associations; liability of health care professionals, with which we are chiefly concerned in this chapter; liability of health care institutions, including managed care organizations; antitrust law; health care financing, both public and private; limitations on reproduction; abortion and fetal–maternal conflicts; wrongful birth, life, and conception; assisted conception; definitions of death; decision making regarding death and dying; and regulation of research involving human subjects.[1(ppxvii-xx)]

If we limit ourselves to one of these galaxies in particular—namely, the liability of health care professionals—we find that such liability can take various forms. For example, health care professionals may be held liable for deceptive or unfair business practices, for breach of contract, or for tortious behavior, with which we shall chiefly concern ourselves here.

A *tortious* act is a wrongful act that "subject[s] the actor to liability under the principles of the law of torts."[3] A *tort* is "a legal wrong committed upon the person or property of another independent of contract."[3] If someone (the plaintiff) sues you (the defendant) in tort, he or she is alleging that you violated some duty that you owed him or her and that the duty in question did not arise contractually.

There are three types or categories of torts: intentional torts, negligence, and strict liability. We shall not concern ourselves further here with strict liability. An *intentional tort* is a "wrong perpetrated by one who intends to do that which the law has declared wrong."[3] Thus, a battery (see Chapter 9) is an intentional tort. Contrast this with *negligence*, in which the wrongdoer fails to exercise sufficient or due care in doing what is otherwise permissible.

Medical Negligence (Medical Malpractice)

Negligence is conduct that falls below the standard of care established by law for the protection of others against an *unreasonable* risk of harm. (We shall have more to say about the concept of reasonableness later.) In order to prevail in a medical negligence action, a plaintiff must establish four elements: (1) that the defendant health care practitioner owed him or her a duty, (2) that the defendant health care practitioner breached that duty (i.e., that the defendant did not meet the standard of care), (3) that the plaintiff suffered some harm or damage against which the law provides protection, and (4) that it was the defendant health care practitioner's breach of duty that caused the harm or damage suffered.

Duty

The question of whether a particular defendant owed a legal duty to a particular plaintiff is a question of law for the court (judge) to decide, not a question of fact for the jury.[4(p128)] In terms of the duty element, American law distinguishes between acts (*feasances*) and omissions (*nonfeasances*).[4,5] Once a person acts, he or she is under a legal obligation to act reasonably. Stated otherwise, in the doing of an act (feasance), the actor owes a general duty of due care to those around him or her. If the actor improperly does something that he or she had a right to do, a *misfeasance* is said to have occurred.

On the other hand, with a few exceptions that we shall discuss later, the law does not require a person to act even when inaction might seem unreasonable. There is, in other words, no general duty of due care that applies to instances of nonfeasance.

> Suppose A, standing close by a railroad, sees a two-year-old babe on the track and a car approaching. He can easily rescue the child with entire safety to himself, and the instincts of humanity require him to do so. If he does not, he may, perhaps, justly be styled a ruthless savage and a moral monster; but he is not liable in damages for the child's injury, or indictable under the statute for its death. . . . The duty to do no wrong is a legal duty. The duty to protect against wrong is, generally speaking and excepting certain *intimate relations* . . . a moral obligation only, not recognized or enforced by law.[6] (Italics added)

"Intimate relations," of course, lie at the very heart of medical practice. Let's consider, therefore, exceptions to the no-duty rule. There are five such exceptions that we shall discuss here. These exceptions create duties to act when not acting would be unreasonable.

The first exception is the existence of a special relationship between the plaintiff and the defendant. For our purposes here, the most important such special relationship is the health care provider–patient relationship. Once a provider–patient relationship has come into existence and before it is lawfully terminated, the health care professional is legally obligated to behave reasonably vis-à-vis his or her patient whether that behavior consists of action (feasance) or inaction (nonfeasance). Thus, it stands to reason that if one of my patients suffers a cardiac arrest in my waiting room and I fail to tend to him because it was not his turn, the law will not accept (nor, likely, would the other patients in my waiting room) my argument that because this was an instance of nonfeasance I owed him no duty of care. Because of the special relationship existing between the patient and the health care professional, the law imposes on the health care professional an affirmative duty to act reasonably.

The second exception to the no-duty rule is the existence of a law creating an affirmative duty to act. An example of such a law is the Vermont rescue statute, the text of which reads as follows:

§ 519. Emergency medical care

(a) A person who knows that another is exposed to grave physical harm shall, to the extent that the same can be rendered without danger or peril to himself or without interference with important duties owed to others, give reasonable assistance to the exposed person unless that assistance or care is being provided by others.

(b) A person who provides reasonable assistance in compliance with subsection (a) of this section shall not be liable in civil damages unless his acts constitute gross negligence or unless he will receive or expects to receive remuneration. Nothing contained in this subsection shall alter existing law with respect to tort liability of a practitioner of the healing arts for acts committed in the ordinary course of his practice.

(c) A person who willfully violates subsection (a) of this section shall be fined not more than $100.00. (1967, No. 309 [Adj. Sess.], §§ 2–4, eff. March 22, 1968.)[7]

Many readers will probably recall that the violation of just such a statute provided the premise of the final episode of the NBC sitcom *Seinfeld*. In that episode, Jerry, George, Kramer, and Elaine are sentenced to a year in prison after they witness an overweight man being carjacked at gunpoint but make no attempt to help. This, according to the story line, was in contravention of a law then in effect in the fictional town of Latham, Massachusetts.[8]

The third exception to the no-duty rule is the existence of a contract creating an affirmative duty to act, illustrated by the case *Hiser v. Randolph*:[9]

> Mohave County General Hospital is the only hospital serving . . . Kingman, Arizona. It maintains an emergency room. . . . Dr. Randolph and seven other doctors, comprising the medical profession in the Kingman area . . . established a program with the hospital by which each would take turns in manning the emergency room as the "on call physician" for a 12-hour period.
>
> The on call physician was paid by the hospital at a basic rate of $100 for each day or shift served. . . .
>
> [Mrs.] Hiser went . . . to the emergency room at the hospital at 11:45 p.m. on June 12, 1973. She was in a semi-comatose condition and the nurse in charge of the emergency room evaluated her as appearing to be very ill. Mrs. Hiser had [brittle insulin-dependent diabetes]. . . . She had been treated in the emergency

room of the hospital on the preceding day by Dr. Arnold . . . , her regular physician.

. . . Upon being advised as to who the patient was, Dr. Randolph stated that he would not attend or treat Mrs. Hiser, and that the nurse should call Dr. Arnold. When the nurse called Dr. Arnold, he responded by stating that he would not come to the hospital and that the on call physician should attend Mrs. Hiser. The nurse relayed this information to Dr. Randolph, who again refused to see or attend Mrs. Hiser. . . . [Ultimately, the hospital Chief of Staff] Dr. Lingenfelter came to the hospital and attended Mrs. Hiser, arriving at approximately 12:30 a.m. . . . Dr. Lingenfelter stayed at the hospital throughout the night until Dr. Arnold arrived in the morning. Mrs. Hiser died at 11:00 a.m. on June 13.

Mrs. Hiser's widower sued Dr. Randolph. Dr. Randolph's legal defense was that by virtue of his not having acted, and in the absence of a preexisting physician–patient relationship between himself and Mrs. Hiser, the no-duty rule should apply. The court, however, would have none of it. The court conceded that, as a general rule, medical practitioners were free to contract for their services as they saw fit and that, in the absence of prior contractual obligations, they were free to refuse to treat patients even in emergencies. However, the court went on, under Arizona law a hospital (such as Mohave County General Hospital) providing emergency room services is obligated to provide those services to everyone in need. They wrote:

> In our opinion, Dr. Randolph, by . . . accepting payment from the hospital to act as the emergency room doctor "on call" personally became bound "to insure that all patients . . . treated in the Emergency Room receive the best possible care." . . .
> . . . Under these circumstances, the lack of a consensual physician-patient relationship before a duty to treat can arise has been waived.[9]

The fourth exception to the no-duty rule concerns the voluntary assumption of duty by the defendant. Once the defendant voluntarily begins to act (for example, to render assistance to the plaintiff), he or she must proceed with reasonable care and may not discontinue efforts if doing so would leave the plaintiff worse off than when assistance was begun.[4(pp117-201)]

In *Zelenko v. Gimbel Bros*, a woman became ill while in the defendant's department store.[10] The defendant's employees brought her to the store infirmary, where she was left for six hours without medical care, as a result of which she died. The court assumed that the defendant owed no duty to render assistance to the woman (i.e., assumed that had the defendant done nothing, the no-duty rule would have applied). This is another way of saying that there was no special relationship between plaintiff and defendant, and that there was no law creating a duty on the part of the defendant to act. Yet the plaintiff prevailed in the case because, having voluntarily undertaken to render assistance, the defendant was obligated to exercise due care in doing so.

The fifth exception to the no-duty rule is the defendant responsibility exception. Under this exception, the defendant will owe a duty of warning or assistance if the plaintiff's danger or injury is the result of the defendant's conduct. Originally, this exception applied only when the plaintiff's danger or injury was the result of the defendant's wrongful conduct (misfeasance or malfeasance). When the danger or injury resulted from the defendant's innocent conduct, the exception did not apply. This version of the exception yielded results that were problematic. Consider, for example the case of *Union Pacific Railway v. Cappier*.[11] In that case, the defendant railway was found to have non-negligently run a locomotive over the plaintiff, who had been walking on the tracks. The court decided that the railway owed no duty to render assistance to the victim. The more modern view holds that the defendant owes a duty of care to the plaintiff whenever the defendant's conduct—even if innocent—results in danger or injury to the plaintiff. Thus, state hit-and-run statutes routinely require drivers involved in an accident in which another is injured to render reasonable assistance.[12]

It should be noted here that Good Samaritan laws are not an exception to the no-duty rule, because they do not create a duty to act where none existed prior to the laws in question. The Good Samaritan doctrine holds that

> One who sees a person in imminent and serious peril through negligence of another cannot be charged with contributory negligence, as a matter of law, . . . in attempting to effect a rescue, provided the attempt is not recklessly or rashly made. . . . This protection from liability is provided by statute in most states.[3(p478)]

Consider, for example, the New York State Good Samaritan Act, which reads in part:

> [A]ny person who voluntarily and without expectation of monetary compensation renders first aid or emergency treatment at the scene of an accident or other emergency outside a hospital, doctor's office or any other place having proper and necessary medical equipment, to a person who is unconscious, ill, or injured, shall not be liable for damages for injuries alleged to have been sustained by such person or for damages for the death of such person alleged to have occurred by reason of an act or omission in the rendering of such emergency treatment unless it is established that such injuries were or such death was caused by gross negligence on the part of such person. Nothing in this section shall be deemed or construed to relieve a licensed physician, dentist, nurse, physical therapist or registered physician's assistant from liability for damages for injuries or death caused by an act or omission on the part of such person while rendering professional services in the normal and ordinary course of his or her practice.[13]

Good Samaritan laws exist to encourage bystanders (and health care professionals in particular) to render assistance to persons to whom they owe no legal duty. They do so by shielding such good Samaritans from liability in negligence. They do not shield the Samaritan whose behavior is reckless or intentionally tortious (e.g., performing chest compressions as a part of CPR by jumping up and down on the chest of a cardiac arrest victim of whom, it so happens, one is not fond). Good Samaritan laws are thus best thought of as being exceptions to an exception—specifically, to the fourth exception discussed earlier (the voluntary assumption of duty).

Let's recap here by revisiting the railroad hypothetical employed by the court in *Buch v. Amory Mfg. Co.*

> Suppose A, standing close by a railroad, sees a two-year-old babe on the track and a car approaching. He can easily rescue the child with entire safety to himself, and the instincts of humanity require him to do so. If he does not, he may, perhaps, justly be styled a ruthless savage and a moral monster; but he is not liable in damages for the child's injury, or indictable under the statute for its death.[6]

As we now know, however, if A and the toddler stand in some special relationship (exception 1)—for example, parent-child—then A may have a legal duty to rescue. If the episode takes place in Vermont or in *Seinfeld*'s fictional town of Latham (exception 2), A may owe a legal duty of rescue. If A is a babysitter or nanny who is being paid to watch the toddler (exception 3), he or she may have a legal duty to rescue. If two persons—A and B—are in a position to rescue the child and A waves B off like an outfielder ("I got it, I got it!"), then pulls out at the last instant, leaving B with no chance to rescue the child (exception 4), it is likely that A will be found to have owed the child a duty of rescue. Finally, if A is responsible for the toddler being on the tracks to begin with (exception 5)—for example, having malevolently placed the child there—then A owes the child a legal duty of rescue.

Standard of Care

Once it is established that the defendant health care practitioner owed the plaintiff a legal duty, the issue becomes "Did the defendant breach that duty?" Asked otherwise, "Did the defendant's conduct fall below the standard of care?"

In negligence cases in general, the *standard of care* is "that degree of care which a reasonably prudent person should exercise in same or similar circumstances."[3(p977)] One of the best enunciations of the standard of care as it applies specifically to medical negligence cases is from the 1898 New York case *Pike v. Honsiger:*

> The physician is under an obligation to exercise the same degree of knowledge, skill, diligence and care that the ordinary competent practitioner would exercise under the same or similar circumstances. The physician is under the further obligation to use his best judgment in exercising his skill and applying his knowledge.[14]

If you look closely at the first sentence of this selection, you'll see that essentially what has happened is that the word "practitioner" has been substituted for the word "person."

Generally, juries decide whether or not the standard of care has been met as a question of fact. Considering the complexity of medical practice, however, and the fact that most juries are not made up of health care practitioners, how are the "reasonably prudent persons" who presumably compose the jury supposed to know what an "ordinary competent practitioner" would do under the same or similar circumstances?

Custom-Based Standard of Care

The traditional rule in medical malpractice cases has been referred to as the *custom-based standard of care*.

> In most negligence actions, the defendant's compliance with industry customs is simply one factor for the jury to consider. . . . Since the late nineteenth century, courts have treated physicians quite differently. Medical customs are not merely admissible; they define the physician's legal standard of care. . . .
>
> . . . Under the custom-based standard of care, . . . the jury determines what the customary practice *is*. It does not decide what the custom *ought* to be. The law assigns the normative judgment to the medical profession.[15]

Under the custom-based standard, expert witnesses testify as to how "ordinary competent practitioners" customarily behave under circumstances similar to the case in question. Not surprisingly, the testimony of the plaintiff's experts usually supports the plaintiff's position, whereas the testimony of the defendant's experts usually supports the defendant's position.

There are, however, a number of exceptions to the general rule that what is medically customary establishes the standard of care in medical malpractice cases. We discuss six such exceptions here.

Reasonable Physician Standard of Care

First of all, there has been a recent retreat from the custom-based standard in some states, with movement toward a *reasonable physician standard*.

> Gradually, . . . state courts are abandoning the custom-based standard of care. Thus far, a dozen states have expressly refused to equate reasonable care with customary practices. . . . These states now use a "reasonable physician" test. Another nine states, although not explicitly addressing the role of custom, have also endorsed the "reasonable physician" test. In these states, . . . the jury decides whether the physician behaved reasonably, not whether she complied with custom. Although experts still battle in the courtroom, they argue about what physicians *should* do, not what physicians *ordinarily* do.
>
> In addition to the states that have moved to a reasonability standard, several other states have case law that is too ambiguous or inconsistent to classify con-

fidently. As a consequence, the fraction of states that unambiguously endorse the custom-based standard of care has fallen from a clear majority to a shrinking plurality.[15] (Footnotes omitted)

Statutes Establishing the Standard of Care

A second exception is when a statute establishes the standard of care. You may recall that we previously discussed the Baby K case[16] in Chapter 5 in the context of medical futility. To recap, Baby K was a female anencephalic infant born in October 1992 in Virginia. Because of perinatal respiratory distress, she was intubated and mechanically ventilated. Baby K's mother, Mrs. H, was told that no treatment existed for anencephaly and that no therapeutic or palliative purpose was served by continued mechanical ventilation. Nevertheless, she refused to consent to a do-not-resuscitate order.

The treating physicians consulted the institutional ethics committee, which concluded that ventilator support was futile and should be stopped after allowing Mrs. H a "reasonable time." Mrs. H rejected the committee's recommendation, and rather than pursuing legal action, the hospital took advantage of a window of opportunity—a period during which Baby K was not ventilator dependent—to transfer Baby K to a nursing home in November 1992.

Unfortunately, Baby K required readmission to the hospital in January and again in March 1993. Because it was expected that she would continue to experience episodes of respiratory distress requiring admission, intubation, and mechanical ventilation, the hospital finally commenced legal action, and a guardian was appointed to represent Baby K. The guardian agreed that ventilator support should be withheld from Baby K when she experienced respiratory distress. The hospital requested a declaratory judgment that the withholding of ventilator support would not be illegal.

In July 1993, the U.S. District Court for the Eastern District of Virginia held that, under the federal antidumping law (the Emergency Medical Treatment and Active Labor Act, or EMTALA), "the hospital would be liable . . . if Baby K arrived there in respiratory distress . . . and the hospital failed to provide [the] mechanical ventilation . . . necessary to stabilize her acute medical condition."[16]

EMTALA requires that hospitals provide stabilizing treatment to any person who comes to an emergency department in an "emergency medical condition," where "emergency medical condition" is defined as "acute symptoms of sufficient severity . . . such that the absence of immediate medical attention could reasonably be expected to result in . . . serious impairment to bodily functions, or serious dysfunction of any bodily organ or part."[17] EMTALA, the court wrote, "does not admit of any 'futility' . . . exceptions."[16]

Apart from the implications of the Baby K case for the doctrine of medical futility, the effect of the court's holding was to interpret the EMTALA statute as establishing the legal standard of care for the physicians and health care institutions involved in the case.

Judicial Risk–Benefit Balancing

A third exception to the rule that medical custom establishes the standard of care is when a court (or judge) establishes the standard of care on the basis of judicial risk–benefit balancing. Perhaps the most notorious case illustrating this exception in the medical context was *Helling v. Carey*.[18] In that case, a thirty-eight-year-old plaintiff who suffered visual loss as a result of undiagnosed open angle glaucoma brought an action against the defendant ophthalmologists alleging negligence on their part. During trial, both the plaintiff's and the defendants' medical experts agreed that the "standards of the profession for that specialty in the same or similar circumstances do not require routine pressure tests for glaucoma upon patients under 40 years of age."[18] Under the custom-based standard, the court should have upheld the trial court's verdict in favor of the defendants. Instead, the Supreme Court of Washington wrote:

> The issue is whether the defendants' compliance with the standard of the profession of ophthalmology . . . should insulate them from liability. . . .
>
> Justice Holmes stated in *Texas & Pac. Ry. v. Behymer,* 189 U.S. 468, 470, 23 S. Ct. 622, 623, 47 L. Ed. 905 (1903): "What usually is done may be evidence of what ought to be done, but what ought to be done is fixed by a standard of reasonable prudence, whether it is usually complied with or not." In The *T.J. Hooper,* 60 F.2d 737, on page 740 (2d Cir. 1932), Justice Hand stated: "[I]n most cases reasonable prudence is in fact common prudence; but strictly it is never its measure; a whole calling may have unduly lagged in the adoption of new and available devices. It may never set its own tests, however persuasive be its usages. *Courts must in the end say what is required.* . . ."
>
> We therefore hold, as a matter of law, that the reasonable standard that should have been followed under the undisputed facts of this case was the timely giving of this simple, harmless pressure test to this plaintiff and that, in failing to do so, the defendants were negligent.[18] (Italics added)

In effect, the court in *Helling v. Carey* decided what the legal standard of care for ophthalmologists should be. Unlike the situation in the Baby K case, it did so not in reliance on a statute, but rather in reliance on its own balancing of the costs and benefits of testing.

Informed Consent and the Standard of Care

The fourth exception is that medical custom is not uniformly determinative of the standard of care in the case of malpractice actions grounded in informed consent. You will recall from Chapters 8 and 9 that,

> [w]hile about half of American jurisdictions use a "professional malpractice" standard, under which physicians are required to disclose to patients that information which would have been disclosed by a reasonable, minimally competent

physician[,] . . . [a] substantial number of states use the "material risk" or "reasonable patient" standard, which requires disclosure of risks that a reasonable patient would consider to be material in making a medical treatment decision. A small number of jurisdictions take an even more protective approach, requiring disclosure of information that a particular patient (as contrasted with a[n objective,] "rational" patient) would have wanted to make his or her decision.[19]

It should be apparent that, in those jurisdictions that employ either the objective or the subjective patient-centered standard, the custom-based standard is not being followed.

Res Ipsa Loquitur

The fourth exception is the doctrine of *res ipsa loquitur*, which means "the thing speaks for itself."[3(p905)] It is not so much an exception to the rule that medical custom establishes the standard of care as it is an exception to the rule that expert witnesses must be employed to establish the standard of care in medical malpractice cases.

> [*Res ipsa loquitur* creates a r]ebuttable presumption or inference that [the] defendant was negligent. . . . [This presumption] arises upon proof [by the plaintiff] that [the] instrumentality causing injury was in the defendant's exclusive control, and that the accident was one which ordinarily does not happen in the absence of negligence. *Res ipsa loquitur* is [a] rule of evidence whereby [the] negligence of [the] alleged wrongdoer may be inferred from [the] mere fact that [the] accident happened.[3(p905)] (Italics added)

In the medical context, *Ybarra v. Spangard* illustrates the application of the doctrine.[20] In that case, the plaintiff underwent an appendectomy. Preoperatively "he had never had any pain in, or injury to, his right arm or shoulder." Postoperatively, however, he awoke with pain between the neck and right shoulder that worsened and ultimately resulted in an inability "to rotate or lift his arm, and developed paralysis and atrophy of the muscles around the shoulder."[20] Experts testified that the injury was one that normally results "from trauma or injury by pressure or strain, applied between his right shoulder and neck," but not that anyone in the operating room behaved uncustomarily. The plaintiff also established that the injury must have been caused by at least one of the operating room physicians, or a nurse under their control, although he could not establish which one of the defendants was responsible. The Supreme Court of California held that the doctrine of *res ipsa loquitur* could be applied.

Contract and the Standard of Care

The fifth exception to the rule that medical custom establishes the standard of care is when a patient sues a physician for breach of contract. These actions are grounded not in tort law but in the law of contracts, and they tend to arise when physicians make promises to patients regarding the outcome of treatment.

Thus in *Hawkins v. McGee,* 84 N.H. 114, 146 A. 641 (1929), the defendant doctor was taken to have promised the plaintiff to convert his damaged hand by means of an operation into a good or perfect hand, but the doctor so operated as to damage the hand still further. The court . . . asked the jury to estimate and award to the plaintiff the difference between the value of a good or perfect hand, as promised, and the value of the hand after the operation.[21]

A similar outcome was seen in *Sullivan v. O'Connor,* where the defendant surgeon was found to have promised the defendant, a professional entertainer,

to perform plastic surgery on her nose and thereby enhance her beauty and improve her appearance. . . . [H]e performed the surgery but failed to achieve the promised result; rather the result of the surgery was to disfigure and deform her nose, to cause her pain in mind and body, and to subject her to other damage and expense.[21]

In these contract cases, proof that the defendants operated in accordance with surgical custom was irrelevant. It mattered only that a contract existed (a discussion of the elements of which is beyond the scope of this book) and that the defendants did not deliver the results they were found to have promised. In effect, by making promises, the defendants established their own individualized standard of care.

Best Judgment Rule

Before turning to the third element of negligence—causation—we have one more loose end to tie up. Look again at the enunciation of the standard of care in medical negligence cases cited earlier:

The physician is under an obligation to exercise the same degree of knowledge, skill, diligence and care that the ordinary competent practitioner would exercise under the same or similar circumstances. *The physician is under the further obligation to use his best judgment in exercising his skill and applying his knowledge.*[14] (Italics added)

What, you might ask, is the effect of including this second sentence in the formulation of the medical standard of care? The best way to answer this is by considering Case 15-A.

Case 15-A Burton v. Brooklyn Doctors Hospital

Plaintiff Daniel Burton was born six weeks prematurely on July 3, 1953, at Brooklyn Doctors Hospital.[22] He was transferred the next day to New York Hospital.

Just two days earlier, "a national human research study known as the Cooperative Study of Retrolental Fibroplasia [RLF] and the Use of Oxygen was undertaken to determine the role of oxygen in RLF and the effect of its withdrawal or curtailment." The Cooperative Study would

Case 15-A   Burton v. Brooklyn Doctors Hospital (*continued*)

go on to find that "the prolonged liberal use of oxygen was the critical factor in the development of RLF, and that curtailing oxygen to premature infants after 48 hours to clinical need decreased the incidence of RLF without increasing the risk of death or brain damage." The Cooperative Study's conclusions were announced on September 19, 1954, and published in October of 1956, one year and three years, respectively, after the events in question.

Although at the time of Daniel Burton's admission to New York Hospital "liberal exposure to oxygen continued to be routine treatment for premature babies . . . , the view that more oxygen was better had already become suspect. In fact, New York Hospital had, from January 1952 to June 1953, conducted its own study and concluded that 'prolonged oxygen therapy may be related to the production of RLF.' The results of that 18-month study were announced by the hospital on June 16, 1953 [over two weeks before Daniel Burton's admission], at a meeting attended by its pediatricians and ophthalmologists." Because the results of its own study were deemed preliminary and insufficient, the hospital decided to become a participant in the Cooperative Study. This was the situation that existed on July 4, 1953, when the plaintiff entered New York Hospital.

Upon Daniel Burton's arrival, Dr. Lawrence Ross, a pediatric resident, ordered that the plaintiff be placed in an incubator with oxygen to be delivered at 3 to 4 liters per minute. That same evening, Dr. Ross, aware that oxygen had been implicated as a cause of RLF, ordered that oxygen be "reduced as tolerated."

On July 6, Dr. Mary Engle, an instructor in pediatrics and coauthor of the New York Hospital study mentioned earlier, on instructions from Dr. Levine (the chairman of the Department of Pediatrics) and without ever examining the plaintiff or speaking to his parents, entered the following order in his medical record: "Oxygen study: In prolonged oxygen at concentration greater than 50%." As a result of Dr. Engle's order, the concentration of oxygen to which the plaintiff was being exposed was increased over a span of twenty-eight days from thirty percent to a high of eighty-two percent. "Except for faint light perception in his left eye, plaintiff is totally blind and, because his eyes are shrinking, will require enucleation and replacement with plastic ones."

In a lawsuit brought against Drs. Ross and Engle, how should the case be decided?

Analysis

It should be apparent that the principal issue here is whether each of the defendants met the standard of care. Did they "follow sound medical practice in 1953 in permitting plaintiff to be exposed to an increased oxygen environment for a prolonged period, even though it was common practice at the time, when they were aware of the possibility that RLF might result"? Let us consider each of the defendants in turn.

If you apply only the first sentence of the previously discussed enunciation of the medical standard of care to Dr. Engle—"The physician is under an obligation to exercise the same degree of knowledge, skill, diligence, and care that the ordinary competent practitioner would

(*continues*)

Case 15-A   Burton v. Brooklyn Doctors Hospital (*continued*)

exercise under the same or similar circumstances"—the answer would have to be that yes, she met the standard of care, because there was at least a respectable minority of physicians, and quite possibly a majority, who were still proponents of oxygen use in July 1953. However, once you apply the second sentence to Dr. Engle—"The physician is under the further obligation to use his best judgment in exercising his skill and applying his knowledge"—the conclusion you reach is that no, she did not meet the standard of care because even though use of oxygen in premature infants was medically customary at the time, *she knew better*. In other words, she did not follow her best judgment. The appellate court found particularly illuminating the fact that in New York Hospital's involvement in the Cooperative Study, two out of every three babies enrolled in the study were given curtailed oxygen—a tacit admission on the part of the hospital that it believed curtailment of oxygen was preferable.

Dr. Ross, on the other hand, whose order to reduce oxygen was countermanded, did not breach his duty of due care to the plaintiff. In ordering that oxygen be "reduced as tolerated," he was following both his best judgment (subjective standard) and the opinion of at least a respectable minority of "ordinary competent practitioners" (objective standard) who had come to believe that oxygen use in premature infants was detrimental.

The appellate court decided that Dr. Engle and the hospital had failed in their duty to the plaintiff, and that Dr. Ross was not liable.

Causation

The third element in a medical malpractice case involves inquiry into whether the defendant health care practitioner's negligence caused the harm for which the patient is suing. This is a compound inquiry, involving two distinct types of causation: *cause-in-fact* (also known as *scientific causation*) and *proximate causation* (also known as *legal causation*). We discuss each in turn.

Scientific Causation (Cause-in-Fact)

Scientific causation is a question of fact for the jury (or the judge when he or she acts as the finder of fact).

> [T]he plaintiff, in general, has the burden of proof. He must introduce evidence which affords a reasonable basis for the conclusion that it is *more likely than not* that the conduct of the defendant [caused] the result. A mere possibility of such causation is not enough; and when the matter remains one of pure speculation or conjecture, or the probabilities are at best evenly balanced, it becomes the duty of the court to direct a verdict for the defendant.[23]

A number of tests are traditionally employed in determining whether the defendant's conduct caused the plaintiff's damages. The most commonly employed test is the "but for" test. Under this test, the defendant's conduct is the cause-in-fact of the plaintiff's injury if the injury would not have occurred but for the defendant's conduct. Consider, for example, a case in which a passing motorist throws the remains of a lighted cigarette into the plaintiff's front yard, which catches fire and destroys the plaintiff's house. The plaintiff identifies and sues the motorist. Is the motorist's conduct the cause-in-fact of the homeowner's injury? Clearly it is.

Now imagine that the property of the above plaintiff lies between two parallel roads, one running past the front yard and another running past the backyard. Suppose that each of two passing motorists (defendants A and B) throws the remains of a lighted cigarette onto the defendant's property (defendant A into the front yard, defendant B into the backyard). The two separate fires that result simultaneously consume the plaintiff's house. Either fire alone would have been sufficient to destroy the plaintiff's house and property. Is defendant A's conduct the cause-in-fact of the homeowner's injury? The answer under the "but for" test would seem to be no, because the plaintiff's injury would have occurred even absent of defendant A's conduct. Further, it should be apparent that if we subject defendant B's conduct to the same test, we would be left with the same result. Applying the "but for" test of causation in this scenario leaves the unfortunate plaintiff without any remedy in tort and unjustly allows both negligent defendants to avoid liability.

To avoid such inequitable outcomes in cases where, as just described, joint causes are involved, the law has fashioned an alternative test of actual scientific causation, the so-called substantial factor test. Under this test, the defendant's conduct is the cause-in-fact of the plaintiff's injury if the defendant's conduct was a substantial factor in causing the injury. Applying this test, one finds that the conduct of defendant A was a cause-in-fact of the plaintiff's injury, as was the conduct of defendant B.

A third test of scientific causation is illustrated in the discussion of Case 15-B.

Case 15-B   Summers v. Tice

Defendants Tice and Simonson were hunting quail with the plaintiff when both fired in his direction.[24] The plaintiff was struck in the eye and in the lip. "Both defendants were using the same gauge shotgun and the same size shot. The trial judge sitting without a jury found both defendants negligent and found that the plaintiff was in no way at fault. Unable to decide which defendant's shot hit the plaintiff, the judge awarded judgment against both defendants, who appealed."[4(p216)] The obvious question is, How was scientific causation established against each of the defendants?

Analysis

You will recall from the previous discussion that the plaintiff "must introduce evidence which affords a reasonable basis for the conclusion that it is *more likely than not* that the conduct of

(continues)

Case 15-B   Summers v. Tice (*continued*)

the defendant [caused] the result . . . [or else] it becomes the duty of the court to direct a verdict for the defendant."[23] Because "the court was unable to ascertain whether the [two] shots [that struck the plaintiff] were from the gun of one defendant or the other or [whether] one shot [came] from each of them,"[24] it would seem that the court would have no choice but to direct a verdict[25] for the defendants in this case. This is true whichever of the two scientific causation tests discussed earlier we choose to employ. We simply do not know whether Tice or Simonson or both were responsible for the plaintiff's injuries.

On the other hand, we do know that both defendants were found to have fired negligently in the plaintiff's direction (they owed a duty of due care to the plaintiff, which they breached); and we know that at least one, and possibly both, of the defendants caused the plaintiff's injury. That being the case, the directing of a verdict for the defendants would allow at least one of them and quite possibly both of them to unjustly avoid liability.

To avoid this injustice, the court employed yet a third test of scientific causation, which for our purposes here we shall call the "*Summers v. Tice*" test. Under this test, which is employed when *alternative* rather than *joint* causes are involved, "where the plaintiff can show that each of two persons was negligent, [though] only one could have caused the injury, . . . [it is] up to each defendant to show that the other caused the harm." In other words, in such cases courts will shift the burden of proof from the plaintiff to the defendant in the interests of fairness and justice.

You may recall the case of *Ybarra v. Spangard*, discussed earlier in the context of *res ipsa loquitur*. Remember that in that case the plaintiff could not establish which of the defendants was responsible for his injury. In that case, too, the court employed an alternative-causes type of test of scientific causation, writing:

> We . . . hold that where a plaintiff receives unusual injuries while unconscious and in the course of medical treatment, all those defendants who had any control over his body or the instrumentalities which might have caused the injuries may properly be called upon to meet the inference of negligence by giving an explanation of their conduct.[20]

Legal Causation (Proximate Causation)

Legal causation is more difficult to explain to nonlawyers. It is probably best understood as a means of limiting liability in the interest of justice or fairness. The test of legal causation is based on *foreseeability*. The general rule of proximate causation is that a defendant is liable for all of the harmful results that fall within the increased risk caused by his acts; that is, if the defendant's act increases the risk of a particular harmful result occurring, and that harmful result does occur, the defendant's act is said to be the proximate cause of the harm.

Consider the following examples:

> A chauffeur negligently collides with another car which is filled with dynamite, although he could not know it. An explosion follows. A, walking on the sidewalk nearby, is killed. B, sitting in a window of a building opposite, is cut by flying glass. C, likewise sitting in a window a block away, is similarly injured. And a further illustration. A nursemaid, ten blocks away, startled by the noise, involuntarily drops a baby from her arms to the sidewalk. We are told that C may not recover while B may. As to B it is a question for court or jury. We will all agree that the baby might not survive. Because, we are again told, the chauffeur had no reason to believe his conduct involved any risk of injuring either C or the baby. As to them he was not negligent.[26]

The chauffeur's conduct is the proximate cause of A's injury because his act (negligently colliding with another car) increased the risk that nearby pedestrians would be harmed, and in fact a nearby pedestrian *was* harmed. The chauffeur's conduct is *not* the proximate cause of either C's injury or the baby's injury because his act (negligently colliding with another car) did *not* foreseeably increase the risk that persons a block away (as was C) or ten blocks away (as was the baby) would be harmed. As regards B, whether or not the chauffeur's conduct is the proximate cause of B's injury will depend on whether or not the finder of fact (the jury, or the judge acting as jury) believes that the chauffeur's act increased the risk that persons "sitting in a window of a building opposite" would be harmed.

There are a number of exceptions to the foreseeability rule, but we shall mention only one here: the *eggshell-skull rule*. This rule refers to the hypothetical case of the plaintiff whose skull is as thin as an eggshell and is wrongfully struck on the head by the defendant who was unaware of the plaintiff's condition. Under the rule, the defendant is liable for all damages resulting from the wrongful contact, even those (unforeseeable) damages that would not have occurred if the plaintiff's skull were normal. Stated otherwise, defendants must "take their victims as they find them."[5(p105)]

Damages

We begin our discussion of damages by briefly explaining the various types of damages.[1(pp400-408),5(pp164-175)] *Actual* (or *compensatory*) *damages* "replace the loss caused by the wrong or injury. . . . The rationale behind compensatory damages is to restore the injured party to the position he or she was in prior to the injury."[3(p270)]

Unlike compensatory damages, *exemplary* (or *punitive*) *damages*

> are awarded to the plaintiff over and above what will . . . compensate him. . . . [and] are based upon an entirely different public policy consideration—that of punishing the defendant or of setting an example for similar wrongdoers. . . . In cases in which it is proved that a defendant has acted willfully, maliciously, or

fraudulently, a plaintiff may be awarded exemplary damages in addition to compensatory or actual damages.[3(p271)]

Nominal damages are "a trifling sum awarded to a plaintiff in an action, where there is no substantial loss or injury to be compensated, but still the law recognizes a technical . . . breach of the defendant's duty."[3(p272),27]

In general, plaintiffs who prevail in medical malpractice actions are permitted to recover actual or compensatory damages. These include *economic damages* (which include lost wages and medical expenses, both past and future), and *noneconomic damages* (pain and suffering). The plaintiff bears the burden of proving these damages by a preponderance of the evidence. In contrast, neither nominal damages nor punitive damages are generally available to plaintiffs in medical negligence cases.

Because a plaintiff may sue a defendant only once for the same injury, he or she generally asks not only for damages that have already occurred, but also for damages that will occur in the future as a result of the defendant's negligence.

"Under the traditional *collateral source* rule, "a jury, in calculating a plaintiff's damages in a tort action, does not take into consideration benefits—such as medical insurance or disability payments—which the plaintiff has received from sources other than the defendant—i.e., 'collateral sources'—to cover losses resulting from the injury."[19(p429)]

Damage Innovations: MICRA

The Medical Injury Compensation Reform Act of 1975 (MICRA) was a California statute, the purpose of which was to lower medical malpractice premiums. Although the law was multifaceted, we limit ourselves here to mentioning two of its salient provisions. First, Civil Code Section 3333.2 of MICRA limited noneconomic damages in medical malpractice cases to $250,000 or less. This cap on damages attributable to pain and suffering prevented juries from awarding astronomical sums—such as the $163.9 million awarded by a New York jury to a twenty-seven-year-old plaintiff rendered quadriplegic in an accident on the New Jersey Turnpike.[28] Such verdicts raise the cost of medical malpractice insurance and, indirectly, the cost of health care.

Second, Civil Code §3333.1 of MICRA modified the traditional collateral source rule (described earlier) in cases involving medical malpractice. Under §3333.1,

> a medical malpractice defendant is permitted to introduce evidence of collateral source benefits received by or payable to the plaintiff. . . . Although §3333.1 . . . does not specify how the jury should use such evidence, the legislature apparently assumed that in most cases the jury would set plaintiff's damages at a lower level.[19(p429)]

Damage Innovations: "Loss of a Chance" Doctrine

Before concluding our discussion of medical malpractice, let's consider another damage innovation—the *"loss of a chance" doctrine*.

Case 15-C   Gooding v. University Hospital

Mr. Gooding suffered lower abdominal pain and fainted at home.[29] His gastroenterologist, Dr. Borland, directed that he be brought to the emergency room (ER) of Memorial Hospital of Jacksonville. The ER staff failed to take a history or to examine Mr. Gooding in the belief that Dr. Borland, who was in the hospital and aware that Mr. Gooding was coming to the ER, would arrive shortly. Dr. Borland did not respond to repeated paging. Mr. Gooding died about forty-five minutes after arriving at the hospital. The autopsy revealed that he died from a ruptured abdominal aortic aneurysm that caused massive internal bleeding.

Mrs. Gooding brought a wrongful death action against the hospital alleging negligence by the ER staff in evaluation and treatment. The plaintiff's expert witness testified that the inaction of the ER staff violated accepted medical standards, but failed to testify that immediate diagnosis and surgery more likely than not would have enabled Mr. Gooding to survive. The hospital moved for a directed verdict on the causation element. Should the motion be granted?

Analysis

Recall that under traditional evidentiary standards, a plaintiff must prove that it is more likely than not that his or her injury was caused by the defendant's negligence. Mr. Gooding's injury was wrongful death. Has Mrs. Gooding introduced evidence affording a reasonable basis for the conclusion that it is *more likely than not* that the conduct of the hospital caused her husband's death? The answer is no; that evidence would have consisted of testimony on the part of her expert witness that immediate diagnosis and surgery more likely than not would have enabled Mr. Gooding to survive. Therefore, the hospital's motion for a directed verdict should be granted.

In fact, however, the trial court denied the motion, and instructed the jury that they could find for Gooding if the hospital destroyed Mr. Gooding's chance to survive. The jury found the hospital liable and awarded $300,000 in compensatory damages to Gooding's estate. The hospital appealed, and the appellate court reversed the decision of the trial court. Subsequently, the Supreme Court of Florida affirmed the decision of the appellate court. The Supreme Court declined to deviate from the "more likely than not" test for causation, and held that a jury could not reasonably find that but for the negligent failure to properly diagnose and treat Mr. Gooding he would not have died.

The trial court's decision differed from those on appeal because the trial court applied the loss of a chance doctrine whereas the higher courts did not. The doctrine holds that where a physician's negligence reduces the plaintiff's chances of survival—even though the chance of survival was below fifty percent before the negligence—the physician should be liable for the value of the chance that the plaintiff lost. As you might imagine, the policy consideration underlying this doctrine is the protection of the plaintiff whose chance of survival is below fifty percent.

Chapter Summary

Medical malpractice (medical negligence) is a subset of medical liability, which is, in turn, a subset of health law. Along with intentional torts and strict liability, negligence is a tort. Tort law seeks to compensate the victims of wrongdoing, to deter future wrongdoing, and to exact retribution. To prevail in a medical malpractice action against a physician defendant, a plaintiff patient must prove that the defendant physician owed him or her a legal duty, that the defendant's conduct fell below the standard of care (i.e., that the defendant breached his or her duty), that the plaintiff suffered damages, and that the defendant's conduct was the cause of the damages sustained by the plaintiff.

The health care professional owes an affirmative duty of care to all patients with whom he or she has a provider–patient relationship and, in certain cases, to others. The standard of care requires the health care professional to exercise the same degree of knowledge, skill, diligence, and care that the ordinary competent practitioner would exercise under the same or similar circumstances, and to use his or her best judgment in exercising that skill and applying that knowledge. The standard of care in medical malpractice cases is generally established by medical custom, although there are exceptions to this rule.

Proof of causation requires proof that the defendant's conduct brought about the plaintiff's damages (scientific causation or cause-in-fact) and that the plaintiff's damages were foreseeable (legal or proximate causation). Plaintiffs prevailing in a medical malpractice action may recover for actual and future damages, both economic (e.g., medical expenses and lost earnings) and noneconomic (pain and suffering). Modern damage innovations have included limitations on noneconomic damages and the loss of a chance doctrine.

Review Questions

1. What is health law?
2. What are some of the various grounds for medical liability?
3. What are the goals of tort law?
4. What is negligence, and what elements compose it?
5. What is the no-duty rule? List five exceptions to that rule.
6. What is the standard of care in medical malpractice cases, as formulated in *Pike v. Honsiger*?
7. List five exceptions to the rule that medical custom establishes the standard of care in medical malpractice cases.
8. Distinguish between scientific and legal causation.
9. Distinguish and explain the three tests used to establish scientific causation.

10. Explain the policy rationale underlying legal causation.

11. Explain and distinguish among actual damages, future damages, punitive damages, and nominal damages.

12. What is the loss of a chance doctrine, and how does it operate?

Endnotes

1. Furrow BR, Greaney TL, Johnson SH, Jost TS, Schwartz RL. *Health Law.* Vol. 1. St. Paul, MN: West Publishing, 1995:vii.
2. Furrow BR, Johnson SH, Jost TS, Schwartz RL. *Health Law: Cases, Materials and Problems.* 2nd ed. St. Paul, MN: West Publishing, 1995:viii–ix.
3. *Black's Law Dictionary.* Abridged 6th ed. St. Paul, MN: West Publishing, 1991:1036.
4. Franklin MA, Rabin RL. *Tort Law and Alternatives: Cases and Materials.* 4th ed. Mineola, NY: Foundation Press, 1987:117–201.
5. Emanuel S. *Torts.* 3rd ed. Larchmont, NY: Emanuel Law Outlines, 1988:130–163.
6. *Buch v Amory Mfg. Co.,* 69 N.H. 257 (1897).
7. The Vermont Statutes Online. Vt.Stat.Ann., tit. 12, section 519. Available at: http://www.leg.state.vt.us/statutes/fullsection.cfm?Title=12&Chapter=023&Section=00519. Accessed November 10, 2007.
8. Wikipedia. The Finale (Seinfeld). Available at: http://en.wikipedia.org/wiki/The_Finale_(Seinfeld_episode). Accessed November 10, 2007.
9. *Hiser v. Randolph,* 126 Ariz. 608, 617 P.2d 774 (Ariz. App. 1980).
10. *Zelenko v. Gimbel Bros,* 287 N.Y.S. 134 (N.Y. Sup. Ct. 1935).
11. *Union Pacific Ry. v. Cappier,* 72 P.281 (Kan. 1903).
12. Hit and run laws by state. Available at: http://www.deadlyroads.com/state-laws.html. Accessed November 11, 2007.
13. New York Good Samaritan Act, NYS Public Health Law, Article 30—Emergency Medical Services; 3000-a.1. Available at: http://www.cprinstructor.com/NY-GS.htm. Accessed November 11, 2007.
14. *Pike v. Honsiger,* 155 NY 201 (1898).
15. Peters PG. The role of the jury in modern malpractice law. *Iowa Law Rev* 2002;87:909.
16. *In the Matter of Baby K,* 832 F.Supp. 1022 (U.S. District Court, Eastern District Virginia, 1993).
17. 42 U.S.C.A. § 1395dd (1995).
18. *Helling v. Carey,* 519 P.2d 981 (Wash. 1974).
19. Hall MA, Bobinski MA, Orentlicher D. *Health Care Law and Ethics.* 7th ed. New York: Aspen Publishers, 2007:203–204.
20. *Ybarra v. Spangard,* 154 P.2d 687 (Sup. Ct. Cal. 1944).
21. *Sullivan v. O'Connor,* 296 N.E.2d 183 (Mass. 1973).
22. *Burton v. Brooklyn Doctors Hosp.,* 452 N.Y.S.2d 875 (N.Y. App. Div. 1982).
23. Prosser WL. Section 41. In: *Handbook of the Law of Torts.* 4th ed. St. Paul, MN: West Publishing, 1971.
24. *Summers v. Tice,* 33 Cal.2d 80, 199 P.2d 1 (1948 Cal.).
25. "In a case in which the party with the burden of proof has failed to present a prima facie case for jury consideration, the trial judge may order the entry of a verdict without allowing the

jury to consider it, because, as a matter of law, there can be only one . . . verdict." See *Black's Law Dictionary,* p. 316.

26. *Palsgraff v. Long Island Railroad Co.*, 248 N.Y. 339 (N.Y. 1928).

27. One of the most notorious examples of nominal damages came in the lawsuit (an antitrust action) brought by the USFL (United States Football League) against the NFL (National Football League). The USFL sought damages of $567 million (which would have been tripled to $1.7 billion under antitrust law). The jury awarded the USFL only one dollar in (nominal) damages, which was tripled under antitrust law to three dollars. Ultimately, the USFL received a check for $3.76 in 1990, representing the trebled nominal damages plus seventy-six cents in interest. See http://en.wikipedia.org/wiki/United_States_Football_League and http://www.thisistheusfl.com/index.htm. Accessed November 26, 2007.

28. Perez-Pena R. Queens jury awards record judgment in suit on a turnpike accident. *New York Times*, July 22, 1993. Available at: http://query.nytimes.com/gst/fullpage.html?res=9F0CE5DB1438F931A15754C0A965958260. Accessed December 7, 2007.

29. *Gooding v. University Hosp.*, 445 So.2d 1015 (Fla. 1984).

Chapter 16

My Brother's Keeper? Allocating Legal Responsibility Among Medical Providers

Yahweh asked Cain, "Where is your brother Abel?" "I do not know," he replied. Am I my brother's guardian?" "What have you done?" Yahweh asked. "Listen to the sound of your brother's blood, crying out to me from the ground. Now be accursed and driven from the ground that has opened its mouth to receive your brother's blood at your hands. When you till the ground it shall no longer yield you any of its produce. You shall be a fugitive and a wanderer over the earth."

—Genesis 4:9

Chapter Learning Objectives

At the conclusion of this chapter the reader will be able to:

1. Define, recognize, and differentiate among *direct liability, derivative liability, vicarious liability,* and the liability of multiple tortfeasors whose acts combine to cause an *indivisible harm*

2. Define and recognize *corporate negligence* and explain how it relates to derivative liability

3. Define and recognize the concept of *respondeat superior* and explain how it relates to vicarious liability

4. Define and recognize *apparent* or *ostensible agency* and explain how it relates to vicarious liability

5. Define and recognize the *borrowed-servant doctrine* and explain how it relates to *respondeat superior* and vicarious liability

6. Define and recognize the *captain-of-the-ship doctrine* and explain how it relates to *respondeat superior* and vicarious liability

7. Define and recognize the *nondelegable duty doctrine*, explain the policy considerations that underlie it, and explain how it relates to vicarious liability

8. Explain what a partnership is and how it relates to vicarious liability

9. List the elements of a joint enterprise and be able to recognize a joint enterprise and understand how it relates to vicarious liability

10. Define, recognize, and differentiate between *individual* and *common liability* and explain how they relate to the indivisible harm concept

11. Define, recognize, and differentiate between *joint and several liability* and *several liability* and explain how they relate to common liability

The focus of the text so far has been on the relationship between the health care professional and the patient. Their interaction, however, does not take place in a vacuum. Often other health care professionals or health care institutions are involved in the care of the patient. These others might be midlevel providers, such as physician assistants, or they might be subspecialists; the institutions might be, for example, hospitals. This chapter concerns itself with the following question: how does the law apportion—among multiple defendants—legal responsibility when things go wrong? Asked otherwise, when do I, as a health care provider, need to be concerned that the behavior of other health care providers might put me at risk? In exploring this question we shall introduce a number of new concepts.

We begin by asking you to consider the following:

> [I]f two drivers negligently inflict harm that can be apportioned, each would be liable only for what he or she had done. For example, if plaintiff had fainted in the street and D1, approaching from the east, had negligently failed to stop and had run over plaintiff's leg, and at the same time D2, approaching from the west, had negligently failed to stop and had run over plaintiff's arm, each defendant would be liable for the respective harm done to the limb that each had run over.[1]

By analogy, it would seem reasonable to hypothesize that the following rules govern the allocation of responsibility among defendant health care providers:

1. A physician is liable for his or her own negligence.

2. A physician is *not* liable for the negligence of another.

Indeed, besides deriving logically from the scenario just described, on their faces these rules seem intuitive and self-evident. We shall apply our posited rules to actual legal cases to see if they are predictive of the outcomes. To the extent they are, we shall retain them; to the extent they are not, we shall modify them or derive exceptions to them.

Consider Case 16-A.

Case 16-A   Maltempo v. Cuthbert

The plaintiff, Mr. Maltempo, was a twenty-one-year-old male with insulin-dependent diabetes mellitus.[2] He was arrested, and in jail his medical condition deteriorated. His family attempted to reach their family doctor, but instead reached Dr. Cuthbert, who was the covering physician.

Case 16-A Maltempo v. Cuthbert (*continued*)

The family said to Dr. Cuthbert that Mr. Maltempo was "in very bad shape and jail personnel did not believe he was sick." Dr. Cuthbert reportedly told the Maltempos that he would "look into the matter and call them if there were any problems." The doctor proceeded to call the jail; upon being told that Mr. Maltempo was under the care of the jail doctor (Dr. Freeman), Dr. Cuthbert pursued the matter no further. The following morning Mr. Maltempo aspirated and died en route from the county jail to the state prison. Maltempo's widow sued Dr. Cuthbert for negligence and recovered $45,000. How did Maltempo prevail?

Analysis

The outcome of the case is understandable in light of the material discussed in the preceding chapter. Dr. Cuthbert's statement that he would call the Maltempos if there were any problems was, in essence, a voluntary assumption of duty,[3] and his promise to do so served to establish the standard of care in this case (think back to *Hawkins v. McGee*, discussed in Chapter 15). Whereas Dr. Cuthbert argued that his conduct did not fall below the standard of care because it would have been unethical for him to interfere with Dr. Freeman's treatment, the court distinguished between interfering with the treatment being rendered by another physician and merely inquiring as to Maltempo's condition. Finally, Dr. Cuthbert tried arguing that Dr. Freeman, and not he, had caused Maltempo's death, but the court rejected this, writing: "The fact that others were subsequently negligent and could have prevented the boy's death may mean that there were multiple causes; it does not vitiate the causal relationship between Cuthbert's negligence and Maltempo's death." In other words, Dr. Cuthbert's wrongful acts and omissions were a cause (in both a factual and a legal sense) of Maltempo's death. Dr. Freeman's intervening acts and omissions, even assuming they were negligent, did not "break the chain of causation" because the negligence of other medical providers is foreseeable. Had Freeman instead shot and killed Maltempo based on some old grievance between them, that intervening act would likely have been found to be unforeseeable and would likely have released Dr. Cuthbert from liability.

Direct Liability

Case 16-A illustrates *direct liability*. The liability of each of the drivers (D1 and D2) in the chapter-opening scenario was also direct, because each was liable only for the consequences of his own tortious acts. Now compare *Maltempo v. Cuthbert* with that scenario. Think of Cuthbert as D1 and Freeman as D2. In this case, rather than negligently driving over the plaintiff's leg, Cuthbert has negligently failed to help the plaintiff (perhaps by shouting to D2 to "look out!") after promising to do so. As a result, Freeman (D2) runs over the plaintiff's arm, and Cuthbert is made to pay for the injured arm as a result.

Assuming for the sake of argument that the jail doctor was negligent (the opinion does point out that "[t]he other defendants, the sheriff and the jail doctor and nurse, all settled with [the] plaintiffs for a total of $80,000"[2]), his liability is direct, because it springs from the consequences of his own acts and omissions.

Perhaps it is not as evident on first glance, but Cuthbert's liability is also direct, because he, too, is being held liable for the consequence—Maltempo's death—of his own wrongful acts and omissions. Simply stated, it was wrong for Cuthbert not to check on the condition of Maltempo *because he (Cuthbert) said he would.* Had Cuthbert, when contacted by the Maltempo family, simply told them that Mr. Maltempo was under the care of another physician and that he (Cuthbert) could not attend to him while he was incarcerated, it is likely that Cuthbert would have avoided liability. Instead, by saying he would "look into the matter and call [the Maltempos] if there were any problems," he essentially assumed a duty and set the standard of care for himself, which he then proceeded to breach. He "caused" Maltempo's death in two ways. First, "his assurances . . . lulled the Maltempos in believing that their son was being cared for, and effectively prevented them from seeking other emergency help."[2] Second, his failure to make substantive inquiries regarding Maltempo's condition arguably delayed medical treatment. In other words, had he inquired a little more deeply into the medical condition of the prisoner, he might have discovered that a serious situation existed and Maltempo might have been saved.[4]

Thus, in the interest of clarity we can restate (with changes underlined) the rules posited earlier as follows:

1. A physician is liable for <u>the foreseeable consequences of his or her own wrongful acts or omissions.</u>

2. A physician is *not* liable for <u>the consequences of another's wrongful acts or omissions.</u>

Consider the following case.

Case 16-B   Morey v. Thybo

In this case, Mrs. Thybo employed Dr. Morey as her obstetrician, and he was in sole charge of the case from June 5, when her membranes ruptured, through June 11.[5] On June 11, the Thybos also employed Dr. Rice, "an oldtime friend." Drs. Morey and Rice had no personal or professional relationship or acquaintance. Dr. Rice concluded that delivery would be impossible without the use of instruments. By agreement of Drs. Rice and Morey, during the delivery of the child and the placenta Dr. Rice used the instruments and Dr. Morey administered the anesthetic. Postpartum, Mrs. Thybo alleged that Dr. Rice used unsterilized forceps, failed to remove all of the afterbirth, and negligently tore and lacerated her vagina. Mrs. Thybo sought to hold Dr. Morey liable for Dr. Rice's malpractice. Is there any legal basis for charging Dr. Morey with Dr. Rice's acts or omissions?

Case 16-B Morey v. Thybo (*continued*)

Analysis

The court began its analysis by pointing out that Drs. Morey and Rice were "[t]wo physicians, independently engaged by the patient and serving together by mutual consent."[5] (This is important because, as we shall see shortly, the relationship between the doctors will determine whether any exception to the second of our previously posited rules is applicable. For now, accept it as a given that no exception is applicable.) In such cases, the court wrote, "[e]ach, in serving with the other, is rightly held answerable for his own conduct, and *as well for all the wrongful acts or omissions of the other which he observes and lets go on without objection, or which in the exercise of reasonable diligence under the circumstances he should have observed.* Beyond this, his liability does not extend [italics added]."[5] In the end, the appellate court decided that Dr. Morey neither observed nor should have observed any of the wrongful acts or omissions of Dr. Rice, and that therefore he should not be held liable for them. The court, in so deciding, found no evidence "that Morey knew of and acquiesced in the use of unsterilized forceps." In answer to the question of whether he should have known, the court answered, "Not unless . . . he ought gratuitously to have entertained a suspicion that an apparently learned and skillful surgeon was about to commit a gross medical offense, and to have followed up the suspicion by inquiring whether his brother had forgotten to sterilize his hands and his instruments. No such unreasonable burden is imposed by the law." With regard to the plaintiff's allegations regarding Dr. Rice's failure to deliver the afterbirth and his negligently tearing and lacerating her vagina, the court found that "Morey, from his position, could not know of them for himself; and . . . he was not negligent in inferring [that the afterbirth had been removed in its entirety and] that no lacerations requiring repair operations had been inflicted."[5]

Unlike Case 16-A, in this case the plaintiff blatantly attempted to hold Dr. Morey liable for the consequences of Dr. Rice's negligence. The court said no and said, in essence, that if Dr. Morey were to be held liable for the consequences of Dr. Rice's negligence, it would have to be because of a wrongful omission on Dr. Morey's part—a failure to object to any negligence that he either observed or should have observed.

Applying lessons learned in *Morey v. Thybo,* we can modify the posited rules as follows:

1. A physician is liable for the foreseeable consequences of his or her own wrongful acts or omissions.

2. A physician is *not* liable for the consequences of another's wrongful acts or omissions, <u>unless the physician observes or should observe those wrongful acts or omissions and fails to object to them.</u>

Derivative Liability and Corporate Negligence

In the landmark case *Darling v. Charleston Community Memorial Hospital,* an eighteen-year-old suffered a broken leg playing football.[6] Dr. Alexander, an independent contractor (not a hospital employee) on emergency call that day, placed the leg in a plaster cast. Shortly thereafter, the patient complained of pain and swelling, and discoloration of the toes were noted. Three days after the fracture, Dr. Alexander "split the sides of the cast with a Stryker saw; in the course of [doing so] the plaintiff's leg was cut. . . . Blood and other seepage were observed . . . , and there was a stench in the room, which one witness said was the worst he had smelled since World War II."[6] The patient ultimately required an above-the-knee amputation.

In an action against the hospital, the hospital was held directly liable (i.e., was adjudged to have itself been negligent) on either or both of two grounds: (1) for failing to "have a sufficient number of trained nurses for bedside care of all patients at all times capable of recognizing the progressive gangrenous condition . . . and of bringing [it] to the attention of the hospital administration and of the medical staff" and (2) for failing "to require consultation with or examination by members of the hospital surgical staff skilled in such treatment; or to review the treatment rendered . . . and to require consultants to be called in as needed."[6]

The hospital's liability in this case is an example of what is called *derivative liability:*[7]

> Unlike cases involving pure vicarious liability, cases of derivative liability, such as the wrongful hiring of an incompetent employee, *involve wrongful conduct both by the person who is derivatively liable and the actor whose wrongful conduct was the direct cause of injury to another.* The liability is derivative because it depends upon a subsequent wrongful act or omission. As one court explained in a negligent entrustment setting:
>
> > Obviously, an owner who is negligent in entrusting his vehicle is not liable for such negligence until some wrong is committed by the one to whom it is entrusted. Even if the owner's negligence in permitting the driving were gross, it would not be actionable if the driver was guilty of no negligence. The driver's wrong, in the form of legal liability to the plaintiff, first must be established, then by negligent entrustment liability for such wrong is passed on to the owner.
>
> *Derivative liability is thus predicated on the tortious conduct of the defendant personally.* However, like vicarious liability, there is no liability without the subsequent tortious conduct of another.[8] (Internal footnotes omitted; italics added)

In *Darling,* the hospital itself behaved wrongfully by understaffing itself with nurses or by failing to supervise the quality of medical care being delivered by its medical staff, or both. Nevertheless, the hospital's wrongful acts and omissions would not have given rise to a legal action if not for the negligence of Dr. Alexander; thus, the hospital was held legally responsible for harm caused, at least in part, by the conduct of Dr. Alexander.

Understand the following two points regarding derivative liability: (1) the derivative liability of a defendant such as Charleston Community Memorial Hospital depends on that defendant having himself or itself behaved wrongfully (i.e., an innocent defendant cannot be held derivatively liable), and (2) derivative liability is one of "a number of circumstances where one person is held legally responsible for harm caused[,] at least in part, by the conduct of another."[8] We shall encounter others later in this chapter.

Finally, yet another point to note here is that in this case an institution (the hospital), as opposed to a physician, was held liable. The hospital's liability in this case illustrates the doctrine of *corporate negligence*. Under the doctrine of corporate negligence, "hospitals can . . . be found liable for some act of negligence on their part with respect to patient care decisions made by independent doctors."[9] Corporate negligence is a subtype, if you will, of derivative liability. Other types also exist.[10]

We can use this opportunity to restate our rules in a way that takes into consideration the existence of derivative liability and the possibility of institutional negligence as illustrated by the *Darling* case. Thus, we can say:

1. A <u>health care provider</u> is liable for the foreseeable consequences of <u>his, her, or its</u> own wrongful acts or omissions.

2. A <u>health care provider</u> is *not* liable for the consequences of another's wrongful acts or omissions, <u>unless</u>

   a. <u>the provider observes or should observe those wrongful acts or omissions and fails to object to them, or</u>

   b. <u>derivative liability applies.</u>

Now consider Case 16-C in light of all you have learned so far.

Case 16-C Yorston v. Pennell

The plaintiff, Yorston, accidentally shot himself in the leg with a nail gun.[11] He was brought to the hospital and became a patient of Dr. Pennell, an attending surgeon on the medical staff but *not* a hospital employee. Also involved in the care of the patient were Dr. Hatemi, the surgical resident, and Mr. Rex, a surgical subintern, both of whom were hospital employees. Mr. Rex was instructed to do the admitting history and physical examination (H&P) by Dr. Hatemi. During the course of the exam, the patient advised Mr. Rex that he was allergic to penicillin, but Mr. Rex neglected to note this in his written H&P. Subsequently, Dr. Hatemi, on the instructions of Dr. Pennell, operated on Yorston. Postoperatively, in reliance on Rex's H&P, Hatemi prescribed 600,000 units of penicillin to Yorston, who experienced an allergic reaction. Yorston sued Dr. Pennell and won a judgment. How did Yorston prevail?[12]

(continues)

> **Case 16-C Yorston v. Pennell (*continued*)**
>
> **Analysis**
>
> Was Dr. Pennell liable directly (i.e., under the first of the hypothetical rules formulated earlier), perhaps for not adequately supervising Rex and Hatemi? In fact, the case was not submitted to the jury on that theory. If we know this, and we know that Yorston prevailed anyway, then liability in this case must be grounded in some exception to the second of the hypothetical rules.

Vicarious Liability (Imputed Negligence)

Unlike any of the cases we discussed previously, Dr. Pennell's liability is completely divorced from any wrongdoing on his part. His liability is said to be *vicarious;* the negligence of someone else is being *imputed* to him. In vicarious liability, "[t]he person who is being held responsible for the conduct of the tortfeasor has engaged in no wrongful conduct personally, but is liable because of his or her relationship with the actor who engaged in the wrongful conduct."[8] Stated otherwise, " '[i]mputed negligence' [or vicarious liability] means that, [where A is negligent and B is not,] by reason of some relation existing between A and B, the negligence of A is to be charged against B, although B has played no part in it, . . . or indeed has done all that he possibly can to prevent it."[13] In the cases we discussed before *Yorston v. Pennell*, a defendant's liability was contingent upon some wrongful act or omission on his part. Not so here, where Pennell's liability is not contingent upon any wrongful act or omission of his own, but rather on the wrongful acts or omissions of others.

The *Respondeat Superior* Doctrine

The specific type of vicarious liability at work in *Yorston v. Pennell* is known as *respondeat superior,* which translates as "let the master answer" or "let the higher up answer." *Respondeat superior* most commonly applies in the employer–employee context—that is to say, the employer is vicariously liable for the acts of the employee. (The employee is liable as well, although in his or her case liability is direct.) The policy rationale underlying the doctrine is that the employer, having both a "deeper pocket" than the employee and a right to control the employee, is better situated both to pay for the plaintiff's damages and to prevent future potential plaintiffs from being damaged.

Closely related to the *respondeat superior* doctrine are two special rules governing liability of hospital employees such as nurses or resident physicians. These are the borrowed-servant doctrine and the captain-of-the-ship doctrine.

The Borrowed-Servant Doctrine

The *borrowed-servant doctrine* is particularly relevant if one thinks more closely about *Yorston v. Pennell*. Recall that Dr. Hatemi and Mr. Rex were hospital employees. They were not employees of Dr. Pennell. Why, then, should Dr. Pennell—as opposed to the hospital— be held vicariously liable under the *respondeat superior* doctrine for their negligence? The answer is that Hatemi and Rex were the *borrowed servants* of Pennell:

> A long established, widely accepted rule of law is that a general employee of one employer may become a special employee or "borrowed servant" of another. (Under this rule, a nurse employed by a hospital may become a special employee of a physician or surgeon with staff privileges.) Is the special employer liable for the negligence of the borrowed servant? The proper test, under the doctrine of *respondeat superior*, is whether the special employer has the right to control the actions of the borrowed servant.[14]

The Captain-of-the-Ship Doctrine

The *captain-of-the-ship doctrine* is a stricter, more extreme (and largely discredited) form of the *respondeat superior* doctrine. The captain-of-the-ship doctrine essentially holds "that the surgeon's mere presence in the [operating room] makes him or her legally responsible for everything that happens there, regardless of whether he or she has any ability to control the actions of others."[15]

Thus, the hypothetical rules we proffered earlier require further amendment. They should read as follows:

1. A health care provider is liable for the foreseeable consequences of his, her, or its own wrongful acts or omissions.

2. A health care provider is *not* liable for the consequences of another's wrongful acts or omissions, unless

   a. the provider observes or should observe those wrongful acts or omissions and fails to object to them, or

   b. derivative liability applies, or

   c. <u>one of the following forms of vicarious liability applies:</u>

      i. <u>*respondeat superior.*</u>

Apparent or Ostensible Agency

Another exception to the second of our hypothetical rules concerns the doctrine of apparent or ostensible agency. *Agency* is "a relationship between two persons, by agreement or otherwise, where one (the agent) may act on behalf of the other (the principal) and bind the principal by words and actions."[16] Stated otherwise, principals may be held vicariously liable for the acts of their agents. *Respondeat superior* is a form of agency, because the employee (agent) may bind the employer (principal). The concept of agency is complicated and largely beyond the scope of the present chapter. We discuss it only briefly here.

There are a number of different types of agency. *Actual agency* "exists where the agent is really employed by the principal." [16] Thus, an employee is an *actual agent* of the employer. Alternatively, an *apparent* or *ostensible agency* "exists where one, either intentionally or from want of ordinary care, induces another to believe that a third person is his agent, though he never in fact employed him."[16(p760)] Under this doctrine, for example, emergency room physicians (and other hospital-based physicians such as radiologists and anesthesiologists) are sometimes held to be *apparent* or *ostensible agents* of the hospitals in which they work, "regardless of the specifics of the arrangement with the hospital,"[9(p454)] because patients may wrongly, though reasonably, believe that they work for the hospital. Reformulating our hypothetical rules to take apparent or ostensible agency into account, they read as follows:

1. A health care provider is liable for the foreseeable consequences of his, her, or its own wrongful acts or omissions.

2. A health care provider is *not* liable for the consequences of another's wrongful acts or omissions, unless

   a. the provider observes or should observe those wrongful acts or omissions and fails to object to them, or

   b. derivative liability applies, or

   c. one of the following forms of vicarious liability applies:

      i. *respondeat superior*

      ii. the doctrine of apparent or ostensible agency.

Nondelegable Duty

In the case of *Jackson v. Power*, the sixteen-year-old plaintiff was seriously injured when he fell from a cliff and was brought to the emergency department at Fairbanks Memorial Hospital (FMH), where he was evaluated by Dr. Power.[17]

> Dr. Power's examination revealed multiple lacerations and abrasions of the . . . face and scalp, multiple contusions and lacerations of the lumbar area, several broken vertebrae and gastric distension, suggesting possible internal injuries. Dr. Power ordered several tests, but did not order certain procedures that could have been used to ascertain whether there had been damage to the patient's kidneys. Jackson had, in fact, suffered damage to the renal arteries and veins. . . . This

damage, undetected for approximately nine to ten hours . . . , ultimately caused Jackson to lose both of his kidneys.[17]

Jackson sued for negligence in diagnosis and treatment, and sought to hold FMH liable for Dr. Power's negligence.

By now you should be asking yourself, on what basis? Let's go through the possibilities. Was Jackson claiming that FMH had been (directly) negligent in selecting, retaining, or supervising Dr. Power? No, Jackson made no such claim. Was Jackson claiming that FMH was vicariously liable under the doctrine of *respondeat superior*? No, Jackson conceded that Dr. Power was an independent contractor and not an employee of FMH. Was Jackson alleging that Dr. Power was an apparent or ostensible agent of FMH? In fact, that had been one of Jackson's arguments at his jury trial. The jury, however, had found against Jackson on that question, and the appellate court did not disturb that finding. And yet Jackson prevailed in his appeal. How?

The appellate court in *Jackson* based its decision on the concept of a *nondelegable duty*. As the name implies, some legal duties are so important that they may not be delegated. As applied in *Jackson v. Power*, the nondelegable duty argument goes as follows: "the public policy supporting hospital responsibility is so strong that, as a matter of law, the hospital may not avoid responsibility by delegating the function to an independent contractor."[9(p456)] The court wrote:

> A non-delegable duty is an established exception to the rule that an employer is not liable for the negligence of an independent contractor. . . . We . . . hold that a general acute care hospital's duty to provide physicians for emergency room care is non-delegable. Thus, a hospital such as FMH may not shield itself from liability by claiming that it is not responsible for the results of negligently performed health care when the law imposes a duty on the hospital to provide that health care. . . . FMH is, therefore, vicariously liable as a matter of law for any negligence or malpractice that Dr. Power may have committed.[17]

Reformulating our hypothetical rules to take nondelegable duty into account, they read as follows:

1. A health care provider is liable for the foreseeable consequences of his, her, or its own wrongful acts or omissions.

2. A health care provider is *not* liable for the consequences of another's wrongful acts or omissions, unless

   a. the provider observes or should observe those wrongful acts or omissions and fails to object to them, or

   b. derivative liability applies, or

   c. <u>one of the following forms of vicarious liability applies:</u>

    i. *respondeat superior*

    ii. apparent or ostensible agency

    iii. <u>nondelegable duty.</u>

Partnerships

Another exception to the second rule concerns partnerships. "Partnerships are liable for [the] wrongful and tortious acts of employees and partners committed within the scope of their employment or business."[18] A general partner "participate[s] fully in the profits, losses and management of the partnership and . . . is personally liable for its debts."[16(p773)] In contrast, a limited partner's "participation in the profits is limited by an agreement and [he] is not liable for the debts of the partnership beyond his capital contribution."[16]

> The UPA [Uniform Partnership Act, after which are modeled the statutes (of almost all states) that govern general partnerships] . . . makes partners jointly and severally liable for wrongful acts and omissions . . . (e.g., torts). . . .
>
>   . . . Under joint and several liability, torts committed by the partnership subject all partners to liability in their individual capacities so that innocent partners may be liable for their partners' negligence. Thus, where a jury finds one partner guilty of medical malpractice and a second partner not guilty, judgment is nevertheless entered against the second partner under joint and several liability.[18]

We shall have more to say about joint and several liability later. Briefly, if multiple defendants are jointly and severally liable, they are "responsible together and individually. The [defendant] . . . does not, however, receive double compensation."[16]

Our rules as formulated earlier require further refinement. They should read as follows:

1. A health care provider is liable for the foreseeable consequences of his, her, or its own wrongful acts or omissions.

2. A health care provider is *not* liable for the consequences of another's wrongful acts or omissions, unless

    a. the provider observes or should observe those wrongful acts or omissions and fails to object to them, or

    b. derivative liability applies, or

    c. <u>one of the following forms of vicarious liability applies:</u>

        i. *respondeat superior*

        ii. apparent or ostensible agency

        iii. nondelegable duty

        iv. <u>partnership.</u>

Joint Enterprises

Consider Case 16-D.

Case 16-D O'Grady v. Wickman

In this 1968 case, the plaintiff, Mrs. O'Grady, was admitted to the hospital with severe back pain.[19] Dr. Fabric, a general practitioner who reportedly had never attended her before, became her attending physician. At the request of Dr. Fabric, a number of diagnostic tests were performed, the results of all of which were reportedly negative. Dr. Fabric wrote in O'Grady's chart, "Patient has a tumor of the right ovary and retroflexed uterus. Recommend surgery. May have to do a suspension or removal of uterus." Dr. Fabric then consulted Dr. Wickman, a gynecologist, whose examination of Mrs. O'Grady was limited to vital signs and a "female examination." Dr. Wickman recommended a right salpingo-oophorectomy and left tubal ligation, then performed a right salpingo-oophorectomy and a hysterectomy. Postoperatively, Mrs. O'Grady developed leakage of urine from the vagina, but was discharged from the hospital anyway. She was seen by a Dr. Sall, who diagnosed a vesicovaginal fistula. To add insult to injury, she continued to experience back pain, which was finally diagnosed by an orthopedist as being the result of a limb length discrepancy. The pain was relieved by means of a heel lift. Mrs. O'Grady sued Drs. Fabric and Wickman, both of whom prevailed on a motion for a summary judgment.[20]

Mrs. O'Grady appealed. What is important for our purposes here is that on appeal one of O'Grady's arguments was that there were questions of fact, which if decided in her favor, would have allowed a jury to hold Dr. Fabric responsible for the conduct of Dr. Wickman. Therefore, she argued, summary judgment should not have been granted. The appellate court held in favor of Mrs. O'Grady. How?

First, it is important that you understand the question that is being asked and why it matters. Remember, Mrs. O'Grady is arguing here that Dr. Fabric was *vicariously* liable, so the first of our hypothetical rules is not implicated. The Fabric/Wickman relationship was neither of the *respondeat superior* type nor a partnership, nor did the doctrines of apparent agency or nondelegable duty apply. So how could Dr. Fabric possibly have been responsible for the conduct of Dr. Wickman?

Analysis

The court wrote that one physician is liable for the acts of another when there is "a concert of action and a common purpose existing between the two doctors." The term *joint enterprise* is sometimes used as shorthand for this type of relationship. A joint enterprise may be conceptualized as something like a partnership, but for a more limited time and purpose. A joint enterprise may be defined as "an undertaking to carry out a small number of acts or objectives, entered into by associates each of whom has an equal voice in directing the conduct of the enterprise."[21]

It is important to remember that the court did *not* say that Drs. Fabric and Wickman were engaged in a joint enterprise, but rather said that a jury should have been allowed to decide whether they were.

A case that actually provides us with an example of a joint enterprise is the Colorado case *Bolles v. Kinton.*[22] In that case, the plaintiff, Mrs. Kinton, fell and injured her left hip. She was seen by Dr. Bolles, who summoned Dr. Starks (Dr. Bolles's son-in-law, who lived with Dr. Bolles and shared an office with her, although they were not partners). Together, the two osteopaths diagnosed a contusion, decided that x-rays were unnecessary, and treated the injury accordingly, notwithstanding the fact that the left leg was perceptibly shortened and the left foot everted. Dr. Bolles ceased her connection with the case after a few visits, while Dr. Starks continued to treat Ms. Kinton for seven weeks. Subsequently, other practitioners became involved, x-rays were done, and a fracture of the neck of the left femur was discovered. Surgery, including bone grafting, was required. Mrs. Kinton sued and won a verdict against Drs. Bolles and Starks jointly for $6,250. The court said that this in fact was a joint enterprise and wrote that "a physician cannot discharge a case, and relieve himself of responsibility for it, by simply staying away without notice to the patient."[22]

Reformulating our rules, they now read as follows:

1. A health care provider is liable for the foreseeable consequences of his, her, or its own wrongful acts or omissions.

2. A health care provider is *not* liable for the consequences of another's wrongful acts or omissions, unless

    a. the provider observes or should observe those wrongful acts or omissions and fails to object to them, or

    b. derivative liability applies, or

    c. one of the following forms of vicarious liability applies:

        i.   *respondeat superior*

        ii. apparent or ostensible agency

        iii. nondelegable duty

        iv. partnership

        v.   a joint enterprise.

You will recall our mentioning earlier that there are "a number of circumstances where one person is held legally responsible for harm caused[,] at least in part, by the conduct of another."[8] So far we have discussed three such circumstances: where the provider observes or should observe the wrongful acts or omissions of another and fails to object to them, derivative liability, and vicarious liability. In Case 16-E we encounter a third.

Case 16-E   Variety Children's Hospital v. Osle

At Variety Children's Hospital, Mrs. Osle underwent an operation for removal of a cyst from each breast.[23] Dr. Rader, who was not an employee of the hospital, performed the surgery. The cysts were placed in a single container. The scrub nurse testified that she had asked Dr. Rader if he wanted the specimens separated and sent to pathology, but that he had replied that it would be all right to put them in a single container because they were benign anyway. Dr. Garcia, the pathology resident, knowing that the two specimens came from different breasts, nonetheless failed to keep the cysts separate during the dissection. By dissecting them together, he destroyed their identity. Although only one of the cysts was malignant, it was necessary for Mrs. Osle to have both breasts removed. The pathologist admitted that if the larger cyst had been labeled as such and if the two cysts had been sectioned separately, their identity would have been preserved.

Dr. Rader and Variety Children's Hospital were found *jointly and severally liable* for $100,000. Joint and several liability means, again, that "the plaintiff may sue [the defendants] together or separately and may recover the full extent of his harm against either one—or both if they are sued together."[1(p215)] The court wrote that "the evidence . . . support[ed] a finding . . . that the negligence of Dr. Rader and that of the hospital [acting through Dr. Garcia] were so intertwined as to constitute one cause for plaintiff's injury."[23]

Indivisible Harm

The rule of law applied by the court in *Variety Children's Hospital* was the following: "If two defendants are acting independently and their two negligent acts combined to cause an *indivisible* harm, they would be jointly and severally liable for all the harm [italics added]."[1] Thus, a third "circumstance where one person is held legally responsible for harm, caused at least in part, by the conduct of another . . . [involves] shared culpable conduct such as that of joint tortfeasors . . . responsible for the plaintiff's *indivisible* injuries [italics added]."[8] Strictly speaking, the two defendants in *Variety Children's Hospital* (Drs. Rader and Garcia) were *concurrent tortfeasors*—that is, "those whose independent, negligent acts combined or concurred at one point in time to injure a third party"[16]—as opposed to joint tortfeasors, but no matter. The outcome would remain the same. What is most important about this case is the fact that the harm to the plaintiff was indivisible.

The indivisibility of the harm to the plaintiff in *Variety Children's Hospital* distinguishes it from the negligent drivers scenario with which we began the chapter, in which the harms to the plaintiff (one to his arm and one to his leg) were clearly divisible and attributable to a particular defendant. " 'Divisible injury' refers to a harm with portions or components separable and attributable to discrete tortfeasors in a multiple-tortfeasor injury. The general rule for divisible injury is that each defendant is answerable for the portion [of the injury] caused by that defendant."[24] In other words, the liability imposed in cases involving divisible injuries is said to be *individual*.[25] " 'Indivisible injury' refers to a harm not separable into discrete portions or components attributable to discrete tortfeasors in a multiple-tortfeasor injury."[24] The liability imposed in cases involving indivisible injuries is said to be *common*, or *group*, or *shared*.[25]

How is liability in cases involving indivisible injury "shared"? Traditionally, as we saw in *Variety Children's Hospital*, the liability was shared by imposing on the multiple tortfeasors joint and several liability. As we explained previously, " '[j]oint and several liability' for indivisible injury in multiple-tortfeasor cases refers to a rule whereby each defendant sued and found liable may be held to answer for the entire judgment amount."[24]

Many states have, however, modified the traditional rule of joint and several liability,[24] adopting instead *several liability* in cases involving indivisible injury in multiple-tortfeasor cases. " 'Several liability' for indivisible injury in multiple-tortfeasor cases refers to a rule whereby each defendant sued and found liable may be held to answer only for a share of the entire judgment amount reflecting that defendant's proportion of responsibility among the various parties sharing in that responsibility."[24] Arizona, for example, did so by means of a statute, which reads in part:

> In an action for personal injury, property damage or wrongful death, the liability of each defendant for damages is *several* only and is not joint. . . . [T]he liability of the person who caused the injury shall be allocated to each person in proportion to that person's percentage fault. . . . Each defendant is liable only for the amount of damages allocated to that defendant in direct proportion to the defendant's percentage of fault, and . . . judgment shall be entered against the defendant for that amount. . . . In assessing percentages of fault the trier of fact shall consider the fault of all persons that contributed to the alleged injury, death, or damaged the property, regardless of whether the person was, or could have been, named as a party to the suit.[26]

You will recall that we introduced the case of *Variety Children's Hospital* by suggesting that it was one of "a number of circumstances where one person is held legally responsible for harm caused[,] at least in part, by the conduct of another." In *Variety Children's Hospital*, the tortious conduct of either defendant was probably sufficient to cause substantially the same harm to the plaintiff that their combination produced. That being the case, should we ground liability here under rule 1 as we have posited it? The answer is no, and the reason is that it will not always be the case that the tortious conduct of either defendant will be sufficient to cause substantially the same harm to the plaintiff that their combination produces.

Consider the following case:

> In *Mitchell v. Volkswagenwerk, AG,* 669 F.2d 1199 (8th Cir. 1982), plaintiff was a passenger in a car that left the road. Plaintiff was thrown from the car and

rendered paraplegic by the accident. There was great dispute about whether the paraplegia occurred while the plaintiff was still in the car (in which case the negligent driver would have been liable for it) or whether it occurred after the plaintiff was out of the car (in which case the car's manufacturer might have been liable for it due to a defective door.) The jury returned a verdict for $360,000 against the manufacturer and $210,000 against the driver. The court reversed the judgment entered on that verdict on the ground that plaintiff had suffered an indivisible injury and that, if the jury could not decide when it occurred, the proper approach was joint and several liability for the entire injury.[1]

If the passenger was in fact rendered paraplegic while still inside the car (something we will never know), to hold the manufacturer liable for the injury is to hold it liable for an injury that it did not cause. Recall, too, the case of *Summers v. Tice*,[27] which we discussed in the previous chapter. In that case, although both of the defendants were negligent, only one could have caused the injury to the plaintiff's eye. In its opinion in that case, the Supreme Court of California cited a factually similar, previous case from Mississippi—*Oliver v. Miles*[28]—and, quoting from the opinion in that case, wrote: " 'We think that . . . each is liable for the resulting injury to the boy, although no one can say definitely who actually shot him. *To hold otherwise would be to exonerate both from liability, although each was negligent, and the injury resulted from such negligence* [italics added].' "[1]

In each of these cases—*Mitchell v. Volkswagenwerk, AG, Summers v. Tice*, and *Oliver v. Miles*—a defendant who had himself or itself been negligent was nevertheless held liable not for the consequences of his or its own wrongful acts or omissions, but for the wrongful acts or omissions of his or its codefendants. We know this to be true because in all three cases both defendants were held jointly and severally liable, even though in all three cases the injury could only have been caused by one of the defendants.

Clearly, liability in each of these cases must be grounded in an exception to the second of our rules as posited earlier, which we now rewrite as follows:

1. A health care provider is liable for the foreseeable consequences of his, her, or its own wrongful acts or omissions.

2. A health care provider is *not* liable for the consequences of another's wrongful acts or omissions, unless

    a. the provider observes or should observe those wrongful acts or omissions and fails to object to them, or

    b. derivative liability applies, or

    c. one of the following forms of vicarious liability applies:

        i.   *respondeat superior*

        ii. apparent or ostensible agency

        iii. nondelegable duty

       iv. partnership

       v. a joint enterprise, or

    d. the negligent acts of two health care providers combine to cause an indivisible harm.

Chapter Summary

Physicians and other health care providers—including institutional providers—are liable for the foreseeable consequences of their own wrongful acts or omissions. Such liability is said to be direct. As a general rule, physicians and other health care providers are *not* liable for the consequences of another's wrongful acts or omissions unless an exception to this rule is applicable. Exceptions include the following: (1) where the provider observes or should observe the wrongful acts or omissions of another and fails to object to them, (2) where the negligent acts of two health care providers combine to cause an indivisible harm, (3) derivative liability, and (4) vicarious liability. Vicarious liability may be imposed on a physician or other health care provider, and the negligence of another imputed to him, her, or it on the basis of *respondeat superior*, apparent or ostensible agency, a nondelegable duty, the existence of a partnership, or the existence of a joint enterprise. Where one or more of these exceptions are applicable, a physician or other health care provider may be held legally responsible for the harm caused, at least in part, by the wrongful conduct of another.

Review Questions

1. When multiple tortfeasors are involved, may a physician or other health care provider be held legally responsible for the harm caused, at least in part, by the wrongful conduct of another? If so, when?

2. What is direct liability?

3. What is derivative liability, and how does it differ from vicarious liability?

4. Explain corporate negligence.

5. Name and explain five different types of vicarious liability.

6. Explain the borrowed-servant and the captain-of-the-ship doctrines. How do they relate to *respondeat superior* and vicarious liability?

7. What is the nondelegable duty doctrine? What policy considerations justify it? How does vicarious liability under it differ from vicarious liability under apparent or ostensible agency?

8. What are the elements that constitute a joint enterprise?

9. Explain the difference between individual and common liability. Which is applicable to a situation involving multiple tortfeasors causing an indivisible harm?

10. Differentiate between joint and several liability and several liability and explain how they relate to common liability.

Endnotes

1. Franklin MA, Rabin RL. *Tort Law and Alternatives*. 4th ed. Mineola, NY: Foundation Press, 1987:216.
2. *Maltempo v. Cuthbert*, 504 F.2d 325, 328 (5th Cir. 1974).
3. Recall from Chapter 15 that the fourth exception to the no-duty rule is the voluntary assumption of duty by the defendant. Once the defendant voluntarily begins to act (for example, to render assistance to the plaintiff), he or she must proceed with reasonable care and may not discontinue efforts if doing so would leave the plaintiff worse off than when assistance was begun.
4. Admittedly, Cuthbert's liability seemingly differs in some respects from that of Freeman. It might seem that Cuthbert is being held liable for Freeman's acts or omissions. After all, had Freeman taken better care of Maltempo, the prisoner would not have died and Cuthbert would not have been sued; however, Freeman was not before the court, and neither, it appears, was the issue of liability on his part. The issue was simply whether Cuthbert was liable for Maltempo's injury, and the court determined that he was.
5. *Morey v. Thybo*, 199 F. 760 (7th Cir. 1912).
6. *Darling v. Charleston Community Memorial Hospital*, 33 Ill.2d 326, 211 N.E.2d 253 (Sup. Ct. Ill. 1965).
7. In fact, "a claim based on . . . [derivative liability] . . . is based on [a defendant's] direct negligence." See Martin E Jr. Coverage for vicarious and derivative liability under Texas law. Presented at the 4th Annual Insurance Law Institute, the University of Texas School of Law and the Insurance Law Section of the State Bar of Texas (October 6–8, 1999, Dallas, Texas). Available at: http://www.haynesboone.com/FILES/tbl_s12PublicationsHotTopics%5CPublication-PDF60%5C575%5C10_06_1999_Martin.pdf. Accessed April 5, 2008.
8. Underwood WD, Morrison MD. Apportioning responsibility in cases involving claims of vicarious, derivative, or statutory liability for harm directly caused by the conduct of another. *Baylor Law Rev* 2003;55:617, 620.
9. Hall MA, Bobinski MA, Orentlicher D. *Health Care Law and Ethics*. 6th ed. New York: Aspen Publishers, 2007:436.
10. Regarding derivative liability,

   > Several well-established categories of liability meet this definition of derivative liability. One category includes those cases where the defendant's negligence affirmatively enabled a third person's foreseeable and culpable conduct to cause the plaintiff's injuries. This category would include, for example, a case where a trucking company negligently hired, retained or supervised a habitually intoxicated truck driver who injured the plaintiff as a result of driving while intoxicated. It would also include claims that a defendant had negligently entrusted a vehicle or some other dangerous instru-

mentality to another, such as a pawn shop that negligently sold a Saturday Night Special to a violent and underage youth, who then used the handgun to gun down a police officer. Another category of cases meeting this definition of derivative liability includes cases where the defendant negligently interfered with the plaintiff's safety measures and thereby created an unreasonable risk of harm resulting from the foreseeable criminal, intentional or negligent intervention of a third person. Yet a third category would include cases where a defendant unreasonably fails to take necessary steps to warn of, or reduce the risk of, foreseeable criminal intervention, such as a property owner whose unlawful failure to secure its property permits a foreseeable crime of violence to occur on the premises. (Internal footnotes omitted.)

See Underwood WD, Morrison MD. Apportioning responsibility in cases involving claims of vicarious, derivative, or statutory liability for harm directly caused by the conduct of another. *Baylor Law Rev* 2003;55:617, 620.

11. *Yorston v. Pennell*, 397 Pa. 28; 153 A.2d 255 (Sup. Ct. Pa. 1959).
12. The first question that might occur to you is, Why did Yorston sue Dr. Pennell instead of Hatemi and/or Rex? The answer is that he could not sue them (or at least could not prevail in a lawsuit against them) because the hospital and its employees (including Hatemi and Rex) were protected under the doctrine of charitable immunity. Not so Dr. Pennell.
13. *Crowell v. City of Philadelphia*, 531 Pa. 400, 407, 613 A.2d 1178, 1181 (Sup. Ct. Pa. 1992), quoting Keeton WP, et al., eds. *Prosser and Keeton on the Law of Torts*, §69. 5th ed. St. Paul, MN: West Publishing, 1984.
14. Havighurst CC, Blumstein JF, Brennan TA. *Health Care Law and Policy*. 2nd ed. New York: Foundation Press, 1998:626.
15. "Captain of the ship" doctrine continues to take on water. Available at: http://findarticles.com/ p/articles/mi_m0FSL/is_4_74/ai_80159549. Accessed January 10, 2008.
16. *Black's Law Dictionary*. Abridged 6th ed. St. Paul, MN: West Publishing, 1991:40.
17. *Jackson v. Power*, 743 P.2d 1376 (Sup. Ct. Alaska 1987).
18. Partnerships. In: Furrow BR, Greaney TL, Johnson SH, Jost TS, Schwartz RL, eds. *Health Law*. Vol. 1. St. Paul, MN: West Publishing, 1995:319–333, p. 325.
19. *O'Grady v. Wickman*, 213 So.2d 321 (Fla. App. 1968).
20. "[A]ny party to a civil action [may] move for a summary judgment . . . when he believes that there is no genuine issue of material fact and that he is entitled to prevail as a matter of law." See *Black's Law Dictionary*, p. 1001.
21. *Lyon v. Ranger III*, 858 F.2d 22 (1st Cir. 1988), quoting Keeton W, et al., eds. *Prosser and Keeton on the Law of Torts*, §72. 5th ed. St. Paul, MN: West Publishing, 1984:517.
22. *Bolles v. Kinton*, 83 Colo. 147, 263 P. 26 (1928).
23. *Variety Children's Hospital v. Osle*, 292 So.2d. 382 (Fla. Ct. App. 1974).
24. Hager MH. What's (not!) in a restatement? ALI issue-dodging on liability apportionment. *Conn Law Rev* 2000;33:77, 79.
25. Kilgard R. Cleaning up after multiple tortfeasors: part one—the prerequisites for common liability. *AZ Attorney* 1999;35:26.
26. See Kilgard R. Cleaning up after multiple tortfeasors: part two—the nature of the common liability. *AZ Attorney* 1999;35:32 , citing Arizona Revised Statutes §12-2506 (2008).
27. *Summers v. Tice*, 199 P.2d 1 (Sup. Ct. Cal. 1948).
28. *Oliver v. Miles*, 144 Miss. 852 (1926).

Section V

Humanities in Medicine

Chapter 17

Introduction to Medical Humanities

Humanities are the hormones of medicine.

—William Osler, "The Old Humanities and the New Science"

Chapter Learning Objectives
At the conclusion of this chapter the reader will be able to:

1. Understand the inadequate state of medical education and medical practice prior to the twentieth century

2. Recognize the accomplishments made by the adoption and implementation of Flexner's report in 1910

3. Realize that medicine has been associated with those considered educated or learned

4. Know the rationale behind the emphasis on science in medical education

5. Understand what medical humanities contributes to medicine and how it currently is included in professional courses today

Medical humanities, with its emphasis on stories and perspective, became part of medical education in the mid-1970s, more than fifty years after Abraham Flexner's recommendations about medical education were implemented. This chapter offers a brief review of Flexner's role and contributions to medicine and of subsequent developments that explain why medical humanities programs were added to the curriculum and what they are intended to accomplish.

Medical Humanities

The humanities and arts provide insight into the human condition, suffering, personhood, our responsibility to each other, and offer a historical perspective on medical practice. Attention to literature and the arts help to develop and nurture skills of observation, analysis, empathy, and self-reflection—skills that are essential for humane medical care.[1]

Because medical humanities has become an important part of medical education in recent years, the following three chapters provide information about that discipline and examples of the kinds of literature and art that might be chosen for discussions in courses for health care professionals. Each of these chapters relates to one of the three major stages

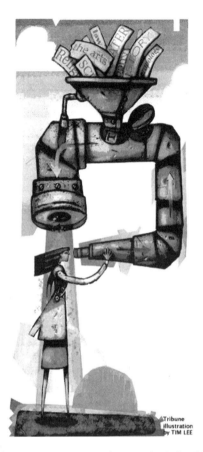

Permission for use granted by Masters' in Bioethics and Medical Humanities, University of South Florida College of Medicine.

in the human journey from birth to death—reproduction and childbirth, midlife, aging and the end of life.

Before moving to stage-of-life explorations, this introductory segment reviews the development of medical training in this country, the unintended omission and later restoration of medical humanities, and the role and importance of *perspective* for gaining knowledge, affirmation, and identification for the purposes of connecting with and understanding the untidy constructs of reality that identify and inform our lives.

Medical Education: The Background

In the latter part of the 1800s, the fledgling America Medical Association (AMA) recognized the irregular and lax conditions associated with medical education occurring across

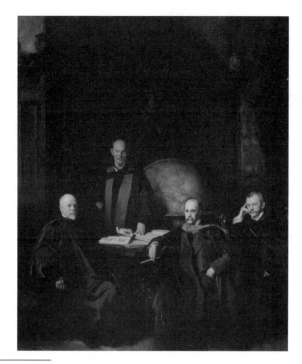

Figure 17-1 *The Four Doctors,* by John Singer Sargent, 1905, depicts the four physicians who founded Johns Hopkins Hospital. The original hangs in the William H. Welch Medical Library of Johns Hopkins University.

Reprinted with permission from the Alan Mason Chesney Medical Archives, The Johns Hopkins Medical Institutions.

the country and the need for reform measures. A handful of progressive institutions— Harvard, the University of Pennsylvania, and Johns Hopkins (Fig. 17-1)—had followed the biomedical science and hands-on training model set by schools in Europe, but many other training "institutions" in the United States were for-profit and proprietary, with only marginal interests in curriculum development. Inadequate and often exploitive, the schools had become embarrassing and unacceptable to those who championed medicine's higher purposes and who were determined to establish higher norms.

As medical historians know, Abraham Flexner, a highly regarded nonphysician educator, was asked in 1909 by the Carnegie Institution to study the specific conditions of medical education. After traveling across the United States and Canada and noting, primarily, the obvious weaknesses and deficiencies of the then current system of medical education, Flexner called for professional standards that would establish systematized, experiential, and universally applied medical education. Not surprisingly, his comprehensive report, presented in 1910 and known as the Flexner Report, confirmed concerns expressed by the AMA, outlined the need for standards, and served as a transformational event for medical education and the monumental advancements that were to follow.

A Disproportionate Shift from Liberal Arts to Science

Although the Flexner Report continues to be recognized for its standardization measures and contributions to restructuring, few realize that Flexner and medical leaders of that period had a tacit understanding about the qualifications of those entering medicine. Flexner's report *did* place an appropriate and necessary emphasis on scientific principles and training standards, but he and others *assumed* that medical students would continue to have the strong liberal arts backgrounds that had informed Osler, Welch, and other medical leaders of the time. Because these great men, usually in European settings, had studied works by Euripides, Shakespeare, Swift, and Molière, as well as the biomedical sciences, they represented and defined "educated" or learned men. In successive decades, the focus on the previously omitted sciences was strengthened—and then became dominant. Although the Flexnerian model accomplished what had been needed, the almost exclusive emphasis on the sciences tended to divert interest from the liberal arts into the realm of the newly emphasized areas. Students choosing a career in medicine therefore prepared for admission into medical schools by focusing on previously unavailable or poorly presented courses in biology, chemistry, and other sciences.

This background matters if we are to understand the recent role of humanities in the curriculum for physicians, nurses, and other health care professionals. World War II served as a showcase for the dramatic accomplishments derived from the imposed Flexnerian standards. Science and technology collaborated in ways that seemed to produce miracles on the battlefield. In contrast to medical capabilities in the Civil War and World War I, Americans were dazzled by pharmaceutical successes and new surgical procedures that saved lives. Physicians, whose historical stature in society often had been one of denigration and scorn (as seen in works by Chaucer, Shakespeare, Molière, Dickens, and Shaw), gained great admiration and respect. Funding became available for postwar hospital construction (the Hill-Burton legislation, for example) and for expanded training programs for physicians, nurses, and other health care professionals. Within a few decades the standards imposed by Flexner's landmark study had produced such remarkable and tangible results that the period between the late 1940s and the 1960s came to be recognized as medicine's Golden Age.

> The traditional rite of passage for a clinician begins with a . . . period of fact acquisition. Two years of medical school are tacked onto four years of college preparation for the refinement of that body of facts. Although latitude exists for other explorations, the emphasis is on the scientific method: hypothesis, testing, experimental design, results and conclusions.[2]

Physicians who had been shaped, in large part, by Flexnerian standards demonstrated measurable achievements and began to enjoy decades of unprecedented successes and authority. By the 1970s a number of complex events had had a profound effect on medicine and would lead to reconsiderations about training and eventual transformations. Prompted by several factors, widely accepted patterns of paternalistic behavior began to face gradual challenges, prompted by several factors, including the growing numbers of college graduates, an increased workforce of better-educated women, substantial minority group gains, informational age technologies, ethical dilemmas, and globalization trends. Each of these factors contributed to an erosion of absolute—and predominantly male—medical authority. With rising costs, questions about scarce resources and distributive justice, and greater interest in informed decision making, conversations about health care enlarged to include other health professionals, of course, but also other persons affected by and interested in health care institutions and practices, including ethicists and those with backgrounds in the humanities.

With a growing presumption by more educated and more articulate patients that physicians needed to listen to patients and their stories, the expanding discourse led to the consideration and inclusion of humanities and ethics in the health care curriculum. Many critics of medicine believed that physicians had become too focused on science, too controlling, too detached, and too arrogant. As noted by Burnside and others, fact acquisition defined the initial and formative patterns of medical training. In 1983, Bernice Wenzel observed that "medicine as practiced by the highly skilled physicians produced by modern schools is said to be medical science, not the art of healing. The patient is considered a laboratory object rather than a human being. . . . The medical curriculum is dehumanizing."[3]

Restoration of Medical Humanities to the Curriculum

Beginning in the 1970s, pastors at hospitals, medical school deans, and others interested in health care began addressing the concerns expressed by Wenzel and others. By the 1990s the curriculum in most medical schools included required or elective courses in medical humanities and ethics. Currently, in lecture formats and small group sessions, visual and verbal selections are presented that explore a wide range of concerns about human understanding and caring skills. Examples from literature range from the works of physician-writers Anton Chekhov, Susan Onthank Mates, and Richard Selzer to those of nonmedical writers and artists such as Ernest Hemingway, Ted Kooser, Dannie Abse, Lucille Clifton, and Frida Kahlo.

As shown in the next few chapters, verbal and visual accounts of illness can provide health care professionals with concrete and powerful lessons about the lives of sick people. Fiction and film, for example, about great suffering and ordinary stresses can demonstrate medicine's power, implications, and frustrations. Narratives or stories about patients *and* about health providers can widen both the lens and the perspective for understanding the complexities of the human condition. Course texts are usually chosen from the traditional literary canon, possibly Leo Tolstoy, Mikhail Bulgakov, William Carlos Williams, and Hemingway, and from among the works of contemporary and culturally diverse writers such as Ted Kooser, Walker Percy, Perri Klass, Jon Mukand, Jane Kenyon, and Sara Gruen. Novels, short stories, film, poetry, and drama can convey both the concrete particularity and the metaphorical richness of the health care predicaments of sick people and their care providers.

In recent years of teaching literature to students and faculty, medical humanities professionals have clarified conceptual frameworks and identified the means by which these studies can contribute to and strengthen the competencies needed by health care professionals. The role of literature and the arts is likely to enrich the profession and individuals therein. The inclusion of medical humanities in the curriculum may improve critical reading and appraisal, history taking, communication skills, "surrogate experience," the understanding of the role of the health care professional, ethics, and self-expression. All of these skills are central to our understanding of good medical practice.

Medicine and Literature: Useful Allies

> For there will be the arts
> and some will call them
> soft data
> whereas in fact they are the hard data
> by which our lives are lived.[4]

In its various forms—novels, poetry, theater, film, and music—the humanities contribute to a fuller, more considered understanding of what being human means. Stories and images describe how we manage or respond to events in our lives such as episodes of sickness, struggles with disappointment, miseries, and joys. Throughout history, literature and medicine have been synergistic allies, complementary agents for approaching truth and well-being. Not surprisingly, from Homer to Tolstoy to Jean-Dominic Bauby, visual and verbal stories that reference human dilemmas, whether within a strict medical context or not, define who we are as human beings. We recognize parts of the story as our own.

Many physicians who are better known as writers (W. Somerset Maugham, Anton Chekhov, Friedrich Schiller, Mikhail Bulgakov, Oliver Wendell Holmes, William Carlos Williams, etc.) have employed the observing, listening, and interpreting skills learned in medical training to create great stories and poems. In his pursuit of writing *and* medicine, Chekhov referred to himself as "chasing two hares at once."[5] In his poem "The Cure," Williams described his own writing compulsions in this way: "For when I cannot write I'm a sick man / and I want to die."[6]

In one of his best-known poems, about a red wheelbarrow (poem XXII), Williams slyly and provocatively emphasizes the importance of observing ordinary details in life—and medicine—that might be underestimated.

> so much depends
> upon
>
> a red wheel
> barrow . . .
>
> . . . .
>
> beside the white
> chickens[7]

Listening matters, he suggests—observing, imagining, and wondering, not upon wheelbarrows or white chickens exactly, but on the marginalized, neglected, or overlooked. Throughout his career in medicine, he depended on his observations of patients for the stories he would write:

> The relationship between physician and patient, if it were literally followed, would give us a world of extraordinary fertility of the imagination which we can hardly afford. There's no use multiplying cases, it is there, it is magnificent, it fills my thoughts. . . .[8]
>
> The poem springs from the half-spoken words of such patients as the physician sees from day to day. He observes it in the peculiar, actual conformations in which its life is hid. Humbly he presents himself before it and by long practice he strives as best he can to interpret the manner of its speech. In that the secret lies. This, in the end, comes perhaps to be the occupation of the physician after a lifetime of careful listening.[8(p362)]

Here and elsewhere Williams is revealed as a full-time observer, listener, and interpreter, a discoverer of the ordinary and the unexpected. Health care professionals, he believed, are located on the front lines, in the trenches—precisely where small and large dramas of life occur. Dr. Robert Coles, who had been influenced by Williams, paid tribute to his mentor by noting that physicians are in fact, "all day listener[s]."[9] The formation of the story, they both concur, is the privilege—and the soul—of medical practice.

In addition to physician-writers, a burgeoning list of other health professionals have joined the roster of good writers, such as nurses (Judy Schaefer, Courtney Davis) and physical therapists. Just as important, and embraced eagerly within the context of medical humanities, are non–health care professionals, who have and continue to script stories about the human condition. Charles Dickens, for example, had no particular association with health care. His stories, however, cast a strong light on social abuses and their effects on individuals and society in the same way that Käthe Kollwitz's bold prints and sculptures provide powerful denunciations of war and its atrocities. Unlike a factual account of history in a lecture session or the listing of symptoms in a physician's office, these stories suggest a way for distanced readers or listeners to think about events, establish order, and find meaning in their own lives. Poems by Emily Dickinson and Robert Frost stir our ability to *imagine* from a distance, but also nudge our feelings about the story as it relates to ourselves and those we know. How can we not wonder about Frost's character stopping his horse in the woods or how the roads we have not taken in some way affect our own lives? Not precisely the stuff of medicine . . . or are they?

Medical humanities programs and courses utilize these kinds of nontraditional tools and genres to explore elusive qualities that characterize and define not just the patient, but also the physician and the society they both share. Directly or indirectly, the tools focus on medical settings and circumstances, aspects of the human journey from birth to death, and various voices and perspectives. By exercising the emotions and the intellect, the contents of these courses are intended to complement information and skills learned in basic science courses and texts *and* to contribute to better care practices.

In these stories words have been chosen or discarded with care, phrases tested and edited. Similarly, the visual artist or photographer has selected, etched, and cropped. Collectively, the constructed stories twist and turn to reveal contradictory feelings, competing philosophies, and familiar events, but in entirely new ways. In their various forms, styles, and sounds, stories bind us together, help us feel connected to others as we experience the full range of human emotions, and reassure us that others have faced the same difficulties we face. We are not alone. If the story is effective, we are engaged, taken in, and possibly changed.

Many students are caught off guard by required humanities courses. They expect basic science classes (anatomy, physiology, biochemistry, and so on) and are surprised by nonscientific materials and approaches for considering diverse cultures and contexts of illness and care. Occasionally, the interdisciplinary terrain mapped out by the medical humanities courses may be seen as an abyss, but more often it is regarded as an unexpected and welcome vista. The approach is relational or multifaceted rather than decisional or authoritarian, moving away from what Patti Lather called the "lust for absolutes, for certainty in our ways of knowing" long dominant in patriarchal constructs.[10] The various forms of narrative used in medical humanities courses move students away from textbook description and analysis and force them to discover connections, to re-vision ways of knowing what they know. The classes stir participants to deconstruct their own conclusions and preferences, to stretch beyond boundaries, and to raise new questions. To include such courses or to expect health professionals to have some background in the liberal arts is, as was noted earlier, not a new idea at all, only one that was de-emphasized when another need—scientific standardization—was indeed essential.

In spite of students' complaints about nonmedical materials, their impatience with nonphysician lecturers, and their occasional display of unattractive arrogance, fiction and art do get under their skin; they are remembered and recalled unexpectedly and involuntarily.

Perspective: What We See, What We Hear

> For you will learn to see most acutely out of
> the corner of your eye
> to hear best with your inner ear
> For there are late signs and early signs
> For the patient's story will come to you[4]

When we read books, see films, attend plays, and visit museums, we agree generally that literature and the arts provide enjoyable, provocative, and instructive activities for reflecting upon uncertain, slippery dimensions of human life that extend beyond the scientific text. In various forms, selections from medical humanities, such as *The Crying Game, The Sea Beyond*, Mapplethorpe's photographs, and *Water for Elephants*, challenge, confirm, and confound our assumptions about people and behavior. Rather than providing crisp answers and firm direction, stories tend to explore beneath the surface, to raise questions, and to produce a sense of wonder. They are most powerful when they orchestrate perplexity, fail to confirm what we already know, and lead to temporary disorientation and new ways of seeing.

Perspective in medicine has always been important, but the focus primarily has been physician dominated within a paternalistic framework. As discussed earlier, in recent years that perspective in medicine has shifted so that paternalistic practices and their adherence to *detached objectivity* have given way, somewhat, to broader ways of seeing and interpreting medical events and patient circumstances. An emerging appreciation for the *subjective* voice—that is, the voice of the patient, the family member, or someone other than the health care professional's detached orientation—has become important. The professional's role continues to be strong, but less authoritative, having evolved into a more engaged relationship with patients and others involved in the health care experience. Increasingly, the patient, who once relied entirely on oversight and management by health professionals, is better informed and more prepared to ask specific questions about procedures and medications. If passive in the past, he or she is likely to be more forthright and articulate today. If paternalistic medicine was modeled on objective assessments and routine practices, contemporary patients and care providers exhibit new behaviors and expectations.

To understand the role and weight of perspective, let us consider two visual, nonmedical examples. In the early 1900s a number of young painters, such as Paul Cézanne, Pablo Picasso, and Georges Braque, sharpened their artistic skills by creating variations of different subjects to demonstrate nuances of style. Not surprisingly, one or more women bathing was one of the most popular subjects for this aggressive and talented group of young men. One of several contributions by Braque to that subject, now located at the

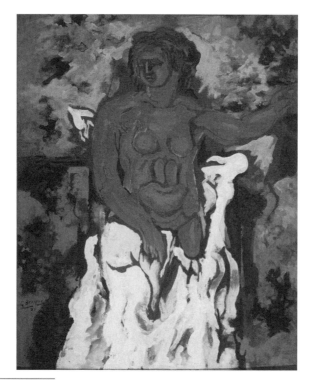

Figure 17-2   Georges Braque, *Bather,* 1922. Oil on board support, 670 × 543 mm. London, Tate Collection.

© Tate, London 2008. © 2008 Artists Rights Society (ARS), New York/ADAGP, Paris.

Tate Gallery in London, is entitled *Bather* (Fig. 17–2). The viewer's gaze settles on the partially covered woman and assesses, rather easily, her physical appearance: monumental, muscular body; dark skin; and classic features. As indicated by the painting's title, the portrayal is objective or impersonal: we know nothing about the woman in the picture. With no access to her history or to her undoubtedly complex story, the viewer sees only what the painter has chosen to reveal.

Instead of accepting the bathing woman as the gazed-upon object that she has been defined as since her creation by Braque in 1922, a contemporary poet, Carol Ann Duffy, has provided another perspective by allowing the woman to speak. Rather than accepting Braque's clever representational achievements, the first stanza of Duffy's ironically titled poem, "Standing Female Nude," reveals the opposite: a subjective voice, a model who does have something to say about herself, the artist, and the artwork.

Six hours like this for a few francs.
Belly nipple arse in the window light,
he drains the colour from me. Further to the right,
Madame. And do try to be still.
I shall be represented analytically and hung
in great museums. The bourgeoisie will coo
at such an image of a river-whore. They call it Art.[11]

By speaking, the subject steps out of the frame and acquires a revisionist dimension, a level of interest and depth. The formerly static body in towel draping is no longer inert. The model's coarse words present an irreverent dismissal of the painter and an account of her own grim circumstances. Six hours of posing for a few francs provided the means for her to get by.

Duffy, of course, is familiar with the story of Braque and his poor artist friends in Paris struggling to interpret and express currents of modernity. If one artist portrayed a nude in new ways, others borrowed from that interpretation to offer their own versions. What mattered was the art. What matters for Duffy is the subject—*this* subject. Until Duffy came along several decades later, this particular model was rendered unimportant, inconsequential. The objectified woman had no story, nothing to say. If the model's new subjective voice is heard by a viewer of the painting, the effect will be an insidious, altered appraisal. The new perspective has produced a new story, a radical change. In refusing to limit her own response to the particulars of the painting, Duffy has wondered, instead, about the historically inconsequential woman.

A second visual example is an installation piece, *Ilusione optica*, by contemporary artist Felice Varini (Fig. 17–3), which provides an ambitious illustration of the numerous points

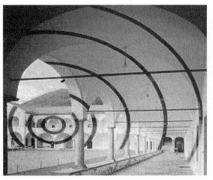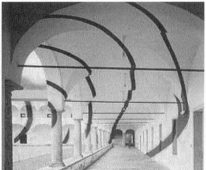

Figure 17-3A and B   Felice Varini, *Ilusiones.*

Courtesy of Felice Varini.

of view associated with perspective. Varini paints color on buildings, walls, floors, and windows in geometric patterns, but the viewer sees the colored surfaces merge to form the shape *only if* he or she is positioned in an exact spot or focal point. If the viewer moves ever so slightly away from that singular vantage point, the visual perfection of the geometric shape is lost. Then, the intended coherent whole dissolves into disconnected fragments. The installation is fractured, composed of random lines or huge splotches of color. When the participating viewer physically returns to the correct focal point, the intended image is again revealed.

Patients are more than inert objects in beds, and medical providers are not detached observers. Both are as multifaceted as Varini's colorful shards. When freed from scripted conversations and routine expectations, both patients and care providers may reveal useful discoveries and connections that could contribute to better understandings of problems and practices. Varini's optics and Duffy's imagined voice serve as reminders of the importance of perspective and its role in shaping stories and interpretations.

When the Pulitzer Prize–winning play *Wit* opened in New York City a few years ago, the audience was mesmerized by the inability of the brilliant professor of literature and the similarly brilliant research physician to speak *to* each other. Vivian Bearing, *Wit*'s fifty-year-old protagonist, is a highly respected professor of English literature whose work has centered on seventeenth-century poet John Donne. Accustomed to the intellectual rigors associated with Donne's poetic intricacies, she is uncompromising in research and teaching. Upon admission to the hospital's oncology unit with stage 4 metastatic ovarian cancer, Bearing encounters a research unit and team that is similarly rigorous and uncompromising. In unrelated spheres of study, she and Harvey Kelekian, the physician in charge of her experimental chemotherapy program, share a passion for aggressive probing and rationality. Both have been intensely focused on their work and demonstrate a shared arrogance in their separate searches for knowledge and excellence. Neither has bothered with compassion or kindness in their pursuits and relationships. He begins with a thud: "You have cancer." A few lines later, she is engaged in mental gymnastics relating to the words he uses, such as "insidious," "treacherous," "antineoplastic," and "pernicious."

Dr. Bearing's academic status is unequaled; she is at the pinnacle of her profession. Now, dressed in the hospital-issue gown, the formerly proud woman must submit to the realm of medicine. In this setting, she feels more like a piece of meat or a bug than a human being. Her first words are to the audience, in which she mimics the routine, vapid language patterns of health care workers while serving to draw viewers into the world she currently inhabits: "Hi, how are you feeling today? Great. That's just great." For Vivian, an erudite wordsmith, the line demonstrates medicine's reductive capabilities, its power to diminish. The question is an empty formality. Because the answer, "great," completes a meaningless hospital ritual, her presentation of both question and answer establishes the situation she is in and demonstrates the unexpected transformation of language—her tool—from power to meaninglessness. When the research physician advises her that the experimental treatment will not stop the cancer but will "make a significant contribution to our knowledge," the audience is aghast. No human connection has been established.

Human beings define themselves and others by the stories they tell and the perspective they choose to present. Selections from medical humanities help us to expand our limited experiences, cultivate our sympathies to human problems and concerns, and develop an aversion to denials about ourselves and our neighbors. By listening to stories and putting fragments together, we may come to understand "Why We Tell Stories":

> Because each of us tells
> the same story
> but tells it differently
>
> and none of us tells it
> the same way twice[12]

Review Questions

1. What were the circumstances of medicine that inspired Abraham Flexner's study, and what was the eventual impact of his study and report?

2. Why was the focus on science emphasized and what was the result of that emphasis? What major event demonstrated the success of Flexner's implemented plan? How did that plan affect, eventually, all health professionals?

3. What kind of study characterized the "learned" man or woman, and how has that changed?

4. Consider the realities of health care in the following timeframes:

    a. Immediately after the Flexner Report and through World War I

    b. After World War II

    c. Before and after the implementation of Medicaid and Medicare

5. Why has medical humanities been added to the curriculum for health professionals, and what does it offer that is not included in traditional medical training? More important, how does it complement traditional courses in medicine and what does it contribute to patient care understandings and skills?

6. Provide and discuss at least one example from literature, film, or art that was not included in the chapter (e.g., *The Diving Bell and the Butterfly*).

7. Find Felice Varini on the Web. Select some of his installations to discuss how they reflect the way we receive and interpret information. What if we were totally rational and never colored outside the lines?

Endnotes

1. Aull F. New York University School of Medicine medical humanities mission statement. Available at: http://medhum.med.nyu.edu/. Accessed September 1, 2008.
2. Burnside J. Visual arts and skill acquisition. In: Berg G, ed. *The Visual Arts and Medical Education*. Carbondale, IL: Southern Illinois University Press, 1983:63.
3. Wenzel B. Medical education in transition. In: Berg G, ed. *The Visual Arts and Medical Education*. Carbondale, IL: Southern Illinois University Press, 1983:6.
4. Stone J. Gaudeamus igitur: a valediction. In: *Renaming the Streets*. Baton Rouge: Louisiana State University Press, 1985:23.
5. Anton Chekhov to Alexei Suvorin, 11 September 1888. In: *Anton Chekhov's Life and Thought: Selected Letters and Commentary*. Heim MH, Karlinsky S, trans. Berkeley: University of California Press, 1973:107.
6. Williams WC. The cure. In: *The Collected Later Poems*. New York: New Directions, 1950:23.
7. Williams WC. XXII. In: Litz AW, MacGowan C, eds. *The Collected Poems of William Carlos Williams: Volume One, 1909–1939*. New York: New Directions, 1996:224.
8. Williams WC. The practice. In: *The Autobiography of William Carlos Williams*. New York: Random House, 1948:360.
9. Coles R. *The Call of Stories: Teaching and the Moral Imagination*. Boston: Houghton Mifflin, 1989:14.
10. Lather P. *Getting Smart: Feminist Research and Pedagogy with/in the Postmodern*. New York: Routledge Press, 1991:6.
11. Duffy CA. Standing female nude. In: Abse D, Abse J, eds. *Voices in the Gallery: Poems and Pictures*. London: The Tate Gallery, 1986:122.
12. Mueller L. Why we tell stories. In: *The Need to Hold Still*. Baton Rouge: Louisiana State University Press, 1980:62-63.

Chapter 18

Reproduction and Childbirth

Female bodies, and especially pregnant and newly maternal bodies, leak, drip, squirt, expand, contract, crave, divide, sag, dilate, and expel.

—Rebecca Kukla, *Mass Hysteria*

Chapter Learning Objectives
At the conclusion of this chapter the reader will be able to:

1. Understand historical contexts and the restrictions placed on women

2. Recognize how the release of restraints led to new words, vocabularies, and stories about women and their bodies

3. Recognize the authenticity of the subjective voice and its complementary role in medicine

4. Consider the importance and power of stories that define and shape women's experiences

5. Understand that the emphasis on subjectivity has led to parallel benefits for men, disabled persons, and others

Selections from medical humanities are useful for approaching, however briefly, the pervasive pattern of restrictive social and religious contexts associated with reproduction and childbirth throughout history and for understanding the gradual—and then dramatic—release of those restrictions after the mid-1800s. Other related but previously restricted topics include the death of a child or mother, miscarriage, abortion, and birth defects.

In an effort to understand the emerging voices of women and their radically new explorations and sounds, this chapter begins with a short review of the circumscribed narratives that once dominated descriptions of reproduction and birth, or the "female condition," as portrayed predominantly by male observers. The initial background discussion demonstrates past attitudes about these private matters and explains why emerging voices in contemporary life about these topics can be unexpected and shocking. Inherited attitudes that had prevailed for centuries have been modified or discarded by modern and postmodern storytellers and artists. Although most of these new verbal and visual accounts are welcomed by contemporary audiences, their departure from traditional mores and previously imposed standings of propriety can be provocative and discomforting.

To demonstrate that the new voice of women, like that of men discussing personal aspects of their own bodies and concerns, has implicit and explicit value, this chapter focuses on selections from the large body of writings and art by women *and* some men about women that first began to appear in the late nineteenth century. If women's stories were written for centuries exclusively by men within an overriding theological framework and from positions of power and dominance, it is not surprising to find that more recent narratives by women offer different, even radically different, perspectives about themselves and their bodies. New words in new narratives have burst forth to provide vital, previously omitted insights that are important—and often medically useful. An examination of examples from the medical humanities illustrates how these works differ from and contribute to the materials found in medical textbooks. Women who once depended on private letters, diaries, and journals to speak for themselves about pregnancy and other suppressed or *silenced* circumstances would be shocked to discover the range of personal accounts of femaleness today.

The chapter concludes with more contemporary examples from literature and art about formerly taboo subjects: miscarriage, abortion, birth defects, and child or maternal deaths. None of these topics would have been broached if women had remained bound by previous traditions and expectations.[1] The contrast between centuries of women's restricted history with what has emerged in recent decades reveals a remarkable release of information, words, and emotions about women that can guide and assist care by professional care providers. The content, but also the shapes and sounds, of women's own words may startle some, but most listeners are excited about these voices and the authenticity they bring to both separate and collective experiences—and care options.

The Background: An Inherited Framework

> Unto the woman he said, I will greatly multiply thy sorrow and thy conception; in sorrow thou shalt bring forth children; and thy desire shall be to thy husband, and he shall rule over thee.[2]

Women's place in Western history has been shaped in large part by theological texts, specifically those dealing with Eve and, later, with the Virgin Mary. As readers of the Bible knew and as thundering sermons proclaimed, Eve's disobedience led to humankind's fall from grace and subsequent expulsion from the Garden of Eden. It was clear, as well, that this female progenitor and her successors were destined for subordination to men.

Later, in New Testament stories, the baby Jesus is miraculously conceived and born with no accompanying narrative about painful labor and childbirth. Mary, his mother, represented the supreme model for motherhood, whether escaping into Egypt on a donkey or nursing her newborn child. Especially for the Catholic religion, the portrayals of women as represented by Mary, the epitome of motherhood, and Eve, an insubordinate sinner, offered two polarities: one, an impossible representation of perfection, the other, a relegation to second-class status. Both stories were recounted repeatedly and imposed on captive audiences by theologians throughout the centuries.

In the Middle Ages, from the pulpit and elsewhere, stories about women focused on embedded oppositions: those who were virtuous and those who were not. Christians accepted Eve's intellectual weakness (her failure to resist Satan's temptation), her psychological weakness (her skillful seduction of Adam), and her biological weakness (her suffering pain during childbirth). Mary, the mother of the Christ child, was virtuous and pure. *The Annunciation* by Fra Angelico (Fig. 18-1) is one of many visual representations

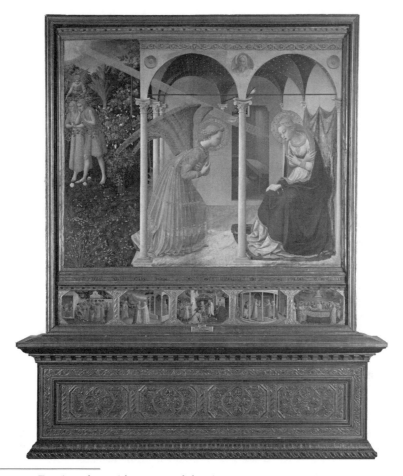

Figure 18-1 Fra Angelico. Altarpiece of the Annunciation. c. 1430–1432. Tempera on panel. 194 × 194.

Museo Nacional del Prado. Reprinted with permission.

that portrays both stories on the same canvas. On the left, the shamed couple is driven from Eden, while to the right, and more central, the Virgin Mary learns that she is with child.

Centuries Pass: No Change

In the seventeenth century, very few women were literate, and the experiences of pregnancy and childbirth were not considered a decent topic for public conversation.[3]

Many centuries passed between Fra Angelico's pictorial portrayal of women and the colonization of New England, but the circumstances of most women's lives were unaltered. Although Puritan Protestants did not portray Mary with the same zealousness as Catholics, the idea of "Eve's curse"—the infliction of pain during childbirth—continued, as did the dictates of confinement or concealment during pregnancy. Pregnant women covered or concealed their growing abdomens during the nine-month period of *confinement*, and restricted their activities. Etiquette and social mores regarding the female body and exposure of genitalia required women to rely upon their circle of women friends for comfort and the local midwife for information and assistance.

In the Puritan colony of Massachusetts, Cotton Mather's solemn words and embedded reference to the high incidence of childbirth mortality underscored the continued power of the biblical curse:

[Mothers] need no other linen . . . but a *Winding Sheet*, and have no other chamber but a *grave*, no neighbors but *worms*.[4]

Already acutely aware of the high rate of death during childbirth within their small communities, pregnant women—and their husbands—must have trembled in fear at this kind of stentorian pronouncement. In another voice and using very different words, Anne Bradstreet in 1650 addressed her own pregnancy and the risks she faced:

All things within this fading world hath end
Adversity doth still our joys attend;
No ties so strong, no friends so dear and sweet
But with death's parting blow is sure to meet. . . .
If any worth or virtue were in me,
Let that live freshly in thy memory
And when thou feel'st no grief, as I no harms,
Yet love thy dead, who long lay in thine arms,
And when thy loss shall be repaid with gains,
Look to my little babes, my dear remains.
And if thou love thyself, or loved'st me,
These O protect from step-dame's injury.[5]

Other writings by Bradstreet show that children were an intense joy to her, but the hovering reality of maternal mortality could not be dismissed.

New Opportunities: The Medical Model

Beginning in the eighteenth century with the use of forceps by male physicians and into the nineteenth and early twentieth centuries, changes began to occur that would shake irretrievably the biblical passage associated with Eve's monumental sin and the lives of women. Gradually, the circle-of-women model was replaced by the new obstetric model that included physician care and relief of pain. As their role in childbirth grew, physicians—and women—overcame prevailing gender issues. By the mid-nineteenth century, middle-class women were becoming more accustomed to male physicians, who, with the use of ether or chloroform, could provide relief of pain. The physician-controlled use of twilight sleep drugs required hospital settings, as did the emphasis on asepsis by Semmelweis and Oliver Wendell Holmes, which resulted in reductions in mortality. Both advances led to a decline in home birthing options. The preference for twilight sleep and a shorter, less painful delivery led to a shift from birth as a natural event supervised by women to a hospital event managed by physicians. This model was to remain in place from the early decades of the twentieth century until today. Nevertheless, some women were dissatisfied with the sterile hospital setting, in which they frequently felt like objects responding to the demands of strangers providing and administering drugs.

A poem by Helen Chasin, "The Recovery Room: Lying-In," offers an introduction to the trend we have been describing. Postpartum reflections generally had not been commonplace or appropriate topics for poetry. It was considered too personal, even tasteless, for a woman to describe the birth experience, but what this speaker presents, however radical, *is* commonplace and familiar to those delivered by doctors in hospitals. Her "pubic seam stitched back," she seems to be "wrapped in scopolamine."[6] The mother in the poem is recovering from a routinized, medicalized labor and birth, events that are hazily recollected. She has been lying in, acted upon, supervised by her physician and unknown others. Although the poem describes an efficiently managed birth without much pain, the account is numbing and uninspiring.

From Private to Public: The Shock of the New

During the time that most women were choosing physician-managed birth with its promise of reduced pain and mortality, events were occurring that would contribute to reconsiderations of such arrangements. The suffrage movement, two great wars, scientific advancements derived in part from Flexnerian standards, and broader educational opportunities were having profound effects on women's lives and on decisions affecting their personal lives. Women writers such as Jane Austen, George Eliot, and Virginia Woolf and male colleagues such as George Bernard Shaw and Henrik Ibsen were among the liberating forces for establishing new grounds for women to reflect upon personal choices and decisions. After centuries of restriction and obliqueness regarding pregnancy and childbirth and of social subservience, women's voices began to sound in the late nineteenth and early twentieth centuries.

As circumstances allowed for more possibilities and options, women became more deliberative and more vocal about their choices and experiences. Whereas obstetricians had cared for their grandmothers and mothers, late twentieth-century women began to reframe their childbearing experiences. Even though physician-managed care still remains the norm, there has been a movement toward more options, as evidenced by the use of fewer drugs in labor and delivery, more midwifery and home births, more homelike hospital birth suites, and more family participation as contrasted with sterile white coat settings. All of this indicates that contemporary women have become far more knowledgeable, articulate, and participatory than their forebears could ever have imagined.

Women are no longer silent and are no longer limited to their private diaries and journals. Women's new energy is conveyed by Hélène Cixous in a parallel she draws between childbearing and writing, urging women to speak of and from themselves so that generative forces of life are released, breaking old patterns and establishing more deeply reflective perspectives:

> She gives birth. With the force of a lioness. Of a plant. Of a cosmogony. Of a woman. She has her source. She draws deeply. She releases. Laughing. And in the wake of the child, a squall of Breath! A longing for text! Confusion! What's come over her? A child! Paper! Intoxications! I'm brimming over! My breast are overflowing! Milk! Ink! Nursing time. And me? I'm hungry, too. The milky taste of ink![7]

As the examples in this chapter show, many women are telling their own childbearing stories in exuberant, kaleidoscopic portrayals, revealing how the universalizing biblical accounts and, later, medical accounts have been replaced by a particular, singular woman telling a story about the personal and intimate details of her own life or her narrative character's life and the meanings she makes of details and circumstances. Women have found their subjective voices and can speak for themselves. It's a whole new world.

There remains, however, a sense of prudishness or discomfort about the human body and sex. Those still influenced by historic protocols of silence about personal matters may be surprised and offended by stories that speak about the physical and psychological specifics of pregnancy. In the medical humanities selections that follow, the emerging voices add relevancy. For most listeners, these voices are regarded as real and welcome.

The Normal Pregnancy: Truth Told Slant

The emerging gendered voice with its new words and new images could be and can remain startling to listeners and viewers still accustomed to inherited interpretations of women in male-dominated cultures. When women decided to talk about pregnancy, the tradition of confinement and concealment ended. Rather than submit to protocols that were not reflective of lived experiences, artists and writers created more accurate, more authentic accounts to describe reproduction and childbirth, including problems along the way. The examples discussed here reject the objective formats of the past. The passive female submitting to medical descriptors and constraints has been replaced. For those in medicine, these accounts reveal the importance of individual perspective and the uniqueness of persons. Each example tells only one story, but it is a story worth hearing—or observing.

Margaret Evans Pregnant by Alice Neel (Fig. 18-2) is straightforward and direct—shockingly so, for some. Although the portrayed woman, or any pregnant woman, normally would not be presented this way, including in a physician's office, Neel's large expressionist work represents the reality of pregnancy. The stretched abdomen and pendulous breasts present more than we, as a society, are accustomed to seeing. (More recently,

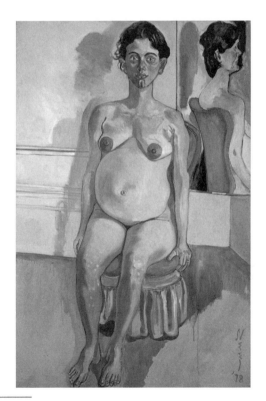

Figure 18-2 Alice Neel, *Margaret Evans Pregnant*, 1978. Oil on canvas, 57 3/4 × 38 in. Private collection.

photographs of the pregnant Demi Moore and Britney Spears provided a similar shock.) During a time when many of the artist's friends and family members were beginning families, Neel "found the subject of generational renewal sufficiently interesting to devote approximately half of her output to the portrayal of parents and children."[8] The subject's eyes look back at the viewer, not at all ashamed or demure—exposed, stripped of veneer. She is, in fact, a pregnant nude. However explained, no neutral response is possible.

"Notes from the Delivery Room," a poem by Linda Pastan, provides readers with another pregnant woman, this time a woman in childbirth whose mind is responding to what her body is experiencing. The woman is reflective, imaginative, alert, and even funny. Nothing like this occurs in medical texts.

> Strapped down,
> victim in an old comic book,
> I have been here before,
> this place where pain winces
> off the walls
> like too bright light
> Bear down a doctor says,
> foremen to sweating laborer,
> but this work, this forcing
> of one life from another
> is something that I signed for
> at a moment when I would have signed anything.
> Babies should grow in fields;
> common as beets or turnips
> they should be picked and held
> root up, soil spilling
> from between their toes—
> and how much easier it would be later,
> returning them to the earth.
> Bear up . . . bear down . . . the audience
> grows restive, and I'm a new magician
> who can't produce the rabbit
> from my swollen hat.
> She's crowning, someone says,
> but there is no one royal here,
> just me, quite barefoot,
> greeting my barefoot child.[9]

Pastan's imagery presents a whimsical, thoughtful, and quietly joyful stream-of-consciousness account of a woman in stirrups in the delivery room. She begins with her appearance, "strapped down / victim in an old comic book," in a place where she has been before.[9] This is not her first pregnancy. Unpredictably, she moves from the comic book image to that of a sweating laborer for the doctor-foreman who is urging her on.

Then, an abrupt change occurs. She becomes more pensive, playful in her thoughts about the cycle of life, including death: "Babies should grow in fields; . . . and how much easier it would be later, / returning them to the earth."[9] We are curious about this thought. Has an earlier child died, we wonder? Without knowing more, the speaker takes the reader back to the delivery table, where she now likens herself to a magician pulling a rabbit out of a swollen hat. The words and images in the poem validate the experience of labor and birth and the immediacy of this woman's own corporeal experience and also, to some measure, that of other women.

Problems: When Things Go Wrong

"[T]he lost baby poem," published in a book entitled *Good Woman* by Lucille Clifton, presents a narrator who speaks directly to the baby she aborted in the distant past. Initially the word "lost" in the title might suggest a miscarriage, but subsequent lines in the short poem reveal the purposeful act of abortion. The narrator remembers the harsh circumstances that led to the decision she was forced to make during the winter of the "year of the disconnected gas / and no car."[10] Rather than apologizing for her actions, the narrator explains the dire circumstances of poverty and helplessness to the "almost body" she sent "down to meet the waters under the city."[10] The poem illustrates the complexities of abortion and underscores on several levels that such a decision is not a simple matter, nor is it over when it is physically over. Clifton's narrator grieves for the conditions that led to the decision and for the loss she never forgets. In memory of the never-realized child whom this "good woman" is addressing with remorse, the speaker concludes with a powerful oath:

> . . . if i am ever less than a mountain
> for your definite brothers and sisters
> let the rivers pour over my head
> . . . .
> for your never named sake.[10]

In terms of abortion discussions and debates, the poem raises a number of issues for medical professionals to consider about poverty, possible disenfranchisement, and the burdens suffered by women. Judgments and absolute assumptions about behaviors seldom reflect the range of possibilities that might have been influential.

In 2007, *Juno,* a fresh, quirky, and enormously popular film about teenage pregnancy, captured the interest of filmgoers. When Juno, a hyperverbal, straight-to-the point teen, tests positive for pregnancy, she suffers no shame or remorse. This teen knows what is up and decides that abortion is her best option. When a pro-life protester outside the abortion clinic describes the fetus's tiny fingernails, Juno bails out and chooses a kind of in-your-face twenty-first-century adoption possibility that Lucille Clifton and her poem's narrator could not have anticipated. This story about a teen-in-charge is not a common story, but it does illustrate a savvy that those under age twenty-five may possess. Old rules and formalities do not apply, and parents, if they are loving and cool, provide support. The story, language, and situation make Linda Pastan and Helen Chasin seem like distant pioneers by comparison. Most medical professionals in training will have seen this film and can use its story for discussion in ethics classes or for understanding how the conditions and conversations about reproduction and childbirth have changed.

Just as stories about birth disorders and their aftermath, such as *My Left Foot* and *Frankie Starlight,* are often included in medical education courses, so too visual images by Frida Kahlo and Marc Quinn have been incorporated to provide more insights into the complexities associated with pregnancy gone wrong. Although unorthodox, the stories, however disparate, can be useful and pertinent to medical professionals who know only some of the vagaries of reproduction and pregnancy, but not everything. Kahlo, one of the most important female artists of the twentieth century, often used art to tell her own complex stories. Many know that she was married to Mexican muralist Diego Rivera, but may not be aware of the terrible trolley injury she suffered that led to a severely damaged spine, traumatic surgeries, several miscarriages, and a childless marriage.

Discussion of miscarriage is usually likely to occur in a private domain, between a woman and the father and close friends or with an obstetrician in a clinical setting. Kahlo's art is more public. In the small but elaborate painting entitled *Henry Ford Hospital, 1932,* Kahlo depicts her own miscarriage, employing the traditional *ex-voto* or *retablo* painting style used in Mexico to depict a tragic event. In images that are frightening, disturbing, and explicit, Kahlo is the patient situated in the bloodied bed. In her hands she holds several umbilical cord-like filaments, each attached to floating objects: a perfectly formed, dead male baby, a slow-paced snail, her uterus, pelvic cavity bones, a piece of medical equipment, and a purple orchid. The city of Detroit, with its productive factories and smokestacks, forms the distant backdrop for this devastating portrayal of personal suffering and loss.

Often, the disappointment of miscarriage is countered by hopes for another pregnancy, but Kahlo's enormously complex painting warns against these assumptions and simplistic conclusions. The conditions of her life and world, unknown to the health professionals caring for her in Detroit, are depicted in the painting: her trolley-damaged pelvis and uterus, cultural references, her failure to produce contrasted with Rivera's artistic successes in Detroit, her emptiness, her loss. Like Linda Pastan's narrator, this patient is not passive or inert. However personal, untidy, and iconoclastic, she has a story to tell.

In 2005 male sculptor Marc Quinn created a twelve-foot sculpture of a visibly disabled woman to be located temporarily on the fourth plinth in Trafalgar Square in London (Fig. 18-3). Entitled *Alison Lapper Pregnant,* the arresting piece of white Carrera marble produced a strong response from viewers who were more accustomed to seeing heroes on

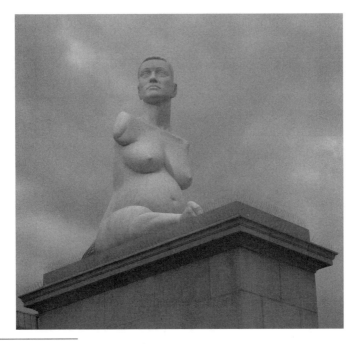

Figure 18-3 *Alison Lapper Pregnant*, by Marc Quinn.

Courtesy of Fabio Ferrari, USF College of Medicine.

horseback or great admirals on columns in their public spaces. Alison Lapper, the model, was born with phocomelia, a condition that presents with flipper-like or amphibian-like appendages at birth. In spite of her bone malformations and shortened limbs, Alison Lapper thrived and was, when the sculpture was executed, eight months pregnant.

The sculpture and its prime location in central London, just in front of the National Gallery, gave voice to an issue, disability and motherhood, that seldom receives this kind of prominent venue. What is customarily invisible became highly, even unavoidably conspicuous, so that viewers drawn to the sculpture offered spontaneous comments to families and strangers. Many found it inappropriate and were outraged by its presence. Occasionally, children were led away. Others expressed very strong support for this example of disability "uncloseted." People came face to face not just with the immovable force but with the spoken reactions of others gathered in groups around the sculpture. The impressive column of Admiral Nelson can invite viewers to comment on its height, but that traditional monument generates none of the animated discussion that was evoked by the vexingly visible monument some yards away.

The Memory Keeper's Daughter, a 2005 novel, has had the impact of bringing readers into the world of Down syndrome (trisomy 21). Like viewers of the sculpture of Alison Lapper in London, readers of this novel come into direct confrontation with health care issues and ethical dilemmas. The vibrancy of both of these stories about disability poses problems for those who would discount or marginalize those human beings outside the boundaries of "normalcy." As a child growing up, Dr. David Henry, the story's protagonist, had endured the heartache of watching his beloved sister die from a birth defect, an experience that contributed to his choice of profession. Years later, his own wife goes into labor during an unusually severe snowstorm. Upon arrival at the small hospital, only he and Caroline, the nurse he had called in advance, form the skeleton staff. These highly unusual emergency conditions require that he and his nurse attend to his wife's delivery alone. There seem to be no complications, and a baby boy is delivered. Because the birth occurs in 1964, prior to the development of amniocentesis, the attendants are surprised by the unexpected arrival of a second infant, a girl, who they both identify immediately as a Down syndrome child. Without seeking professional counsel and without informing his anesthetized wife or initiating any discussion with the nurse, David paternalistically decides to spare his wife and himself the grief of loving a child he assumes will not live very long. He hands the baby over to Caroline and directs her to place the child in a special institution. The nurse disappears into the snowstorm and eventually to another city to raise the child, Phoebe, as her own.

In the long story spun by the author about Dr. Henry's family and Caroline's new family, readers follow a tangled thread on its twisted and knotted course. Along the way readers discover more than they were likely to have known about institutions for rejected children, the development of the rescued and cared-for baby girl, marriage, loss, and suffering. This nonmedical story does not fully explore Phoebe's genetic condition and its characteristic physical features. However, for health care professionals who may deliver a baby with a "problem" and subsequently provide mothers and fathers with medical information about their baby, this story, like all of the humanities stories presented in these chapters, provides information and insights that may be relevant and useful to consider. Whether portrayed with medical accuracy or not, most stories about illness reveal complex features that extend far beyond the hospital setting and transform lives in ways we cannot begin to imagine. As this story shows, external changes can become an integral part of the patient's past and future history.

Loss: Three Stories

We do not expect young mothers to die, but, of course, that does sometimes occur. In a short, provocative poem by John Stone about a mother's death and the delivery of this terrible news to a waiting family, the physician-narrator describes the role and relationship of an empathetic physician toward the stunned family. Four simple, one-syllable words, "I will tell them," register like an incomprehensible blow.

Talking to the Family
My white coat waits in the corner
like a father.
I will wear it to meet the sister
in her white shoes and organza dress
in the live of winter,

the milkless husband
holding the baby.

I will tell them.

They will put it together
and take it apart.
Their voices will buzz.
The cut ends of their nerves
will curl.

I will take off the coat,
drive home,
and replace the light bulb in the hall.[11]

No specific information is revealed about the mother's cause of death; it may not be related to childbirth, but we know that the "milkless husband" is "holding the baby." The family must sort through the news and life as it has just become. The physician, too, must continue with his own life. In this case, readers learn that the physician will go home later to perform an ordinary domestic act: he will "replace the light bulb in the hall."[11]

A woodcut entitled *Die Eltern* (*The Parents*) by Käthe Kollwitz (Fig. 18-4) provides another perspective emphasizing the emotional component associated with a child's death. In some ways, the woodcut visually epitomizes Stone's deadening line, "I will tell them." Not unlike Stone's still-confused family, Kollwitz's "parents" have collapsed into a simple tableau revealing the totality of grief. Father and mother have crumpled to their knees, joined together like a heavy, but inseparable, mass. Such a tragic scene can be familiar to and overwhelming for health professionals, who must recognize the needs of the devastated parents.

Too often, grieving couples who have experienced loss do not and cannot come together; many seek divorce. Health professionals need to maintain a careful balance of detachment and concern, but stories such as those just described and the following by Robert Frost suggest that professional assistance should be available and encouraged. Kollwitz's couple probably will recover, but Frost's couple in the long poem entitled "Home Burial" may not.

Set in rural New England more than fifty years ago, the poem dramatizes a couple's differing responses to the recent death of their child and serves as a microcosm for understanding the dimensions and challenges of suffering. The husband, located at the bottom

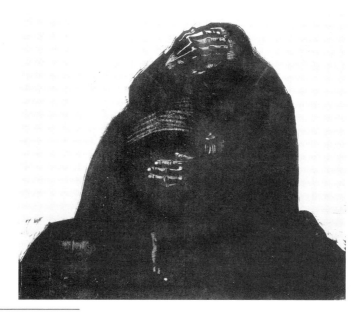

Figure 18-4 Käthe Kollwitz (German, 1867–1945), *Die Eltern* (*The Parents*) from *Sieben Holzschnitte zum Krieg* (*Seven Woodcuts About War*), 1923, published 1924. One from a portfolio of seven woodcuts, composition: 13 3/4 × 16 3/4 in. (34.9 × 42.6 cm); sheet 18 11/16 × 25 11/16 in. (47 × 65.3 cm). Publisher: Emil Richter, Dresden. Printer: probably Fritz Voigt, Berlin. Edition: two editions of 100 each. Gift of the Arnhold Family in memory of Sigrid Edwards.

of the household staircase in the poem, and wife, positioned at the midsection landing, have not come together to discuss what they feel in their shared grief. The mother regards her husband's behavior as cold and uncaring. Appearing unemotional, he has demonstrated a practical stoic attitude toward his child's death. For him, a laboring man, death is an intrinsic part of life. She, on the other hand, suffers constantly. She is enraged and disbelieving about his ability to resume his regular activities and chores. Having remained inside the house to observe the burial from a small window on the staircase landing, she later describes what she witnessed in an angry, accusatory outburst:

> "I saw you from that very window there,
> Making the gravel leap and leap in air,
> Leap up, like that, like that, and land so lightly
> And roll back down the mound beside the hole.
> I thought, Who is that man? I didn't know you."[12]

Earlier, sensing her quiet smoldering, but not quite understanding, the husband had appealed to her for help:

> "My words are nearly always an offense.
> I don't know how to speak of anything
> So as to please you. But I might be taught,
> I should suppose. I can't say I see how.
> A man must partly give up being a man
> With women-folk. We could have some arrangement
> By which I'd bind myself to keep hands off
> Anything special you're a-mind to name.
> Though I don't like such things 'twixt those that love."[12]

This situation is antithetical to that evoked by Kollwitz's powerful woodcut. Frost's couple seems to be locked into their own singular perspectives, with little hope for communication. Although the husband appears willing, this willingness is expressed *after* his wife has witnessed what she regards as a cavalier, even contemptuous burial of their child. She had expected to see his grief. Readers do not know very much about the child, whether a newborn or toddler, but the situation in varying forms is familiar to health professionals dealing with loss.

This and other fictional excursions can help students to examine their own feelings about death, a subject that usually is difficult and uncomfortable. If, like the father, the health professional appears efficient but too detached, the patient may not be helped. A professional who responds with overflowing emotion, on the other hand, fails to provide real assistance as well. The staircase landing, a balanced midpoint for the small but potent drama, suggests an appropriate location for the still-suspended characters—and for health professionals as well. After reading the poem, students will support one or the other character. Most support the husband, but a good discussion will lead to a better understanding of two people whose relationship should have been worked on and improved before this tragic event.

Review Questions

1. Discuss the portrayal of women and their particular health care needs and concerns prior to the twentieth century.

2. In the United States, what events contributed most to the gradual and then accelerated changes affecting women and their health care?

3. Choose any two of the paintings in this chapter and put them into their historic context.

4. What historic restrictions on women have been reduced or eliminated?

5. How comfortable are health professionals in discussions of reproductive anatomy with patients?

6. Frida Kahlo's paintings can be shocking to some viewers. Find four or five of them online that focus on her medical events and consider how they might provide useful insights for health professionals. What is Frida Kahlo's own narrative and how is her art often a reflection of her own personal (medical) experiences?

7. How would you and your classmates or you and your family respond to *Alison Lapper Pregnant* if you had not been introduced to the sculpture in this chapter? Do you think this and other nontraditional, iconoclastic works generate important discussions that might not have occurred if such works were not available? Name and discuss other provocative examples by artists, writers, or filmmakers.

Endnotes

1. Men, who have submitted to self-imposed silence about prostate cancer, erectile dysfunction, and other personal subjects, have been nudged by the new female model, perhaps, but more likely by pharmaceutical broadcast practices, to be similarly expressive. See the poem "Leaning Together in a Storm" by Larry Smith (discussed in Chapter 19).
2. Genesis 3:16 (King James Bible).
3. Kukla R. *Mass Hysteria: Medicine, Culture, and Mothers' Bodies*. Lanham, MD: Rowman & Littlefield, 2005:22.
4. Cited by Hoffert S. *Private Matters*. Springfield: University of Illinois Press, 1989:64.
5. Bradstreet A. Before the birth of one of her children. In: Hensley J, ed. *The Works of Anne Bradstreet*. Cambridge, MA: The Belknap Press of Harvard University, 1967:224.
6. Chasin H. The recovery room: lying-in. In: *Coming Close and Other Poems*. New Haven, CT: Yale University Press, 1968:19.
7. Cixous H. Coming to writing. In: Jensen D, ed. *Coming to Writing and Other Essays*. Cornell S, Jensen D, Liddle A, Sellers S, trans. Cambridge: MA, Harvard University Press, 1991:31.
8. Allara P. "Mater" of fact: Alice Neel's pregnant nudes. *American Art* 1994;8(2):7.
9. Pastan L. Notes from the delivery room. In: *PM/AM: New and Selected Poems*. New York: W.W. Norton, 1982:26. Copyright © 1982 by Linda Pastan. Used by permission of W.W. Norton & Company, Inc.
10. Clifton L. the lost baby poem. In: *Good Woman: Poems and a Memoir 1969–1980*. Brockport, NY: BOA Editions Limited, 1987:60.
11. Stone J. Talking to the family. In: *The Smell of Matches*. Baton Rouge: Louisiana State University Press, 1972:17. Reprinted with permission from Louisiana State University Press.
12. Frost R. Home burial. In: Lathem EC, ed. *The Poetry of Robert Frost: The Collected Poems, Complete and Unabridged*. New York: Henry Holt, 1969:53.

Chapter 19

Midlife

Story allows for distance—a way of observing, experiencing from afar. Often, it's the way to get to the truth.

—Charles Isherwood, "Stories That Tell vs. Storytelling"

Chapter Learning Objectives
At the conclusion of this chapter the reader will be able to:

1. Understand why midlife can be challenging for many

2. Appreciate how the increased numbers of people in midlife will affect medicine

3. Appreciate new characteristics of the midlife population and their expectations for themselves and from medicine

4. Understand why physicians must be prepared to discuss a range of issues with ease and comfort

5. Appreciate midlife concerns about body image, physical decline, and the perceptions of others

6. Understand the multiple responsibilities that may be present in the lives of midlife patients

7. Recognize how images, poetry, prose, and film can provide insights and perspectives for assisting health professionals to understand the complexities of the patient experience

This chapter considers numerous challenges faced by patients—and their care providers—during the middle years of life, a time that can produce tangible concerns about a range of issues that include body changes and sickness as well as intangible concerns associated with disappointment and relationships. Health care providers encountering the problems occurring at this stage of life, both their own and those of their patients, will benefit from medical skills and knowledge but also from the kinds of insights provided by the medical humanities.

Because creative artists expand our capacity for dealing with the uneven textures of patients' lives, fictions and art about midlife with its frequently untidy experiences can be valuable resources for health professionals caring for patients in this life stage. Stories *permit* distance, while eliciting emotional and intellectual engagement and broadening opportunities for creating understanding. Poems, images, and stories increase our ability to recognize and respond to points of view or perspectives that may be unfamiliar and beyond our own values and patterns of thinking.

With large numbers of baby boomers reaching midlife, health professionals can expect more office visits to include concerns about physical and psychological matters for which there are no simple prescriptions. Midlife can be a challenging time for many patients, who may be coping with aging parents and grandparents while raising their own children and sometimes grandchildren; adjusting to an empty nest and interacting with a spouse on a whole new level; questioning, reevaluating and remodeling their lives, careers, and purpose; balancing work and home; dealing with the stresses of financial and retirement issues; adjusting to more leisure time; or coping with their own declining health and ultimate death. Health care visits by people in midlife are often infused with the undercurrents of more life issues than what is readily apparent. The need for care may derive more from worries about menopause, marriage, depression, and mortality than from the pain in the chest for which a patient ostensibly presents. Although flu shots and chest pains matter, this age group also seeks more overt assistance for previously taboo problems such as sexual dysfunction in women or erectile dysfunction in men.

Health professionals should be prepared to approach midlife issues humbly, but also curiously, cautiously, respectfully, and inconclusively, recognizing that the ground can be shaky and that they may know some of the questions but few, perhaps none, of the answers. The stories presented to them may require some "reading between the lines" and helpful questioning while listening intently to patients and observing more than just words.

Women at Midlife

Midlife issues are not a new phenomenon, but for many, this generation does not look or act like its antecedents. Story threads may be more tangled as the boomer cohort struggles to assess and describe confusions clearly and powerfully. Familiarity with classic works (e.g., *King Lear*) and more recent writings, film, and theater productions (e.g., *August: Osage County*) may provide useful insights and pathways for patients, families, and health care professionals.

Onset of menopause, or "the change," once a shameful event for women during which many retreated into the shadowy background, now is regarded differently. Most women are no longer silent about menopause and other traditionally private matters. Contemporary voices address these topics with overdue directness and candor. As suggested by the popularity of *Menopause the Musical*, this time is celebrated in new circles of women and in much of current popular media. In television sitcoms, films, and novels, women are encouraged to embrace the "second half of life." Clothing, job options, and gym conditioning suggest that age forty is the new thirty, and fifty the new forty.

It is curious to consider whether there are two movements underfoot in this regard. Could there be those who actually do embrace this time in their lives, when children are older, financial worries are reduced, and women are more empowered in the workplace? Certainly there are some advantages to growing older—whether it be less social awkwardness, more financial security, or increased self-comfort and confidence. Or is the movement, in part, a response to the now more vocal and socially aware generation of baby boomers who are positive about this normal stage and are engaged in making the second half of life their "best time"? *The Third Age,* a term borrowed from the Tolkien legendarium,[1] has been adopted by some to describe a new phase of life. The analogy designates the First Age of life as *childhood,* the Second Age as *family and career* and the Third Age as *the rest of your life.*

However, popular contemporary women's magazines, such as *More,* that celebrate life after forty often feature women who continue to embrace the trappings of younger women through cosmetic surgery and antiaging serums. Self-acceptance of one's own midlife body can be problematic for some. In addition, other transitions for women at midlife may include dealing with aging parents and facing their mortality—a potential emotional and physical challenge whether a woman is the actual caregiver or is coordinating care from afar. Careers may advance or be interrupted, spouses may become ill, children may leave home, daily routines may become disrupted, and loss of identity may ensue. Reflection and reexamining life to this point and looking into the future can be both exciting and frightening.

Regardless of motive, conscious or otherwise, many women are moving forward in midlife, expecting to be able to combat problems and live with a renewed vigor. As indicated, many will present to health professionals for help with this endeavor.

Men at Midlife

For some men, midlife can also be a difficult and complicated time. Slowly, they are speaking up, sometimes reactively, but more often productively, in earnest conversations among themselves and with women about shared concerns, fears, and partnerships. Although men may never be as vocal as women regarding their emotional needs and concerns, health Web sites, Internet chat rooms, and blogs have become popular forums for addressing such topics as general problems of aging, erectile dysfunction, and prostate enlargement and their treatment. Advertisements for pharmaceutical products that address these concerns have helped bring such topics out of the shadows and into doctor–patient dialogues. Still, conversations are more likely if patients are routinely asked about important health-related subjects such as marital life, job satisfaction, symptoms of depression, and other midlife topics. Men, too, during this life stage may deal with issues of career advancement, life reevaluation, financial security, retirement, and identity loss if the individual was defined by work.

The first *City Slickers* film,[2] in 1991, was inspired by masculine disorientations at midlife and the need for reexamination of values. The hero, played for full comic potential by Billy Crystal, heads West with two buddies to sort out his emotional turbulences. Just as the

Forest of Arden in *As You Like It* enabled Shakespeare's confused characters to make crucial discoveries about life's essential meanings and purpose, so the film's dude ranch setting functions as a modern-day equivalent of Arden, and an age-old remedy. Crystal's rejuvenated character returns to the city a wiser man, better equipped for the challenges ahead. Unfortunately, although self-reflection and renewal are always useful, they cannot guarantee happy endings for problems occurring in life—or in fictionalized accounts of life.

A disturbing portrayal of man in late midlife is presented in the 2002 film *About Schmidt.*[3] In the film, Jack Nicholson portrays the sixty-year-old Schmidt, who must face issues of retirement, his wife's death, strained relationships with his adult child and in-laws, and despair when he has failed to construct meaningful relationships with others. The resulting emptiness, isolation, and pathos is obvious in his actions and inactions: he writes to a young illiterate African child, whose picture he had seen in a fund raising campaign, about insurance and actuarials; he watches television and falls into despair as evidenced by his inattention to hygiene and dress; he uses inappropriate language and makes inappropriate sexual advances toward others. Schmidt-type characters are found in our grocery stores, in our neighborhoods, and in our medical offices. Even professionals who become totally occupied with their work can exhibit the kind of *flatline* behaviors demonstrated in the film.

The greatest benefit, perhaps, from a film such as *About Schmidt* may be for the health professional. Although Schmidt's undesirable life seems impossible for someone in medicine to understand, it serves as a reminder that others have very different stories than our own and that they too need to be respected and cared for. It is also a reminder about the value of making connections and investing in family and friends to remain happy and healthy.

For decades Woody Allen's characters have served as America's favorite neurotics in film portrayals. Yet his real-life behaviors demonstrate that a downhill slide in midlife can occur slowly over a period of years or much more abruptly, as when associated with a major life event such as the loss of a spouse or retirement from an occupation that had given purpose to life. The careful and observant physician must be aware of these and other crises-inducing circumstances, as well as everything in between, and be willing to create a comfortable setting for patients to discuss themselves in the context of these possibly potent and disruptive changes.

Marriage Narratives

It is likely that the full and powerful range of midlife marriage narratives available in the medical humanities represent more useful tools for health professionals than those found in the medical texts. Expressions by articulate writers and artists, who have reflected on these concerns before constructing creative impressions, are familiar and useful as we slip, slide, fall, or, if we are lucky, cruise through this chronological period in our collective lives. When imaginative literature is good, it doesn't go away. Stored in our minds, it moves unpredictably between active and passive states, reappearing involuntarily as an unexpected illuminator or footnote. Hearing an argument between two people, for instance, can evoke a recollection of Edward Albee's unforgettable play *Who's Afraid of Virginia Woolf*,[4] a frightening depiction of what can happen when marriages sour to become pathological and dangerous. In its various forms, fiction helps readers, including health professionals, to understand more fully the complex behaviors of others and themselves.

Frequently, marriages undergo minor or major upheavals that create stress and depression in one or both partners. Couples settle into the routine of children and work and then discover that two or more decades have passed. At midlife, a personal evaluation can lead to serious questions about individual goals and accomplishments. The years of married life may now seem uninspiring, dull, and at times, intolerable; two people living together and sharing a bed and meals, are, in fact, quite separate. Cartoons commonly depict this scene stereotypically: a breakfast table, for example, where the newspaper functions as the metaphoric wall between man and wife.

Marital difficulties or dissatisfaction, unfortunately, have become a common midlife problem that may interfere with well-being and can lead to any number of somatic symptoms. Marital inertia by one or both partners might be consciously recognized and accepted as normal, or it might generate feelings of quiet rage or violence, possibly leading to poor health, destructive relationships, separation, and divorce. In the selected narratives that follow, each example brings a slightly different perspective for recollection when listening to the stories that patients tell. As such, each can contribute to improving the sensitivities and understanding of health professionals for individual patient situations and concerns. The utility of fiction as an outlet or refuge for care providers caring for patients with marriage-related problems at midlife can be illustrated in a brief review of selections focusing on marital stasis or discontent.

American Gothic, the iconic painting by Grant Wood (Fig. 19-1), portrays a stiffly posed, dour-looking couple that can epitomize midlife malaise. Few viewers are inspired by Wood's terrifying image of long-term marriage. And yet, this man and woman are pervasive in our neighborhoods and waiting rooms. There is no warm center in this heartland portrait; instead, there is something disturbingly *gothic* in place. The inert husband—seemingly pitiful and subdued—stands with his head cocked, like a slightly slumped sentry, possibly awaiting some comment from the similarly unhappy-looking woman at his side. Art critics advise that Wood, an irreverent satirist, intended a purposeful taunt, a visual undercutting of marriage as an institution. Instead of portraying idealized harmonies at midlife, this side-by-side pair, in an unfeeling environment containing the cold artifacts of married life, reveals a chilling image of misery. Although there is no explicit reference to a medical concern, the well-known and often-referenced painting does represent an inertia, an unnatural lifelessness that differs from what represents good health and well-being.

Ennui, a painting by Walter Sickert (Fig. 19-2), portrays the kind of complex narrative that could be developed and unraveled in a long novel. Instead, the snapshot-like picture

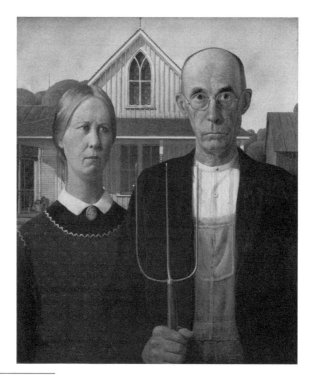

Figure 19-1   Grant Wood, *American Gothic*, 1930. Oil on beaver board, 30 11/16 × 25 11/16 in. (78 × 65.3 cm). Friends of American Art Collection, 1930.934.

Photograph by Bob Hashimoto. Reproduction, The Art Institute of Chicago.

invites an engaged viewer to look for clues and to imagine a plot. Most viewers have the same impression about the figures in the picture: a man and woman, presumably husband and wife, who face in opposite directions in a small room, staring into space. The figures appear disconnected and inert, more like parts of the furniture on which one sits and the other leans than fully human beings. For most, the narrative suggests a sense of deadly boredom between two people, precisely what its translated title, *Boredom,* would have us believe.

The Wood and Sickert paintings provide preparation for the short novel *Ethan Frome* by Edith Wharton,[5] a more fully sketched version of midlife tragedy. Ethan, a bright and talented young man in rural New England full of hopes and expectations, is trapped by poverty and the harsh circumstances of rural life. Barely able to make ends meet hauling wood and tending to menial tasks on his impoverished, "bare as a milk pan" farm, Ethan sinks even deeper into poverty and despair when matched in marriage to a selfish woman with unceasing demands. Soon after the wedding, his wife assumes the role of chronic

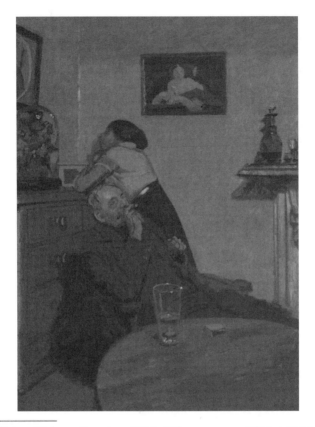

Figure 19-2   Walter Sickert, *Ennui,* c. 1914. Oil on canvas, 1524 × 1124 mm. London, Tate Collection.

sufferer. She becomes unrelenting in her torments, mercilessly draining him of spirit, but worse, of any possibility of happiness and love.

In a cruel twist of plot, the dismal setting is brightened by the miraculous appearance of a vibrant young woman, Mattie, a poor distant relative who will earn her keep attending to the "sickly" wife. Although the stage is set for new hope and escape, the unfolding drama tragically results in even greater despair. Trying unsuccessfully to leave a terrible existence and a truly miserable relationship, Ethan ends up unimaginably worse off than before, his chance for love and freedom with Mattie lost.

Wharton's fictional tale describes loneliness, cruelty, and the human need for love as Ethan, a universal sufferer, is tantalized with the hope of a new life. The profound account of despair, love, infidelity, and tragedy poignantly attends to the strange turns in life, the zigs that ought to zag and vice versa. When stories are as compelling as this one is, they can prepare health professionals for nonjudgmental and compassionate responses.

Films featuring very different accounts of midlife dilemmas are especially useful because of their accessibility and vicarious nature—they are *someone else's story,* not the viewer's. The film *Mr. and Mrs. Bridge*[6] allows viewers to have that vicarious experience with a more passive, but similarly passionless, couple living in more upscale circumstances than the Fromes. The title cleverly references the two important issues developed in the drama: first, an implicit formality or stiffness of address, and, second, the need for a *bridge* to connect the separated couple. The Bridges, played by real-life "Mr. and Mrs." Paul Newman and Joanne Woodward, are rooted in past customs. Mr. Bridge is a strong, forceful, highly opinionated patriarch who treats his wife and children like property. His wife, completely defined by him and those around her, is unable to measure her accomplishments except in terms of what she does for her family. In their prosperous family setting, husband and wife occupy overlapping spaces in the routine and formal house where no one is at ease. Unable to put her finger on an unclear problem, Mrs. Bridge becomes increasingly agitated. Until recently she had attended to the needs of husband, children, and house contentedly and mechanically. Now, she senses a vague emptiness that inexplicably pleads for change. Something is wrong; something is missing.

Mr. Bridge, a lawyer, functions with businesslike efficiency not only at his office but at home as well, where he exhibits the same tedious formalities with his wife and almost-grown children. In one pathetic scene, Mr. Bridge orders Mrs. Bridge not to move from the table at their country club despite tornado warnings. Others find shelter, but the Bridges sit alone and quietly in the club dining room as the building shakes from severe weather around them.

Mrs. Bridge does make tentative attempts to explain her needs and feelings, but her husband becomes visibly uneasy and dismisses her efforts with a careless and insensitive rebuke. Audiences watch sympathetically as Mrs. Bridge confronts her husband in an extraordinary kitchen scene. She struggles awkwardly to express what she feels, while he maintains his customary wall of reserve and distance. Taking the initiative, she has reached out in an effort to bridge the gap between them and to forge a more meaningful future.

American Beauty[7] is regarded by many as one of the most powerful and truly disturbing contemporary films about midlife strife in modern suburbia. The principal characters, Lester and Carolyn Burnham, played by Kevin Spacey and Annette Bening, portray the worst of midlife behaviors. The film is similar to both *Interiors* and *The Four Seasons* in that it deals with a middle-aged man's awakening to his sour and meaningless life. His journey of self-realization includes themes of marriage dissatisfactions, marital infidelity, homosexuality, emotional repression, lies, and mistrust. Although Lester's life and that of his family may be normal and happy from the perspective of those looking in through the white picket fence, that representation is a false but familiar façade. The situation is reminiscent of the routine hospital or clinic question "How are you feeling?" and the requisite response, "Fine," when the questioner is merely saying words without any interest in the response, and the responder is doing the same. The film, however, penetrates into this life and the horrors within.

Married midlife partners who see this movie cannot avoid a separate examination of their own marital status. The interesting part of this phenomenon is that most of them will do this individually, not as a couple, because the topics are too painful and hit too close to home for many viewers. When fictional works such as *American Beauty* reflect real-life elements, they raise sticky questions about a person's own choices and values, however painful this may be. More important, fictional dilemmas, however complex or nuanced, can raise useful questions for viewer self-examination while also suggesting that viewers are not alone in their suffering.

The large number of films about midlife reinforces the importance of stories by writers, artists, and filmmakers, who are the interpreters and record keepers for the society we inhabit. Their stories, in whatever form, tell us what is happening in society and in our lives. As noted, strained relationships and the dissolution of marriage seem to have secured an especially prominent place. Marriages gone wrong and the psychological impact of that failure usually lead one or both members of the couple to medical care pathways.

Changing Bodies

Although marital or sexual boredom, dissatisfaction, and disinterest represent potential problems faced by the midlife patient and his or her care provider, there are many other concerns. Of course, the topic of body image is synonymous with aging. Physical changes occur in midlife when the gradual but inevitable signs of aging first become apparent. Indeed, many may actually define their midlife by changes such as menopause, gray hair, weight and body proportion changes, or signs of physical illness: "I guess I'm getting old; I'm seeing the signs of it." The telltale physical changes of decline bring about an awareness of mortality that previously may not have been in the forefront of our minds, or of a likeness to our parents ("I'm really starting to look like my mother"), or concerns over minor physical ailments, which one might have easily dismissed previously but which now appear as possible harbingers of more serious disease ("I'm getting to that age when I have to start thinking about things like that, you know").

A visual narrative dealing with the theme of reflectivity about the first realizations and the inevitability of the aging process occurs in Suzanne Valadon's painting *The Abandoned Doll* (Fig. 19-3). Having set the stage with numerous props for engaged viewers to consider, Valadon invites them to construct a story or narrative. That the nude, clearly pubescent girl is seated on a bed produces a radical, even startling, departure from domestic scenes created, for example, by Mary Cassatt during the same late-nineteenth and early-twentieth-century period. This painting, like other "progressive" paintings by Valadon,

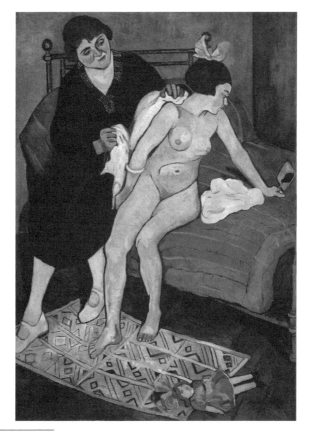

Figure 19-3 Suzanne Valadon, *The Abandoned Doll,* 1921. Oil on canvas, 51 × 32 in. The National Museum of Women in the Arts, Washington, DC. Gift of Wallace and Wilhelmina Holladay.

© 2008 Artists Rights Society (ARS), New York/ADAGP, Paris.

violated subject-matter expectations imposed by the male-ordered world of objectified, gazed-upon, and typically vacuous nudes made popular by male artists.

Valadon (1865–1938), an accomplished artist and free spirit, was one of the emerging group of women who were choosing to step out of traditional boundaries proscribed by inherited rules. With its radical and controversial portrayal of previously unrepresented references to stages of femaleness, *The Abandoned Doll* represents an expression of authentic reality: the consideration of a woman's transition from adolescence to womanhood. The childhood doll has been cast aside, and it is presumed by the viewer that soon the bow in her hair, not unlike the bow on the abandoned doll, similarly will be cast aside by the young woman. The handheld mirror symbolizes adolescent fascination with body changes and appearance The child at this moment is concerned with her appearance and herself. She has the future before her, while her mother, in sharp contrast to her daughter's youth, appears more meditative about the gap between herself, as she moves toward decline and aging, and her daughter. Loss and renewal are captured simultaneously.

It is likely that Valadon's painting served as inspiration for a twentieth-century poem by Sharon Olds entitled "35/10." The poem provides an example of a double focus on shared personal inventory and moral reflection during a mother's ruminative moment. While brushing her adolescent daughter's "dark silken hair," the mother (age thirty-five), who is the narrator of the poem, becomes suddenly aware of her own gray hair in the mirror. She is thus thrust into reflection about the child's (age ten) coming of age at the same time that she is confronting her own progressive aging.

> Why is it?
> just as we begin to go
> they begin to arrive, the fold in my neck
> clarifying as the fine bones of her
> hips sharpen?[8]

This, the mother muses, "is the story of replacement." As her own skin begins to dry and her body "snaps its [reproductive] clasp," the daughter's "purse" fills with "eggs, round and firm as hard boiled yolks." By presenting a poignant narrative about becoming and declining, Olds's narrator puts the reader into the mother's subjective realm, from which larger meanings can be extracted. The engaged or willing reader makes connections between the fictive context and the self to encourage personal examination and an acceptance of life's rhythmic patterns. The reader may draw comfort from the shared experience of aging and the realization of the inevitability of the life cycle. When Valadon's representation of this universal reality and Olds's poetic commentary are considered together, they are likely to generate discussion and reflection about the midlife body as a moving point between the past and the future.

On a daily basis people look into their mirrors to discover subtle and overt signs of physical change. Not surprisingly, this topic has captured the attention of artists and writers whose work can help us negotiate or come to terms with this occasionally terrorizing force. Few would imagine that a poem about a piece of fruit could, in a few short lines, capture so precisely the impact of this shared experience. "The Pear," by Jane Kenyon, appears in a volume whose title, *Let Evening Come,* suggests the need for accepting the inevitability of aging that is illustrated by the poems it contains and their ability to stir connections between their reflective narrators and readers. Unlike any entry in a medical text about aging, this poem's transfixing "moment" turns the personal story inside out to shift the meditative focus from narrator to reader. By eliciting reader contemplation, a double focus is created; the fictive inventory enlarges and deepens unique perspectives about our own physicality in a shared life course.

> There is a moment in middle age
> when you grow bored, angered
> by your middling mind,
> afraid.
>
> That day the sun
> burns hot and bright,
> making you more desolate.
>
> It happens subtly, as when a pear
> spoils from the inside out,
> and you may not be aware
>
> until things have gone too far.[9]

When a narrator, such as this one, reflects on her body as it has become, she is taking stock of where she is in life. At some point most people do the same thing and become quietly stunned to see how far "things have gone." Like her, we may be suddenly "afraid." Without time-lapse photography, aging is an unseen process, as with a pear that has moved imperceptibly past ripeness. Nevertheless, there are moments of confrontation, discovery, and blunt awareness that catch us by surprise. Kenyon's poem produces an empathetic connection between narrator and reader, who are caught together in the sticky filaments of fictional content described by Salman Rushdie:

> [R]eader and writer merge, through the medium of the text, to become a collective being that both writes as it reads and reads as it writes, and creates, jointly, that unique work, "their" novel.[10]

The poet's focus on an ordinary object has produced a strong, unforgettable metaphor for the visualization of midlife that every reader and health professional has had or will experience.

Nora Ephron chronicled the various realizations of aging that begin in midlife in her popular collection of essays, *I Feel Bad About My Neck and Other Thoughts on Being a Woman.* Ephron reflects on the thoughts, looks, attitudes, and day-to-day subjects of contemplation, both trivial and large, affecting modern midlife and aging women. With humor and wit, she is able to relay empathy to her readers, while at the same time acknowledging a need for discovering, enduring, and deciding how each woman is to cope with the changes in her own body and mind. For health professionals treating the ever-growing population of midlife adults, it is important to understand rather than minimize these kinds of concerns. Perceptions, real or imagined, and appearance, as Ephron notes repeatedly in serious and humorous ways, cannot be dismissed during a clinical visit. They do matter.

> The neck is a dead give-away. Our faces are lies and our necks are the truth. You have to cut open a redwood tree to see how old it is, but you wouldn't if it had a neck.[11]

Normal changes of hairlines, skin folds, and wrinkles are one thing, but concerns about illness, real or imagined, are another. Midlife is a time when we begin to acknowledge the reality of our physical frailty. We begin to see family, friends, or colleagues who are diagnosed with real and sometimes terrible diseases. For many, this is an entirely new experience. When in our twenties and told of a death related to breast cancer, we are saddened and move on, but when we are in our forties and are presented with that news, it becomes more personal and real. Self-reflection increases with age and, along with it, health concerns, which may become magnified and frightening.

Health professionals often find fiction, films, and nonmedical essays useful for providing perspectives and insights about patient concerns. Fear of a particular disease such as cancer, especially when suffered by a friend or family member, can cause tremendous stress and anxiety. An example of this is seen in a remarkable and very useful poem by Larry Smith entitled "Leaning Together in a Storm." The story concerns a group of midlife and older men, prostate cancer survivors, who meet regularly as a support group. A young bristly surgeon, obviously not touched by cancer himself, comes to speak to the group, offering slide images and information about therapies, but offering no empathy, support, or gentle kindness to the group of cancer survivors. As the narrator begins, there is a camaraderie in the Cancer Center room among the twelve men in shirtsleeves sipping ice water and making jokes while waiting for the evening's program to begin.

> I am one of them tonight
> meant to acknowledge
> our story within
> our private brotherhood.[12]

Later, when their speaker, a young surgeon, strides into the room, the warm spirit of the meeting changes from an intimate gathering to one that is more brittle:

> We swallow a hundred nightmares
> with smiles and nods.[12]

The poem continues with the narrator and others asking personal questions about sex and intercourse. The speaker, seemingly oblivious to the feelings of the men in his audience, responds with flip answers that are cold, callous, and thoughtless. In the end, the men, as a group, "let it go, trade our feeling for facts we already know."[12]

Health professionals reading the poem may or may not know physicians such as this, but they would understand the importance of sensitivity and caring in such a setting if a healthy relationship between care provider and patient is to be established.

Breast cancer has become a source of fear for many midlife women. This reality and the emotions that the disease evokes in a patient are presented poignantly in Ronna Wineberg's short story "A Crossing." This work explores a health professional as patient, this time Alice, who has found a lump in her breast. She is forced to continue to carry out her patient care duties, but is unable to repress thoughts about the care she may require. When her fears are realized and she must undergo surgery, she approaches the event and preparations leading to it with her customary, matter-of-fact, efficient physician attitude. This has served her well as a doctor, but prevents her from accepting her own illness. She tries to keep her cancer at a distance. She must juggle the busy responsibilities of her midlife concerns—patients and her family—while attending to the preparations for her surgery and her own physical and emotional needs. Alice's world and perceptions are changed forever as a result of her diagnosis. The story provides important insights for us as health professionals, teachers, and as patients. Alice must navigate her own process of acceptance, first briefly resenting her husband's good health, and then finally accepting her diagnosis and illness. Ultimately, she faces her breast cancer with sadness, dignity, and grace, thinking after her surgery, "She wasn't really lucky; she hadn't returned to any world she knew. But it was what she had."[13]

Family Shifts

Another relevant topic for further exploration by health professionals concerns shifts that occur in family care structures. Midlife patients who now care for or are concerned about their own aging parents present frequently with physical and emotional stress. The "sandwich generation" of midlife boomers, tasked with taking care of their own minor children as well as their elderly parents, is often subject to significant emotional, physical, and financial burdens. Many patients fail to acknowledge the toll that these new responsibilities take upon themselves, their spouses, and families, whereas others may feel the need to express their exasperations about these burdens to their own care providers.

Even when financial security is in place, generational tensions cannot be avoided. An obvious illustration occurs in the film *Driving Miss Daisy*,[14] in which a prosperous middle-aged son (Dan Ackroyd) and his very obstinate mother, an aging Jewish widow (Jessica Tandy), deal with the realities and constraints associated with becoming older. Although the tone is light and easy at the onset of the story, the mother gradually declines in health and her determined and valiant struggle for privacy and independence fails. The mother is forced to submit to circumstances she can no longer control. The son is caught between his own wife, who is not especially fond of the starchy old woman, and the mother he cares for and loves. As arranged by the son, the hired chauffeur (Morgan Freeman) begins to assume, over a period of twenty years, the role of family member and trusted friend.

One True Thing,[15] a film based on Anna Quindlen's novel, deals with the unpredictable kinds of burdens, exasperations, and discoveries that frequently happen when grown children have an opportunity to reassess family relationships and childhood experiences. The perspective is that of Ellen (Renée Zellweger), a young woman at a pivotal point in her career as a journalist in New York City. When her mother (Meryl Streep) is diagnosed with an especially pernicious form of cancer, Ellen's world is turned upside down. After unsuccessful efforts to hold on to her hard-earned job and oversee her mother's care from afar, she is pressured by her own feelings and those imposed strongly by her father to leave her promising position in the city. The father's work as a professor and writer—he has been working for more than a decade on his latest novel—prevents him from pitching in as a caretaker. Since childhood, Ellen has held her father, the great novelist, in high regard, a person whose writing achievements she admired and hoped to emulate. Her mother, on the other hand, had quietly supported each family member while efficiently holding the family together. Ellen's preference for her father, she comes to realize, had not been fully examined.

Within a short period after her return home, Ellen is amazed to learn how her mother has sacrificed her life for her family. Characteristically, she had not bothered anyone with the pain she had been experiencing until the cancer had progressed beyond treatment possibilities. The image that Ellen had projected and believed about her family, especially her father, was incorrect, a reflection of immature thinking. As an adult, with a new perspective, she is disturbed to discover that her seemingly charismatic father is and always had been self-centered and selfish. For the first time she recognizes her mother's rich role in the family and the respect with which she is regarded in the community, something she had never bothered to notice before. Ellen's new perspective and interpretation represents a coming of age, however tardy, as she learns about love, responsibility, and adult relationships during the moments surrounding her mother's terrible suffering. Included in the story is an end-of-life ethics problem about the circumstances of her mother's death. Did Ellen assist in her mother's death or was her mother quietly self-sacrificing to the end? And, ultimately, how do the father's life-long patterns, after the death of his wife, her mother, continue to be revealed?

However depressing, these narrative examples and even more recent film representations, such as *The Savages* and *Away From Her*, provide powerful reminders about separate and collective journeys within the range of ordinary experience. Each story and each narrator has a particular point of view or perspective, enabling readers to respond according to their own orientations in life. Health professionals, in fact, may be unprepared for a fuller comprehension of the human capacity for misery and suffering, but exposure to art, literature, and theater by thoughtful and skilled writers can reveal conditions and situations that may have been referred to, but not developed, in an academic text. Storytellers, says physician Edmund Pellegrino, give meaning to what the physician sees and makes him or her see it feelingly. Whatever enriches the doctor's sensibilities must perforce make a better physician.[16]

Whether happily married or happily single, aging will begin in midlife, and unless a person is very lucky, mild illness or more serious physical or psychological diseases can occur. The stories presented in these pages appear to give a lopsided impression of midlife, but the preponderance of thoughtful materials by writers and filmmakers who have focused on indifferent to abysmal relationships suggests that they are, in fact, reflective of real-life situations and that facets of the characters portrayed and the situations depicted will find their way into examining rooms for consideration. The so-called patient story may be an edited version; without a sensitive health professional seeking out omitted footnotes and marginalia, the story is incomplete and the patient may not be helped.

Review Questions

1. How have you thought about midlife prior to reading this chapter? Have there been problems in your family similar to those presented in the discussion?

2. Why should health professionals strive to create a comfortable setting for those in midlife, and why would there be a general sense of both patient and health professional unease regarding this period?

3. Why do films by Woody Allen and a film such as *City Slickers* allow for both insight and distancing? Do stories about inertia, infidelity, and marital malaise generally stick in our minds and assist in articulating difficult issues and concerns?

4. If health professionals tend to expect a clearly defined problem, how do the humanities selections reveal that some problems are difficult to define, grasp, and resolve?

5. Why is midlife a disruptive time for so many people?

6. When you look at the painting *Ennui* and think of your own relationships now and in the future, what details of the painting are most compelling? If the painting were to reflect a modern husband and wife, what might be changed?

7. Do you know anyone who has expressed the sentiments presented in Jane Kenyon's poem "The Pear"? Describe or explain why the poem has a universal quality.

8. Are you concerned about changes in your own body? How are you responding to them? When you have not seen a family member for a long time, have you been aware of your own assessment of the changes you see?

9. More stories are about women or by women, but Larry Smith's poem about men in a support group is a welcome addition. Explain why this poem is important and how it might be useful for health professionals. How did it make you feel about health care providers?

Endnotes

1. Flieger V, Hostetter C, eds. *Tolkien's Legendarium: Essays on the History of Middle-earth*. Westport, CT: Greenwood Press, 2000.
2. *City Slickers* [motion picture]. Directed by Ron Underwood; with Billy Crystal, Bruno Kirby, Daniel Stern. Columbia Pictures, 1991.
3. *About Schmidt* [motion picture]. Directed by Alexander Payne; with Jack Nicholson, Kathy Bates, Hope Davis. New Line, 2002.
4. Albee E. *Who's Afraid of Virginia Woolf?* New York: Antheneum, 1962.
5. Wharton E. *Ethan Frome*. New York: Charles Scribner's Sons Press, 1911.

6. *Mr. and Mrs. Bridge* [motion picture]. Directed by James Ivory; with Paul Newman, Joanne Woodward, Blythe Danner. Miramax, 1990.

7. *American Beauty* [motion picture]. Directed by Sam Mendes; with Kevin Spacey, Annette Bening, Thora Birch. DreamWorks, 1999.

8. Olds S. 35/10. In: *The Dead and the Living*. New York: Alfred A. Knopf, 1983:75.

9. Kenyon J. The pear. In: *Let Evening Come*. Saint Paul, MN: Graywolf Press, 1990:10. Copyright 1996 from the estate of Jane Kenyon. Reprinted from *Otherwise: New & Selected Poems* with the permission of Graywolf Press, St. Paul, Minnesota.

10. Rushdie S. Is nothing sacred? Presented as the Herbert Read Memorial Lecture at the Institute of Contemporary Arts, London, 6 February 1990. In: *Imaginary Homelands: Essays and Criticisms, 1981–1991*. London: Granta, 1991:426.

11. Ephron N. *I Feel Bad About My Neck and Other Thoughts on Being a Woman*. New York: Alfred A. Knopf, 2006:5.

12. Smith L. Leaning together in a storm. [The Writer's Almanac with Garrison Keillor]. October 23, 2006. Available at: http://writersalmanac.publicradio.org/index.php?date = 2006/10/23. Accessed September 6, 2008.

13. Wineberg R. 2005. A crossing. In: *Second Language*. Moorehead, MN: New Rivers Press, 2005:6.

14. *Driving Miss Daisy* [motion picture]. Directed by Bruce Beresford; with Morgan Freeman, Jessica Tandy, Dan Akroyd. Warner Brothers, 1989.

15. *One True Thing* [motion picture]. Directed by Carl Franklin; with Meryl Streep, Renée Zellweger, William Hurt. Universal Studios, 1998.

16. Pellegrino ED. To look feelingly—the affinities of literature and medicine. *Literature Med* 1982;1:19.

Chapter 20

Aging and the End of Life

Deep autumn

My neighbor, how

Does he live, I wonder?

—Basho, seventeenth century

Chapter Learning Objectives

At the conclusion of this chapter the reader will be able to:

1. Imagine a story suggested by the Van Gogh painting in Figure 20-1

2. Recognize and identify the influence of biomedicalization in modern interpretations of aging

3. Consider the role and importance of words, language, and stories in establishing definitions and decisions about the processes and circumstances of aging

4. Recognize the complementary value of stories in poetry, film, and theater as resources for health care professionals

5. Appreciate the role of those in health care who write stories and poems about aging, the end-of-life process, and related ethical issues that provide vital perspectives and insights for colleagues

Aging and end-of-life narratives have increased as our population has aged. Whether verbal or visual, these stories can offer valuable perspectives for health care professionals, patients, family members, and friends. Each narrative provides different information and nuances about a time that most of us expect to experience. Although the focus differs from that of the medical texts, the insights often complement and contribute to what is found in the latter.

When discussing aging and the end of life, the disciplines of medical humanities have an impressive and extremely useful record. From biblical stories to characters in Shakespeare's plays and images by Vincent Van Gogh, Käthe Kollwitz, and Alice Neel, we have depended on the visual and verbal arts for vital information and guidance about these slippery places on the human journey. Just as we learn about the diminishment of a person's body, mind, and power from the aging King Lear, we make similar discoveries

---

Portions of this chapter reflect ideas from *Anticipating deep autumn: a widening lens.* L. LaCivita Nixon, LA Roscoe, 2002. Permission granted from BMJ Publishing Group Ltd.

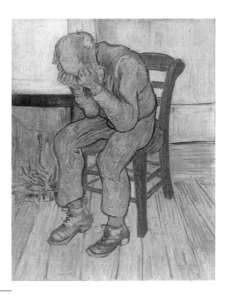

Figure 20-1 Vincent van Gogh, *Old Man in Sorrow (On the Threshold of Eternity)*, May 1890. Oil on canvas. Rijksmuseum Kröller-Müller, Otterlo, Netherlands.

Kröller-Müller Museum, Otterlo, Netherlands.

watching our parents and grandparents move from positions of family or workplace strengths to gradually or dramatically altered circumstances. Most of us are grateful for the insights provided in contemporary accounts of aging in stories such as *Love Letters*, *Driving Miss Daisy*, *A Delicate Balance*, and *Water for Elephants*. All of us, after all, are the stories we hear, the stories we tell. In small and larger ways stories define and connect us on common but separate pathways. Although essential assistance is provided by health professionals, nonmedical narratives can reveal "subtle nuances of color, hue, physiognomy, gait, mannerism, gesture, tremor, form and function—all visible to the eye but needing to be penetrated for meaning."[1] Whereas medicine and science present crucial tools for medical students, humanities courses offer other kinds of perspective that complement the traditional skills associated with medical training.

Contemporary medicine, with its focus on individual pathology, physiology, and biomedical interventions, is a powerful influence and force. The pervasive biomedical model has fostered views of "inevitable decline, disease, and irreversible decay"[2] and, coupled with overwhelming ad campaigns by the pharmaceutical industries, has convinced the public of the "primary and rightful place of medicine in the management of the 'problem' of aging."[2] In the past, religious interpretations about the place of aging in the human life course provided a sense of meaning and possibility, but our recent dependency on medicine for the management and oversight of aging has made it more difficult for aging men and women to seek alternative ways to attach meaning to the process of growing old.

Projections by demographers reveal serious difficulties and challenges: family situations, grim resource evaluations, and inadequate institutional capabilities. The public, frequently overwhelmed by and anxious about uninspiring forecasts, has begun to look beyond medicine for interpretations, meanings, and options. To prolong life and prevent the disabilities suffered by their own parents, many at midlife and beyond are paying closer attention to diet, exercise, alternative medicine, and food supplements, and larger numbers of people are practicing and promoting preventive care. In addition, this generally well educated, more affluent, and influential population cluster, increasingly composed of baby boomers, is dissatisfied with current provisions for older people in society and has begun to advocate articulately and persistently for change. By projecting themselves into their aging parents' lives—with an understanding that their own longevity continues to extend—this cohort is simultaneously euphoric and anxious: they both cling to and abhor their dependence on medicine and technology. Newspaper accounts and gerontological research studies that have raised concerns about isolation, abandonment, and neglect have generated a new interest in choices, decisions, and experiences that have more to do with the values and purpose of human life than mere existence. Now, more people are attentive to subtle winds and tremors at the early stages of what is foreseen as a very long autumn season.

Aging

This chapter considers the role of the humanities in enlarging our abilities to see the multidimensional aspects of aging and alternative ways of attaching meaning to the aging process. The materials included usually do not appear in medical texts but are among those included in medical humanities classes for medical students that increasingly involve participation by basic scientists, clinicians, and other health care professionals. If, since scientific enlightenment, old age has been "removed from its place as a way station along life's spiritual journey and redefined as a problem to be solved by science and medicine . . . [and if the elderly have been] moved to society's margins[,]"[3] the humanities experience is intended to challenge such determinations by restoring a fundamental humanity to older people. The introduction of these materials and the discussion that follows provide health care providers with a greater awareness of a fuller range of aging nuances and prepare them for humanistic responses to stages in the human life cycle that too often are pushed aside as uninteresting.

Age-related writings and visual images by Van Gogh, Neel, Olds, Hemingway, Kooser, and others are discussed to illustrate how fictive representations can and do serve as a moral impetus or stimulus for meaningful reflection about the objective *other* or stranger who may be the person we are treating—but also our mirror image. Physician-writer Walker Percy famously observed that those physicians who listen to their patients often learn not only what is wrong with their patients, but with themselves as well.

The selections may evoke anticipatory insights from artists whose verbal or visual narratives look ahead from midlife in the aging process to subsequent stages; in doing so, these anticipatory writings and paintings demonstrate Richard Rorty's observations about the capacities of fiction to inspire or generate moral guidance about a life stage before it is actually experienced. The role and value of literature and art as tools is woven throughout the discussion as a necessary corollary for nourishing the human spirit in ways that the medical model cannot.

New Stories, New Vocabularies, New Understandings

As a society, we remain fixed on inherited impressions and language, or what Rorty calls the "final vocabulary"—the "set of words which [humans] employ to justify their actions, their beliefs, and their lives,"[4] the familiar, comfortable language that results in rigid patterns of thinking about and describing aging. Given the power and dominance of medicine in our culture to set values and priorities, much of the current discourse about older persons centers on end-of-life matters. Too often lines between being old and dying blur to form a singular image of hopelessness and finality in which older men and women are seen as feebleminded, confined to nursing homes, a burden on their children, "sickly, haggard and bitter—or at best, cute and childlike."[5] A portrait of aging provided by Barbara MacDonald, for example, derives from cultural fixations: "Old is ugly, old is powerless, old is the end, and therefore . . . old is what no one could possibly want to be."[6] On the other hand, many older persons are what Harry Moody calls "wellderly," able to take pleasure in travel, education programs, and leisure activities, who, with reduced obligations, may be enjoying newfound freedoms.[7] Between these extremes realistic portrayals of aging point to complex, multidimensional patterns and textures ranging from good health and active lifestyles to chronic and acute disease marked by varying degrees of disability.

To get beyond the traditional images generated by the biomedical model and its culturally embedded notions and assumptions, Rorty suggests we exercise our "imaginative ability."[4(pxvi)] In his writings about the possibility of a liberal utopia, he suggests that it is "to be achieved not by inquiry but by imagination, the imaginative ability to see strange people as fellow sufferers."[4(pxvi)] He adds that the process of seeing "human beings as 'one of us' rather than as 'them' is a matter of detailed description of what unfamiliar people are like and of redescription of what we ourselves are like."[4(pxvi)] When considering exactly where we need to go in our redescription efforts, Rorty explains that whereas the sermon and the treatise might have been useful tools in the past, they have been replaced gradually and steadily by "the novel, the movie, and the TV program . . . as the principal vehicles of moral change and progress."[4(pxvi)]

By creating characters who are not us, *but who could be*, skilled writers and artists function to enlarge meanings. As Cynthia Ozick observes,

> the writer, an imaginer by trade, will suggest a course of connection, of entering the tremulous spirit of the helpless, the fearful, the apart. . . . The writer will

demonstrate the contagion of passion and compassion that is known in medicine as "empathy," and in art as insight.[8]

Insights such as those provided by visual artists and writers—painters, sculptors, poets, playwrights, filmmakers, and so on—focus on real-life concerns and dilemmas, including old age, and suggest a full range of approaches and meanings for generating personal and public responses. Allowing for distanced entry into a world that may or may not yet be ours, fiction can broaden our understandings about imagined experiences that we, too, are likely to share. Narrative dramas challenge old habits, or what Holstein and Cole describe as dichotomous thinking—"independence versus dependence, freedom versus coercion, body versus spirit, science versus religion"[9]—to forge connections between the objective "they" and the subjective "I." In terms of expanding the levels of reflection, discussion, and constructive responses by individuals and society members, the wider, more inclusive, multilensed narrative can serve as a valuable road map.

Fiction, Art, and Film

> No detail is too small, no sound in the night too muffled,
> to register. From this gradual accumulation of minutiae,
> this keen awareness, poems emerge.[10]

Entering into the lives of older persons by way of fiction and art provides a wide lens for looking at ranges of possibilities and perspectives about a population that is infinitely diverse. In a study about the role and value of humanities disciplines in 1980, the Commission on the Humanities reported that the disciplines make "distinctive marks on the mind: through history, the ability to disentangle and interpret complex human events; through literature and the arts, the ability to distinguish the deeply felt, the well-wrought, and the continually engrossing from the shallow, imitative and the monotonous; through philosophy, the sharpening of criteria for moral decision and warrantable belief."[11] In 1992 Kirk Varnadoe, then director of the Museum of Modern Art, offered similar conclusions when he advised a graduating class at Stanford to "abandon the security of tradition." "Art," he said, "doesn't offer predictable messages," but is most powerful "when it orchestrates perplexity, fails to confirm what you already know, and instead sends you away temporarily disoriented but newly attuned to experience in ways that are perhaps even more powerful because they are vague, rogue, and indeterminate."[12] Varnadoe might have been speaking at a geriatrics conference about the nature of aging and the usefulness of writings such as *Rabbit at Rest* by John Updike, *As We Are Now* by May Sarton, *Old Friends* by Tracy Kidder, and *A Delicate Balance* by Edward Albee. Narratives of aging, like those of lived lives, cannot be packaged into neat containers; those that are most valuable are messy, unfinished, and nonlinear, such as Faulkner's account of Dilsey in *The Sound and the Fury*, the portrayal of eight temporarily "lost" women in the film *Strangers in Good*

Company, and the ongoing critiques surrounding the actions and expectations of the aged father and ruler in *King Lear*.

Fiction was described by Franz Kafka as a liberating force, an ax to the frozen sea around us, a way to begin to "hear voices talking about everything in every possible way" that can be of enormous benefit to humanists and health care providers.[13] In recent decades humanities programs have been added to the traditional medical school curriculum to enable students trained in scientific and clinical aspects of the human body to explore other aspects of the human condition that cannot be measured with ease and precision and to provide an opportunity to "develop a tolerance for ambiguity and . . . [a] realiz[ation] that life is not always, not often, perhaps not *ever* categorized easily into the right answer and the wrong answer."[14] Medical humanist Ron Carson, for example, notes that to

> make sense of ourselves and our world to ourselves and to others, we tell tales—tales of truth, tall tales, tales of wisdom and woe—and listen to tales by others. Stories, with their beginnings, middles, and ends, redeem life from contingency and make it something other than a meaningless succession of events.[15]

In recent years physicians such as Howard Brody, Robert Coles, Audrey Schafer, and Delese Wear have counseled professional colleagues to keep up with medical texts and journals but also with novels, poems, and other genres of literature that contribute non-medical understandings about the human condition. Stories encompassing moral dilemmas and character thought processes and actions during conflict situations usually have an effect on the engaged reader, who is involved, vicariously, as an interested, even concerned participant. In a discussion of moral dimensions in the novels of Henry James, physician Rita Charon underscores this point when she notes that an absorbed or engaged reader is one who will

> lend the full force of his or her imagination and consideration to characters whose actions become transparent and revelatory only in the light of unselfish attentiveness. That is to say, the process of reading James's fictions, exercises and rewards human qualities of goodness that, in the willing reader, may persist into ordinary life.[16]

Whether real or imagined, every telling of a story involves a series of choices about what will be revealed, what will be privileged, and what will be concealed; there are no artless narrations. Powerful stories, even—or especially—those about ordinary moments, do not go away. They remain stored in the receiver's mind until some event prompts recollection, and then return uninvited and unexpectedly for further review, consideration, and personal editing. Consider the confessional thoughts of physician-writer William Carlos Williams, who was seduced not only by the vibrancy of New York City's swirling literary and art currents but also by the humble "words being born" in the mouths of patients to "reveal a glimpse of something . . . dazzling . . . a rare element . . . of mutual recognition."[17] Amazed by what he saw and heard in the examining room or while making a house call, Williams marveled about the power of story: its disturbing intrusiveness, stickiness, and ability to reappear voluntarily in the mind.

Stories and poems can provide little narratives about the human journey as opposed to achieving some sort of grand coherence in our epistemological, ethical, and social views. "Postmodernism," advises Richard Morris, "has generated a distrust of the comprehensive explanations that . . . Lyotard calls 'grand narratives'—vast encompassing megabodies . . . that reduce other stories and historical details to mere satellites within their all-encompassing gravitational field."[18] The emergence of new voices to discuss smaller, previously omitted, and possibly dismissed topics from a subjective perspective generates wider discourse about details of life that are large—and small. Reflection that occurs along separate and collective journeys through life makes it more difficult to separate *them* (those who are old) from *us.* Stories function as connectors or bridges between *them* and *us,* making us more aware of and responsible toward aging's personal and social obligations.

Visual images seldom are easily dismissed. Viewers of Alice Neel's *Self-Portrait* (Fig. 20-2) may discover that the image is deposited in the mind for unexpected recollection

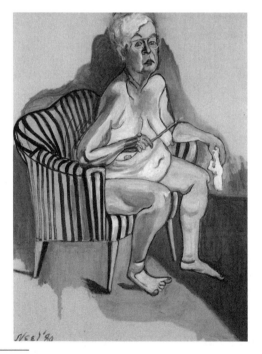

Figure 20-2   Alice Neel, *Self-Portrait,* 1980. Oil on canvas, 54 × 40 in. The National Portrait Gallery, Smithsonian Institution, Washington, DC.

because the painting is so unlike conventional portrayals of women in the male-domi-nated art canon. Many viewers are caught off guard by Neel's reinterpretation of the gazed-upon nude: her figure is mature, not vulnerable, ageless, or passive. Seated in a chair, and without apparent concern for sagging breasts and folds of skin on chin, abdomen, and thighs, the subject looks directly at the viewer through large glasses as an engaged par-ticipant in what has been called the "duality of being, the self as observer and observed."[19]

Viewers conditioned to conventional expectations may be disturbed by the bold depiction of a previously muted reality. More often than not, aging women have been disregarded: "impoverished, disrespected . . . and dismissed . . . as inconsequential and uninteresting."[20] By jolting cultural assumptions, this humanistic portrayal by Neel serves to "transform historically idealized notions of the female body . . . [and] the tension between women's experiences and the socialized roles" that have denied their existence.[21] "Here," says the subject, "is an older, non-nubile, nonreclining female you have avoided, made invisible. Here I am."

In this century, Neel's representational "voice" and those of other women—Eudora Welty's photographic collection of black women living lives of hardship and struggle; Käthe Kollwitz's woodcuts of women, at times fiercely protective and then, when very old and stooped, submissive to an anthropomorphic death; the iconoclastic sounds of Doris Grumbach, Maxine Kumin, May Sarton, Marge Piercy, and Jane Kenyon as they and their narrators speak subjectively about previously unexpressed women's experiences and con-cerns—have revised earlier impressions and conclusions and made visible what had been invisible.[22] It is not surprising that attention has been directed by them to aging's trials, tribulations, and celebrations, and from the discourses they spin no single thread can be followed.

Because people are living longer and because writers and artists are the record keepers for the periods they inhabit, it is not surprising to discover an increase in the depiction of aging during a time when that population has burgeoned. Age-related writings and visual images serve as a moral impetus or stimulus for meaningful reflection about the objective *other* or stranger who may be or *will be* our mirror image. Entering into the lives of older persons by way of story provides an expansive lens for considering the range of possibilities and perspectives about a population that is infinitely diverse. Portrayals of aging can inspire deeper inquiry or generate guidance about a life stage before it is actu-ally experienced.

A Place Called Canterbury, by Dudley Clendinen, provides readers with an intimate and revealing account of aging in a particular place at a particular time, namely, a high-rise retirement community in twenty-first-century Florida.[23] Medical texts and journal articles give physicians critical information about the aging body and treatment options, but Clendinen describes the aging process in other ways that physicians are likely to find useful and compelling. The stories stretch beyond the domain of medicine to reveal con-cerns each of us faces within our lives, notably the changing relationships between parents and children, between spouses, friends, patients, and physicians, and between older people and the physical and sensory world, beginning with their own minds and bodies. There are minor intrigues, plumbing problems, searches for sex, cocktail hour rituals, religious services, considerable confusion, grace, decline, grief—and humor.

Clendinen was fascinated by his mother's new circumstance and by what he came to regard as the "new old age." As a writer, he could not resist the opportunity before him and sought permission to spend more than four hundred, nonconsecutive days living in Canterbury. This very unusual arrangement provided Clendinen with a close-up view of a twenty-first-century phenomenon: the comings and goings of aging people in the final setting of their lives. Canterbury is a well-run camp, and life there is a soap opera. Between the author's exchanges with the witty rabbi and the former jitterbug champs, the enthusiasm generated by a nudity calendar proposal (declined), and the geriatric bib enterprise (thriving), the inhabitants provided Clendinen with an abundance of riches. Whether at lunch in the dining room overlooking the bay, over daily drinks at 5 PM, or in bed in the health center, everyone of this Greatest Generation had a story to tell. This ethnographic page-turner, with its cohort of named characters—the Southern belle, the rabbi who escaped the Holocaust, Emyfish, the ageless New Yorker, Lucile, the warm-hearted fundamentalist, the raunchy atheist, the crusty Yankee, the horny widower, and the maddeningly muddled Wilber—reads like fiction. Whether they were rich or poor, married or widowed, Clendinen listened to them as they spoke and in doing so became a trusted friend and chronicler of the small stories and great events in their collective lives: childhood, the Great Depression, World War II, medical advancements, health care costs, 9/11.

Because the writer's mother spent so many years in the hospital wing, much of the story describes the administrator's extraordinary oversight and the established standards of care that we would hope for all—including ourselves. This serves as a model for all health care institutions. The author's decision to move in and record twelve years of residency provides an important document for medical professionals to read. Seldom do we see such sustained focus on this population: the daily routines, the provisions of care, the behavior of staff, and the details of departure after death.

Memento Mori: The End of Life

Since ancient times, human beings have pondered the mystery of death in various ways, but only in recent decades have scientists been able to use observational skills *and* technology to develop multidisciplinary concepts—many of them subject to lively debate—relating to brain death, or what is generally regarded as the irreversible cessation of all clinical signs of brain function. In conference settings, discussions about coma and brain death frequently focus on clinical experiences, scientific technologies, philosophical insights, and religious values that shape professional, personal, and cultural understandings. Conferees expect to consider the impact of new technologies, responses to them, and the descriptors or neologisms that have been added to the medical vernacular. Discourse often centers on brain death criteria, the formulation of policy, medical and legal defini-

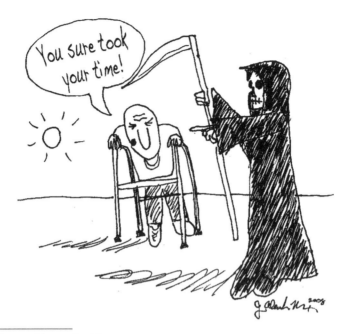

Courtesy of Justin Alexander Nixon.

tions, and case studies. In general, expert speakers present factual information in their search for accuracy and truth about specific circumstances of dying and death.

When Emily Dickinson wrote her well-known imperative, "tell the truth but tell it slant,"[24] she could not have imagined how those words would be cited by medical humanists as a way of describing the materials they use and the work they do in modern medical school environments. Striving to offer thoughtful expertise, scientists, ethicists, and humanists seek truth. Humanists, however, using visual and verbal tools, especially fiction, offer a truth told slant or another lens for understanding and interpreting difficult events and concepts. Frequently, their expertise embodies perspective shifts from the objective realm of science to the subjective realm of the humanities. With the latter, the goal is intended to broaden understanding without trying to nail down a particular truth. Whereas students lean forward in their seats for an absolute answer from the physiology professor, humanities faculty are more likely to frustrate students by suggesting that the *question* is more important than the answer. Understanding complexity, ambiguity, and nuance depends on a moving perspective; the discourse it contributes provides a thickened, less tidy, and valuable kind of expertise.

Fictional lives invite care providers to think about nonscientific and nonmedical elements of dying—unspoken feelings, fears, and doubts within the context of personal lives and sensibilities. In whatever form, stories stimulate the imagination, forcing an evaluation of how we might be thinking, feeling, or reacting in similar circumstances; furthermore, they require the reservation of time and purposeful listening. Consider, for example, the varied insights gained by reading *The Death of Ivan Ilyich* by Leo Tolstoy, "Home Burial" by Robert Frost, "the lost baby poem" by Lucille Clifton, *As We Are Now* by May Sarton, and *Love in the Time of Cholera* by Gabriel García Márquez when exploring the multiple dimensions of dying with students who have spent three months dissecting and memorizing all parts of a formalin-soaked cadaver. Medical humanities faculty provide very different tools of expertise for students to reflect upon life's slippery and complex textures.

Within some stories, differing points of view enable readers to move back and forth with point–counterpoint positions. This occurs in "A Clean, Well-Lighted Place" by Ernest Hemingway, a short story set in a café in which two opposing viewpoints are expressed for readers to follow. The story concerns two waiters, one young, the other older, and an old, only "slightly drunk" man, who comes regularly for brandy in their well-lighted and pleasant bodega. Unnamed, the patron is very old, deaf, and now that his wife has died, alone. Long after other patrons have left, he sits nursing his drink and becomes the topic of discussion for the waiters who await his departure before going home themselves. The younger waiter is openly impatient. When his more reflective and sympathetic partner mentions that the patron had tried to commit suicide last week, the younger man is unmoved and annoyed. "He'll stay all night," he says. "I'm sleepy now. I never get into bed before three o'clock. He should have killed himself last week."[25] Later, when grudgingly responding to a request for more brandy, he pours only a small amount while repeating the offensive remark to the unhearing man, "You should have killed yourself last week." When the shortchanged old man motions with his finger for more brandy, the young waiter rudely overfills the glass, causing the brandy to slop over the rim, down the stem, and onto the saucer. Ignoring or oblivious to the waiter's pettiness, the old man responds to the action with a simple "thank you."[25(p30)]

The young waiter dismisses the old man as an object, a "nasty thing."[25] Distanced and detached, he declares ironically, "I wouldn't want to be that old."[25] Unlike his impatient work partner, the older waiter is more patient and thoughtful about the old man's circumstances. By temperament, experience, and insight, he seems to understand that the clean, well-lighted café is a stand against darkness, chaos, *nada*—the huge, overbearing, inevitable nothingness for the already disabled and very old man whose life is suspended between the lighted café and the darkness of death. The younger waiter misses what the old man lives and the older waiter senses: loneliness and isolation, but with knowledge that some places in the world are salvageable, places where dignity can be retained. The clean, well-lighted café forms a buttress against the nothingness because it is concrete and immediate, rather than abstract. In this short and accessible story, issues relating to dignity, isolation, loneliness, cultural and generational differences, and mortality are easily identified and powerfully portrayed.

The tenderness exhibited by the senior waiter for the old man shows a nobility of spirit that most readers will applaud. Those with parents or loved ones in nursing homes worry about and may have first-hand knowledge about diminishment, disrespect, and loss of dignity. That the old man struggles nightly to reach the lights of the café is important; that one waiter behaves rudely and dismissively is an appalling reminder of what too many aging persons face.

Old men or women may be presented in a very different context by contemporary writers, but the concerns about dignity, isolation, and loneliness remain. Two poetic narratives, one by Paul Zimmer and the other by Ted Kooser, give voice to the real and imagined horrors of advanced aging from the perspective of grown children dealing with one or two fragile or dependent parents. Both are very modern, but represent differing, even controversial, points of view. With the highly newsworthy Kevorkian cases, the Schiavo case, and the Ramon Sampedro case in Spain (*The Sea Inside*), people have begun thinking out loud about end-of-life possibilities, choices, and directives in more informed, more robust conversations. What had been left to natural forces or to paternalistic physicians in past decades is now a matter of discussion about choices and decisions. Increasingly, individuals have outlined with physicians and family members the conditions for prolongation of life or, alternatively, cessation of treatment.

Paul Zimmer's poem "The Tenth Circle" reflects familiar worries that children share regarding aging parents who live alone. The situation in the poem is that if the landlord of the narrator's father's building is aware that any of the elderly tenants have placed more than three calls per month to the switchboard, the landlord is to assume that the resident is no longer capable of independent living and should, therefore, be moved to another health care center. The narrator is concerned about these absolute policy guidelines related to emergencies and how the policy could have an automatic and profound effect on his father's future ability to thrive.

> Dear Dad,
>
> Do not fall for the third time,
> Or if you do, tell no one.
> Hunch over your agony and
> Make it your ultimate secret.
> You have done this before.
> Shrug, tell a joke, go on.
> If an ambulance slips up
> Quietly to the back door
> Do not get on. They mean to
> Take you to the tenth circle
> Where everyone is turned in
> One direction, piled like cordwood
> Inside the cranium of Satan
> So that only the light of
> Television shines in their eyes.

> Dad, call if you need help,
> But don't let them take you
> Easily to this place where
> They keep the motor idling
> On the long black car, where if
> Someone cries out in the night
> Only the janitor comes.
>
> Love, Paul.[26]

In essence the son advises silence about medical events such as a fall: "tell no one." If an ambulance should arrive, do not get in. The strong warnings reflect contemporary health care systems, in which too many nursing home facilities correspond to Dante's *Inferno*, particularly the "Tenth Circle." At that level, everyone faces one direction—"piled like cordwood inside the cranium of Satan."[26] Cries for help are unheard and unanswered.

Illness has always suggested nightmarish qualities, but health care systems have been regarded, with some notable exceptions, as sanctuaries of care. Given recent demographic shifts, care provisions have not kept pace with need. Tremendous concern exists for aging citizens, family members, and care providers about the management of care in the decades ahead. Unfortunately, institutional care realities are frequently so discomforting that the impression created in Zimmer's poem is more real than not. In discussions with students, it is useful to review excerpts from Dante's *Inferno*. Another discussion might focus on the formation of policy statements and how the one described in the poem might generate concern not just from the son, but also from the landlord.

Most children who have cared for an aging parent may have harbored the kind of thoughts contained in the elegiac poem "Father" by Pulitzer Prize winner and former poet laureate Ted Kooser.

> Today you would be ninety-seven
> if you had lived, and we would all be
> miserable, you and your children,
> driving from clinic to clinic,
> an ancient, fearful hypochondriac
> and his fretful son and daughter,
> asking directions, trying to read
> the complicated, fading map of cures.
> But with your dignity intact
> you have been gone for twenty years,
> and I am glad for all of us, although
> I miss you every day—the heartbeat
> under your necktie, the hand cupped
> on the back of my neck, Old Spice
> in the air, your voice delighted with stories.

On this day each year you loved to relate
that the moment of your birth
your mother glanced out the window
and saw lilacs in bloom. Well, today
lilacs are blooming in side yards
all over Iowa, still welcoming you.[27]

Readers may be caught off guard by this love poem with its unconventionally direct thoughts about quality of life issues and family relationships, and some would find the narrator's conclusions, however tempered, as inappropriate and callous, especially those who would want to offer all available medical interventions. Had the narrator's father not died twenty years ago, today would mark his ninety-seventh birthday. In this posthumous apostrophe to his father, the narrator remembers his storyteller voice, his smell of Old Spice, and his fondness for lilacs in spring. The timeliness of the father's death prevented the miseries he as well as the narrator and his siblings might have endured regarding illnesses, clinic and hospital visits, and life-saving interventions. Without specifying the circumstances, the narrator writes that his father died with his "dignity intact."

"Lullaby" by physician-writer Jon Mukand, uses another lens to portray a scene we increasingly recognize from personal experience, read about in the newspaper, or see on television: the comatose patient steadfastly clinging to life. The narrator this time is a physician who reveals his or her innermost thoughts about an unnamed patient whose dying has been prolonged:

Each morning I finish my coffee,
And climb the stairs to the charts,
Hoping yours will be filed away.
But you can't hear me,
You can't see yourself clamped
Between this hard plastic binder:
Lab reports and nurses' notes, a sample
In a test tube. I keep reading
These terse comments: stable as before,
Urine output still poor, respiration normal.
And you keep on poisoning
Yourself, your kidneys more useless
Than seawings drenched in an oil spill.
I find my way to your room
And lean over the bedrails
As though I can understand
Your wheezed-out fragments.
What can I do but check
Your tubes, feel your pulse, listen

> To the heartbeat insistent
> As a spoiled child who goes on begging?
>
> Old man, listen to me:
> Let me take you in a wheelchair
> To the back room of the records office,
> Let me lift you in my arms
> And lay you down in the cradle
> Of a clean manila folder.[28]

The word *lullaby* is commonly associated with infants at bedtime, when parents use soothing songs as helpful inducements for sleep. No child is present in this poem, however—only an old man with kidney failure who has been clinging to life in the hospital. His story is contained in a very thick chart composed of lab reports and notes made by nurses. A clear pattern is in place: each day, the physician-narrator climbs the stairs with coffee mug in hand to face what has become routine and unchanged. But there is more to this story than the chart. Upon close consideration, readers discover more layers in this poem than might be expected.

If the chart is one part of the story, the narrator is another. He or she speaks conversationally to the uncomprehending patient, describing very clearly the simple facts of the situation. It is not quite a conversation but more of a descriptive monologue, a catalogue of this patient's hopeless circumstances and the tenacious forces of life that keep him alive: "heartbeat as insistent as a spoiled child." The information conforms to the decisional ethic pattern or factual presentation of information described earlier, but the manner and style of presentation is more literary, more florid. We are not accustomed to hear physicians talking about "poisoning yourself" or "kidneys more useless than seawings drenched in oil" or insistent heartbeats. Usually physicians are more conservative, more reserved in choice of words and images. The picture presented by this physician in the white coat is less guarded; the words and images reveal a responsive, concerned, distressed physician whose role has become that of an observer.

The third and final story occurs in the last stanza of the poem: six lines that form the lullaby alluded to in the title. Frustrated by an inability to intervene in a situation that is futile, the narrator composes words that direct the old man to his final sleep. The image is one of escape from the prison the physician sees daily. "Let me take you," the narrator whispers, from this bed to a wheelchair, and from there to the records office. There the narrator can "lift you in my arms and lay you down in the cradle of a clean manila folder." The helpless physician is touched by the pathos of the scene and imagines how the old man can be rescued from the tragedy the physician is forced to observe.

In Closing

When serious consideration is given to older people—what aging is, what it means for them, for us, and for the human adventure—we begin to understand that no single thread can be followed and no single story will suffice. In unique ways each person presents an implicit obligation to listen to his or her story so that we can hear different voices, complexities, and nuances relating to the subjective worlds and interpretive experiences of aging that transcend our inherited assumptions. By submitting to the pull of the text we are engaged in roles required of us as readers; we give substance to the imagined world and the psychological life of its inhabitants. As we have discussed, the humanities—literature, art, theater, film—extend our perceptions, intensify our reflections, and enlarge our feelings about our own experiences and those of others. We are stirred at first by the situational context and then, centripetally, by direct and indirect relation to our families, friends, neighbors, and selves. Using fiction, the narrowly focused lens of medicine can be enlarged to suggest other nonmedical ways of seeing, describing, interpreting, and deciding about aging and dying. With uncanny ability, writers, poets, and artists evoke curiosity and concern about recognizable motivations and consequences of human life so that those

> who have no pain can imagine those who suffer. Those at the center can imagine what it is to be outside. The strong can imagine the weak. Illuminated lives can imagine the dark. Poets in their twilight can imagine the borders of stellar fire. We strangers can imagine the familiar hearts of strangers.[8(p283)]

Review Questions

1. Using examples from the chapter or from a work that was not included, explain what the following statement means: "Story allows for distance—a way of observing, experiencing from afar. Often, it's the way to get to the truth."

2. The image at the beginning of the chapter is by Vincent Van Gogh. What can you imagine about this old man? What kinds of care needs might he require?

3. What cultural assumptions have you made about aging people, ranging from patients to neighbors to family members? Have any of those assumptions been incorrect?

4. Why does Alice Neel's *Self-Portrait* catch most viewers off guard? How did you respond to it? Is there anything to be learned from the painting? Why would the painter paint herself in this manner?

5. Conduct a discussion with peers about the poems by Kooser and Zimmer and the cartoon captioned "You're late." What do they have in common, and how can they contribute separately and collectively to self-reflection? Also, how do they show, separately and individually, that our assumptions about people can be incorrect?

6. Are you more like the younger waiter in the Hemingway story "A Clean, Well-Lighted Place" or like the older waiter? Explain fully.

7. As a health professional, how do you evaluate the physician-narrator in Mukand's provocative poem "Lullaby"? What have you experienced or felt that is similar?

Endnotes

1. Pellegrino E. Visual awareness: the visual arts and the clinician's craft. In: Berg G, ed. *The Visual Arts and Medical Education.* Carbondale, IL: Southern Illinois University Press, 1983.
2. Estes CL, Binney EA. The biomedicalization of aging: dangers and dilemmas. *Gerontologist* 1989;29(5):594.
3. Cole TR, Winkler MG. *The Oxford Book of Aging.* Oxford, England: Oxford University Press, 1994:3.
4. Rorty R. *Contingency, Irony, and Solidarity.* Cambridge, England: Cambridge University Press, 1989:73.
5. Nemeth M. Amazing greys. *MacLean's,* January 10, 1994, 26.
6. Macdonald B, with Rich C. The power of the old woman. In: *Look Me in the Eye: Old Woman, Aging, and Ageism.* San Francisco: Spinsters Ink, 1983:91.
7. Moody H. Cited by Rosenthal J. The age boom. *New York Times Magazine,* March 9, 1997, 42.
8. Ozick C. *Metaphor and Memory.* New York: Alfred A. Knopf, 1989:266.
9. Holstein MB, Cole TR. Reflections on age, meaning, and chronic illness. *J Aging Identity* 1996;1:20.
10. Rehak M. Poetic justice. *New York Times Book Review,* April 4, 1999, 15.
11. Commission on the Humanities. *The Humanities in American Life: Report of the Commission on the Humanities.* Berkeley: University of California Press, 1980:12.
12. Varnadoe K. Commencement. *New York Times,* June 15, 1992, A11.
13. Rushdie S. Is nothing sacred? Presented as the Herbert Read Memorial Lecture at the Institute of Contemporary Arts, London, 6 February 1990. In: *Imaginary Homelands: Essays and Criticisms, 1981–1991.* London: Granta, 1991:429.
14. Jones AH, Banks JT, Greene M, Levin G, Perusek D. Teaching literature in medical schools. In: Wear D, Kohn M, Stocker S, eds. *Literature and Medicine: A Claim for Discipline.* McLean, VA: Society for Health and Human Values, 1987:74.
15. Carson R. The moral of the story. In: Nelson HL, ed. *Stories and Their Limits: Narrative Approaches to Bioethics.* New York: Routledge Press, 1997:233.
16. Charon R. The ethical dimensions of literature: Henry James's *Wings of the Dove.* In: Nelson HL, ed. *Stories and Their Limits: Narrative Approaches to Bioethics.* New York: Routledge Press, 1997: 97–98.
17. Williams WC. The practice. In: *The Autobiography of William Carlos Williams.* New York: New Directions, 1951:361.
18. Morris DB. *Illness and Culture in the Postmodern Age.* Berkeley: University of California Press, 1998:11.
19. Wolff J. *Feminine Sentences: Essays on Women and Culture.* Berkeley: University of California Press, 1990:295.
20. Healy S. Growing to be an old woman: aging and ageism. In: Alexander J et al., eds. *Women and Aging: Anthology by Women.* Corvallis, OR: Calyx Books, 1986:61.
21. Bauer D. Alice Neel's female nudes. *Women's Art J* 1994;15(Fall):26.

22. Because the foundations of the patriarchal worldview were based on objective perspectives with little room for or encouragement of personal self-reflection, few male writers have been subjective in scope. In recent years male writers and artists such as Stephen Dunn, Raphael Campo, William Matthews, Donald Hall, Tim O'Brien, Lucien Freud, and Robert Mapplethorpe have moved beyond inherited borders of propriety to speak subjectively about personal matters.

23. Clendinen D. *A Place Called Canterbury*. New York: Viking Press, 2008.

24. Dickinson E. Tell the truth but tell it slant. In: Johnson TH, ed. *The Complete Poems of Emily Dickinson*. Boston: Little, Brown and Company, 1997:506–507.

25. Hemingway E. A clean, well-lighted place. In: *The Snows of Kilimanjaro and Other Stories*. New York: Charles Scribner's Sons, 1961:31.

26. Zimmer P. The tenth circle. In: *The Great Bird of Love*. Springfield: The University of Illinois Press, 1989:51. Copyright 1989 by Paul Zimmer. Used with permission of the poet and the University of Illinois Press.

27. Kooser T. Father. In: *Delights and Shadows*. Port Townsend, WA: Copper Canyon Press, 2004:36. Copyright © 2004 by Ted Kooser. Reprinted with the permission of Copper Canyon Press, www.coppercanyonpress.org.

28. Mukand J. Lullaby. In: Mukand J, ed. *Sutured Words: Contemporary Poetry About Medicine*. Brookline, MA: Aviva Press, 1987:384. Reprinted with permission.

INDEX